*The International Library of Psychology*

# CO-OPERATION, TOLERANCE, AND PREJUDICE

*Founded by C. K. Ogden*

*The International Library of Psychology*

# SOCIAL PSYCHOLOGY

In 7 Volumes

| | | |
|---|---|---|
| I | Personal Aggressiveness and War | *Durbin et al* |
| II | The Psychology of Politics | *Eysenck* |
| III | Dynamic Social Research | *Hader et al* |
| IV | The Group Approach to Leadership-Testing | *Harris* |
| V | Co-operation, Tolerance, and Prejudice | *Lowy* |
| VI | Man and His Fellowmen | *Lowy* |
| VII | The Symbolic Process and its Integration in Children | *Markey* |

# CO-OPERATION, TOLERANCE, AND PREJUDICE

## A Contribution to Social and Medical Psychology

SAMUEL LOWY

Introduction by Robert H Thouless

Routledge
Taylor & Francis Group
LONDON AND NEW YORK

First published in 1948 by
Routledge

Reprinted in 1999 by
Routledge
2 Park Square, Milton Park, Abingdon, Oxon, OX14 4RN

Transferred to Digital Printing 2007



*British Library Cataloguing in Publication Data*
A CIP catalogue record for this book
is available from the British Library

Co-operation, Tolerance, and Prejudice
ISBN 0415-21120-4
Social Psychology: 7 Volumes
ISBN 0415-21134-4
The International Library of Psychology: 204 Volumes
ISBN 0415-19132-7

# CONTENTS

# INTRODUCTION

The type of prejudice with which this book deals is that kind of belief-system which accompanies an irrational hatred for some group of other people. This is a somewhat narrower use of the word " prejudice " than the dictionary might justify, but there does not seem to be any other word which Dr. Lowy could more conveniently have chosen ; and, in what follows, I shall be using the word " prejudice " in this restricted sense.

That such group-prejudices can be very serious in their consequences has been clearly demonstrated by the rise to power of Naziism and the consequent world war. Before these events, it was possible for a popular essayist in this country to display prejudice against Jews without being treated very seriously. His views were likely to produce generally neither conviction nor condemnation ; they were regarded rather as an amusing personal idiosyncrasy than as anything likely to lead to serious consequences. This view is no longer possible. We have seen how literary and theoretical expression of race prejudice can become a driving force behind behaviour of an incredibly awful kind. Extermination camps and massacres must be taken seriously. So also we must take seriously the mental driving forces behind them.

So we are led to ask the question which Dr. Lowy poses in this book : " What are the causes of prejudice and what can be done to abolish or to reduce it ? " If we wish to be clear-sighted in this matter, we must not be over-optimistic about the efficiency of any steps we can suggest to get rid of prejudice. It is much easier for the relatively clear-sighted few to understand the nature of a social evil than it is for them to devise any practical means by which it can be removed. Still more difficult is it to put into operation such practical means as they may succeed in devising. It remains, however, a duty for all who see clearly the pathological nature of prejudice to attack it by every means in their power. Medical science does not relax its efforts against disease because the complete abolition of disease seems to be an unattainable ideal.

There seems to be four main ways in which prejudice has been or can be attacked. It may be attacked on the conscious level in either of two ways : (1) intellectually, as an erroneous system of thought, or (2) morally, as a wrong attitude towards other people. Now, following on the work of Freud, we may also (3) try to get behind the conscious aspects of prejudice and study psychoanalytically its deeper or unconscious sources. Lastly (4) we may consider the social changes necessary to make the environment in which men live one in which there is less likelihood that they will develop irrational hatreds against other men.

The first two of these are the ways of dealing with prejudice which most of us are inclined to try first. We are likely only to explore the possibilities of other methods when the limitations of these more obvious ways have become apparent by the incompleteness of their practical success. We are, for example, using method (1) if we try to show the absurdity of anti-semitism by pointing out that charges against 'the Jews' are true only of some and not of all Jews and that they are also true of some Gentiles, and then go on to enquire whether the anti-semite has even valid statistical evidence that they are true for a larger proportion of Jews than of non-Jews. Or, if the anti-semite defends his prejudice against Jews by asserting their guilt of the death of Jesus, we can ask whether the modern Englishman is also guilty of the murder of Thomas à Becket or of the burning of Joan of Arc.

These are attempts to overcome a prejudice by attacking it on the conscious level by showing it to be an erroneous system of belief. It is a matter of common observation that such an attempt is likely to be wholly unsuccessful if it is applied to an extremely prejudiced person. His probable reaction will be a violently emotional repudiation of our arguments which may take some such form as abuse of the "liberalism" of those who disagree with him, and the assertion of a fresh system of charges against the "liberals". It is clear that, in attacking his reasons, we have failed to attack the real grounds for his opinions, and we may be led to suspect that behind those opinions there are irrational forces of which he himself is not aware.

The reality and importance of the irrational forces behind strongly held opinions is now widely recognized as a result of the work of Freud and the psychoanalysts. There is indeed a tendency for the pendulum to swing too far from the first reliance on the conscious level of the attack on prejudice to the opposite position of denying that the method of dealing with it on the conscious level has any effect at all. Here, as elsewhere, Dr. Lowy seems to me to show an excellent balance of judgment. While making full use of the psychoanalytic point of view in the attempt to understand the unconscious and irrational forces behind prejudice, he does not neglect the necessity for also dealing with it on the conscious level as an erroneous system of thought, that is, as one which can be weakened by showing that the reasons for believing it are bad just as it could be strengthened if the holder of it could be convinced that the reasons for holding it were good. This intellectual attack on the conscious level is precisely what Dr. Lowy is doing in his Appendix I where he shows that the reasons for holding the beliefs of anti-semitism are not good reasons. This appendix would obviously be of no use to the strongly prejudiced anti-semite; in him it would only arouse a strong emotional reaction against acceptance of the facts stated. For the less prejudiced, it would be of value, for the opinions of the ordinary man are liable to be unsettled by well attested facts antagonistic to those opinions.

Such a factual treatment of the beliefs embodied in a prejudice may be most valuable in the education of children. The ground may be prepared in early education for the formation of a particular prejudice by a selection of the facts favourable to that prejudice. On the other hand, the formation of that prejudice may be guarded against by an unprejudiced teacher aware of the danger, by an impartial presentation of the facts. A prejudice often formed in school-days by the English child is that against Roman Catholics by the selection of facts in protestant history books. There is little in the later social environment to reinforce this prejudice and in the average child it wilts through lack of social reinforcement and in the absence of a suitable mental predisposition for its growth may completely disappear. In a personality whose development is, for some reason, favourable to prejudice formation, this early prejudice may last through life and he may engage in anti-Roman religious polemic based on the attitudes developed in the times of the Marian persecutions and the Spanish Inquisition as if these were present-day realities.

I think it is a reasonable hope that in English schools there is relatively little selection of facts favourable to the formation of anti-Jewish prejudice. I can, at any rate, remember nothing of the kind in my own school-days although there was plenty of material for the growth of a prejudice against Roman Catholics and a certain amount for formation of prejudice against the French. Even in this country, however, the story of the crucifixion of Jesus and the study of *The Merchant of Venice* require careful handling by the teacher. Dr. Lowy describes how his fellow pupils in a grammar school (not British) were frequently unable to speak a friendly word to him after their feelings had been worked on by a vivid presentation of the life of Jesus by their religious instructor. We here see the ground prepared in school education for the formation of a prejudice. Clearly the opposite bias could have been given to the Scripture lesson by emphasis on the fact that Jesus was a Jew instead of on the fact that his persecutors were Jews. Better still, because more rational, the teacher can aim at making it clear that neither the nationality of Jesus nor that of his persecutors have anything whatever to do with a reasonable valuation of a Jewish individual at the present day.

The usefulness of dealing with a prejudice merely as an erroneous system of thought has another limitation besides that of not removing the irrational and unconscious forces behind prejudice. On the merely factual level one can deal with only one prejudice at a time. Little has been gained if education shows the factual baselessness of anti-semitism but leaves the minds of those educated free to form similar prejudices against negroes, Germans, or Russians. It is indeed easy to criticize anti-semitism now because there is a popular bias against it in consequence of its association with Naziism. This makes it easy and convenient to take anti-semitism as a typical prejudice for the purpose of illustration of a discussion on prejudice. But it must not be forgotten that this is not the prejudice most likely to endanger world peace in the immediate future. In this respect prejudices against Germans and against Communists are much more dangerous and there is some risk that these prejudices may grow up unchecked while we are concentrating our attention on the undermining of anti-semitism. Because these prejudices are more immediately dangerous, having more serious present-day practical implications, they are more difficult to discuss factually. Social approval also makes a prejudice difficult to deal with factually ; in some countries the factual discussion of prejudice against negroes is virtually impossible because this prejudice has behind it the strong force of social approval.

It follows that even the attack on prejudice on the conscious level must go beyond the criticism of particular prejudices as factually erroneous. Education against prejudice must also build up a general sentiment antagonistic to prejudice formation. It is often charged against religion that it has provided motives for prejudice. If, at its worst, religion has done this, it has also, at its best, provided an atmosphere unfavourable to prejudice formation. The religious conception of all men as brothers equally valuable in the sight of God leads to the idea that hatred of men of other races is a sin against God. If moral conceptions based on religion have had less influence on men than the moralists could wish, they have certainly not been without influence. There is no reasonable doubt that many men whose own mental stresses in combination with their social situation would have led them to hate or despise Jews or negroes or Germans have not done so because they believed that it would be morally wrong and displeasing to God if they did.

Condemnation of an undesirable mental attitude as " sinful " seems to many people to be now out of date, but the same idea may be found in phraseology not bound up with traditional religious ideas. When Dr. Lowy refers to prejudice as " pathological " and as a kind of " paranoia ", this amounts to much the same thing. It is a moral judgment whose effect is [1] to create a sentiment against prejudice ; the modern man tries to avoid the pathological as his grandfather tried to avoid sin. This does not, of course, imply that this condemnation of prejudice is a mere device to induce a reaction of avoidance. On the contrary, its value as a stimulus to the avoidance of prejudice depends, for the reasonable man, on the adequacy of the grounds on which it is asserted. The theoretical analysis on which this condemnation of prejudice is based leads to a psychological result which is the same as that of the condemnation of prejudice as sinful ; it provides for the relatively unprejudiced person a motive for avoiding prejudice. It thus plays a part in creating a social atmosphere unfavourable to prejudice formation. This condemnation of prejudice is what I have referred to earlier as the moral attack on prejudice as a wrong attitude towards other people.

Like the criticism of prejudice as an erroneous system of

[1] The author of this book admittedly desires to convince the critical reader that prejudice is not simply one of a variety of opinions, but literally a paranoiac belief. Obviously, such an attempt at persuasion must be based on a firmer ground than the author's dislike of prejudice, in particular if he might be suspected of having weighty personal reasons for wishing a diminution of such aggressive attitudes. Should he have failed in proving, by his psychological analysis, that the phenomenon under discussion has really the characteristics of a paranoia-like belief, no amount of emphasis employed to make prejudice a disreputable attitude, deserves indeed the serious attention of the reader in his capacity as scientist. The fact that prejudice of a particular type is felt as painful by the group of those who are its target is, perhaps, sufficient justification for a Government interfering with the unlimited freedom of such aggressors. But unless we feel sure that this aggression is based in fact on a delusion, we cannot expect satisfactory results. It might still be argued that people ought to be allowed to have and voice their opinion ; the practical consequence of this liberal attitude, in the long run, cannot be anything but factual aggression with all its demoralizing effects on widespread social spheres. The writer of the *Introduction* makes his point clear in the sentences that follow. (S. L.)

beliefs, the moral criticism of prejudice is an attack on the conscious level. Both are of practical importance and both are limited in their usefulness by the fact that they are ineffective against the strongly prejudiced person. The convinced anti-semite will be no more willing to accept the proposition that his attitude is sinful or pathological than to accept a reasoned refutation of the alleged factual grounds for his prejudice. It is indeed essential to the nature of prejudice that the prejudiced person regards his prejudice as morally right and as a healthy mental attitude. A suggestion that it is otherwise will make him angry but will not change his attitude.

So we are led to consideration of the third method of attack, by the psychoanalytical study of the deeper unconscious sources of prejudice which is the central theme of Dr. Lowy's book. Here he is dealing with a matter that is both difficult and controversial and it is not to be expected that all of those who are competent to discuss this problem will agree in detail with his solution.[1] In brief, this solution is that irrational hatred of groups of other people is the outward projection of the prejudiced person's resentment against the various factors in his social situation which impose restrictions on his behaviour. If we accept this solution of the problem, the practical problem arises as before. What is to be done about it to reduce prejudice to a minimum ?

There seems to be one obvious answer : that by the application of the process of psychoanalysis to the prejudiced person, we can make him aware of the deep-seated cause of his prejudice, and that when the source of the prejudice becomes conscious he can deal with his resentment in a rational way instead of discharging it on such " scapegoats " as Jews, Roman Catholics, or negroes. About the success of this way of dealing with the difficulty Dr. Lowy is, rightly I think, not very optimistic. It is true that successful psychoanalysis is, to a considerable extent, a solvent of prejudice. It is also true that a person who has acquired the psychoanalytical point of view will be relatively distrustful of strong emotional

[1] The author feels that apart from his solution, in essence there are two possible conceptions on prejudice. The one is to consider it entirely justifiable ; the other is to assume that prejudice contains an indubitable nucleus of truth but associated with an exaggerated passion that has to be disapproved on account of social expediency. If, however, we decide to regard the subject's psyche as the sole or main source of prejudice, then we have classed the phenomenon as a delusion. The writer of the *Introduction*, in a private letter, has added that he does not mean to say that some experts " would not agree with the main outlines of the solution, but that they might dispute as to whether this or that factor in one's environment was the important one bringing about the tendency to form prejudiced attitudes ".

The author of this book invites suggestions capable of improving his theory. (S. L.)

reactions such as group hatreds because he will have learned to suspect that they may be expressions of unconscious and irrational forces and that they are likely, therefore, to be unreliable guides to action. His acceptance of any kind of psycho-analytical explanation will reinforce the effect of the moral criticism of prejudice ; he will tend to regard prejudices as untrustworthy as well as pathological or sinful.

But important and useful though it is to create a relatively unprejudiced nucleus of clear-sighted people, this does not do much to solve the problem of the strongly prejudiced. The strongly prejudiced are necessarily resistant to the psycho-analytic point of view since this point of view leads to the idea that prejudice is the product of irrational forces whereas it is essential to the nature of prejudice that its owner regards it as really based on the apparently reasonable grounds he urges in its defence. So he rejects the psychoanalytical point of view. If he were subjected to the actual process of psychoanalysis and not merely to the general influence of psychoanalytical ways of thinking, the prognosis would be little better. A psychotic paranoiac is not curable by psychoanalysis, and if prejudice is, as Dr. Lowy suggests, a "paranoia of the normal", then it may be expected to be resistant to the analytical process for much the same reasons. The prejudiced person does not regard his prejudice as a symptom of mental disease, so he cannot co-operate in a process of psychoanalysis aimed at its removal.

The psychoanalytical interpretation of prejudice suggests to Dr. Lowy, however, another way of dealing with the problem of prejudice which holds out greater hope of practical results. If we regard prejudice as a reaction of the personality to certain types of restriction in the social environment, then it follows that we may hope to find ways of changing the social environment which will reduce such kinds of restriction to a minimum. An ideal society is not merely one in which every individual has adequate food, shelter, and security. These are the essential foundations of a satisfactory social system which are not yet secured for every individual. But, in addition to these things, men need a social setting in which healthy mental development is favoured and in which stresses liable to lead to pathological mental reactions such as the formation of prejudice are reduced to a minimum.

Obviously a certain number of restrictions on the individual are a necessary consequence of social and family life, but equally obviously social restrictions bear unnecessarily hardly on some individuals and there is a possibility of lightening their burden and therefore the degree of resentment which may find its discharge in pathological directions. If the restrictive nurse or parent is followed by a restrictive schoolmaster and a restrictive superior in office or workshop, and if the cumulative effect of these restrictions is to drive the individual to react with attitudes destructive of tolerance and co-operativeness, then it becomes necessary to consider whether we should not aim at a greater freedom in nursery, school, and place of work which will help to produce an individual with more of the qualities which make him a mentally healthy, tolerant, and co-operative member of society. Dr. Lowy suggests as the general formula for the ways in which such desirable social changes may be made that they should act on the hypothesis that all individuals are equally significant for society. When individuals all have this sense of their significance for society, it is hoped that the tendency to prejudice formation will be reduced to a minimum.

This seems to me to be a book which not only makes a useful contribution to psychological theory but also contributes a valuable practical step towards the understanding and therefore to the diminution of prejudiced attitudes. I think that it deserves the serious attention of all who are engaged in considering how we may make a better world, free from irrational hatreds and from the wars and persecutions which follow from them.

R. H. THOULESS.

# FOREWORD BY THE AUTHOR

*This work is addressed to the expert psychologist and sociologist—a mere appeal to the public promises only limited results. There is a need for the creation of a social psychology utilizing psychoanalysis but going beyond its concepts. The dynamic significance of social attitudes is at least as great as that of the psychoanalytical complexes.—There is no possibility of preventing the emergence of infantile complexes whether libidinal or aggressive.—The only feasible way is the fostering of improved social attitudes through a general and indirect approach.—The new social science of the future.—The necessity of being realistic and not increasing weakness in the weak.—Education must not pretend that the world is uncomplicated and badness is the exception.—Prejudice in its various forms.—Statistical and analytically descriptive modes of presentation.—Some of the discussions in this work are likely to remain of interest even in future periods.*

## I.

The theme of this small volume has at all times held the uppermost interest of all people who do not merely live their existence but, if we may say so, consciously think their life. The world-wide crisis of to-day gives added significance to all attempts, literary and experimental, contributing to the knowledge of social life. Nevertheless, the necessity for discussions as contained in this work has not arisen merely in view of contemporary events. The proper time for dealing with the problems, both scientifically and in the practical sphere, ought to have been the period before 1914, and certainly immediately after 1918. To-day much is no longer available that was at the disposal of mankind in the past. In material resources, in the number of enthusiastic politicians and scientists, as well as in the trust and goodwill of the masses, our generation has become comparatively poor. Human minds in general have lapsed to a level of the dark Middle Ages. No person in the present has remained unaffected by recent events ; we have seen that undesirable things, deemed impossible on a large scale in modern times, may, in fact, very easily materialize even in a civilized society. There is now less genuine horror of evil than there had been previously for centuries. For this reason it is possible that the present generation is well-nigh unable to tackle the problems of the human world in the manner that would characterize a more enlightened and peaceful society. However, the need of the present is so great, and the desire of the masses so explicit, that some benefit may accrue to the world from scientific discussion of the kind presented here.

This work is in fact not destined primarily for the general public but for the reader already initiated into general and social psychology. For this reason little allowance has been made, either in exposition or in particular content, for the needs of popular scientific literature.

It is the considered opinion of the writer that a further increase in enlightened human attitudes can hardly be attained in society through the direct literary appeal to the individual. All that it is possible to do through public education has proved to be limited. The mental factors determining tolerance and spontaneous co-operation are largely beyond conscious grasp and control. Those forces responsible for the creation and spread of prejudice are obviously even less so. Consequently, a popular work on the problems dealt with here could hardly have any significance beyond satisfying the general reader's desire for a more or less interesting literary product. Its only practical effect would be to convince the convinced and to please the vast number of helplessly passive participants in the contemporary social drama. The poor always agree with sermons on charitable beneficence.

The results of any research, or of any suggestions aiming at the stimulation of further research, are best utilized by those who, though limited in number, are fully capable of grasping them. In virtue of their distinguished position in a cultured society they are entrusted by their fellow-men with the particular task of thinking more deeply on behalf of the rest, or rather of guiding in some degree the thinking of the rest. It is no good hiking without a map, or exploring what may prove ultimately to be a barren wilderness. The members of the general public, each of them an expert only in the domain of his occupation, deserve from the social scientist the help given through the selection of the probable, or at least of the possible, and rejection of what appears merely an interesting product of phantasy.

The writer feels that in his approach here, as well as in his more popular work, *Man and his Fellowmen*, there is a challenge to the young scientist to look out for possible improvements in psychology. The individual concepts referred to in these works are those of contemporary science ; but they have been given in the course of their discussion, though to varying extents, a modified content ; and their composition into the picture of whole problems might mirror the future outlines of an improved social science. The scientist is not only justified but is performing a real duty in trying something novel where the previous attempts have left conspicuous gaps.

It appears to me advisable that after an excursion lasting five decades into analytical psychology, with its astonishingly strange logic, we should return to the realm of customary thinking, whilst still utilizing the fascinating results of this modern mode of research in our new-old type of approach. It is as if a traveller has brought home from various foreign countries a number of selected objects, and intends now to build a house for himself, which in its outline will be similar to other houses in his native country, but will be improved by a number of novel devices and ornaments.

It is feasible, and even necessary, to create a human psychology embracing the viewpoints of customary logic to a greater extent than psychoanalysis in its classical form can afford. It is not an allowance to unscientific thought or to the natural self-deception (psychological scotoma) of people never analysed that accounts for this necessity. The fact is that the individual's personality is governed by psychological rules of both types, by those intelligible with the help of common-sense logic as well as by those to which the postulates of modern analytical psychologies apply. And the same double rule exists with regard to life in its social aspect. Thus, the competitive complex as outlined in the present work, the phenomena of envy and jealousy in themselves, and further the striving for power, or alternatively the readiness to yield meekly with a view to gaining approval—these and other conscious tendencies are genuinely distinct forces and not merely negligible secondary ones. Their dynamic significance is no less than that of the subconscious psychoanalytical complexes and the processes peculiar to them. Replacement, condensation, ambivalence, repression, deflection, and projection are habitual mechanisms of the human mind ; so are the various illogical attempts to safeguard the feeling of prestige and avoid defeat, as explained in Adler's *Individual Psychology*. But all the other, that is, the logical forces manifested by the personality, a few instances of which we have enumerated above, are of the same practical importance, and equally deserving of the attention of the social psychologist.

It is not simply with a view to stating the obvious and

unquestioned that all this is said here. Social psychology, a doctrine that is really capable of initiating practical progress, requires in fact a viewpoint that is somewhat different from that of psychopathology and psychotherapy. First of all, it appears that for the problems of social size the emphasis either lies equally on both types of mental processes referred to above or perhaps there is a slight bias in emphasis on the " conscious " forces. This is so for two reasons. In the social aspect of the personality, as I feel, these conscious or " logical " forces are in fact more to the fore than the psychoanalytical complexes proper, though the role of the latter must not be overlooked. But, what is even more important, the viewpoint of the practical sociologist and social reformer *has* to be focused more on the group of tendencies that we have called, inaccurately, the logical one.

Let it be assumed that there exist in fact, and in the development of each individual, such things as an oral and anal phase as well as an early Oedipus complex, and that there occurs in psychoneuroses a regression to these phases ; though, quite sincerely, I myself cannot clearly estimate the extent and the role of these forces, in spite of having attained therapeutic results through psychoanalysis just as much as all average psychotherapists. Let it even be hypothetically admitted that the infant, in his anger at not being fed quickly enough, destroys in his mind the cruel mother or her breast ; here I am even less capable of forming any opinion. But where, it may be asked, is the possibility of guarding efficiently against the development of complexes associated with such early processes, and against various characterological and psychoneurotic complaints alleged to be associated with such disturbances ? The optimistic lay psychologist, reading so much about *trauma* and *fixation* and *repression*, believes that with a knowledge of these phenomena nothing can be easier than prevention. No more is needed than a careful psychoanalytically founded education, and everything must turn out right. As if it were, indeed, possible to turn the educators and parents themselves into regulated machines, capable of constantly presenting an optimal conduct. As if, further, it were possible to avoid the impact of the broader environment on the child's mind. As if, finally, it were possible to balance accurately the physiology of the neurohormonal system so as to eliminate the various disturbances in the smooth maturation of the libido, to avoid the creation of the Freudian " Fixierungspunkte " (points of fixation), and to guard against aggressive and self-destructive tendencies becoming too strong.

The edifice of social psychoanalysis—the application of Freudian tenets to social problems—proved to be perfect wisdom in theory but a definite failure, a real folly in practice. With this psychology it is possible at the best to improve or cure a number of psychoneurotics, to do miracles in serious cases ; though hardly to prevent on a large scale the occurrence of psychoneuroses. This, however, is not the path leading towards improvement of the human personality in all respects.

There is another way, the only promising way, of beneficially influencing the growth of the minds and of trying to improve the individual and social aspect of the personalities of the average masses. The general spirit permeating the immediate and the broader environment of the maturing youth, the actual significance accorded to the individual, the amount of appreciation or obstruction he meets, the real attitude toward dutifulness or selfishness immanent in the actual life of society and the legal administration, these and a great number of other environmental phenomena are factors moulding the personality down to the deep subconscious spheres. It is apparent that environmental influences of the above kind have profound effects on all mental processes, the psychoanalytical complexes included.

Here is a tangible approach to the tasks of prevention and improvement. Here are factors the working of which can, to an appreciable extent, be measured and probably modified. Here a genuine possibility presents itself of " strengthening the ego-structures ", of decreasing the persistence of " Oedipal " constellations, of deciding the balance between libidinal processes and destructive tendencies in favour of the former ; and, a matter of still greater significance, a possibility of improving the faculty of tolerance and increasing the enjoyment in co-operation.

If psychology is ever allowed to play a substantial part in advising on administrative matters, then serious, objective young sociologists should have an excellent field for utilizing and elaborating suggestions such as are being made in this and similar works.[1] But only a science of a type that does not appear remote from average manifest life, and only scientists whose way of thinking is in fact appropriate to feasible social programmes can claim and hope for recognition. I am quite aware that the neglect of modern psychology on the part of influential members of the administrative class springs largely from a resistance peculiar to most people who have never been analysed. But what are we going to reply if it be retorted that psychologists who *have*

[1] Cf. K. Horney, *The Neurotic Personality of our Time.*

been analysed, and who are undoubted experts on the therapeutic aspect of our domain, do not always show the desirable measure of objectivity, tolerance, and community with other ordinary mortals? They are, of course, just as much products of a general public spirit, and children of contemporary philosophy, as everyone else. It can only be a new generation that will be able to create a fresh outlook in psychology. Only a new generation will be fitted to impart to society and its administrative bodies guiding principles of modern knowledge, which will, admittedly, only be possible of creation because of the pioneer work of the first psychoanalytical generation and its close followers. The present work, however, is addressed to the younger student of psychology whose mind has not yet been conditioned too much by the doctrines of current medical psychology; this field is as much in need of a thorough overhaul as anything else that is human.

In the new psychology, which cannot but be a social science in the fullest sense, everything valuable and interesting so far discovered or suggested will have its place, but in a somewhat modified setting. The significance of any particular element varies according to its associations with other elements. This is true of abstract concepts just as of concrete objects. Through becoming a social science, the particular concepts of analytical and individual psychology will assume a new content. This development, as all who are acquainted with the facts know, started some time ago, and far-seeing minds within the psychoanalytical movement long ago spoke of "character analysis". The first impulse, as far as I am able to judge, was given by the inaugurator of Individual Psychology, *Alfred Adler*, though much has been found and will yet be discovered that goes far beyond his system. *Wilhelm Stekel's* name is known only to the medical psychoanalyst; but the study of his works betrays considerable insight into the principles which, in the opinion of the present writer, ought overwhelmingly to dominate future research. *W. McDougall's* name will remain associated with the notion of Social Psychology. In psychiatry in the narrower sense the name of *A. Meyer* is associated with the social aspect of psychotic happenings. I am, indeed, convinced that the various psychoneurotic manifestations are capable of description and better understanding in terms of social psychology; and what is more important, treatment of psychoneuroses at an early stage can be shortened if the analyst knows more about the human mind than the transformations of the libido and the phenomenon of moral conflict.

## II

Before embarking on the discussion of the particular phenomena, the author wishes to say a few words of a more general character. Works of enlightenment are read largely by persons of a more or less refined character. The seeking of information on problems of general well-being suggest the presence of a social sense. It may appear unfortunate that many of those who would need guidance in their activities, private or public, have no interest at all in improving their outlook. It is not the psychotic who reads works on the symptoms of the psychoses. It is not the criminal who studies carefully the social and psychological implications of crime. Psychopaths are as a rule content with their personality. Persons imbued by prejudice and irrational hatred will argue that such phenomena do not exist at all; or if they do exist, they themselves are certainly not beset with these mental anomalies.

This work does not appeal to these noxious elements of society. Nor even has it in view a substantial co-operation on the part of the masses of individuals who make the social community.

The discussion to follow will show clearly why this attitude has been taken by the author. But it is fair if the reader knows in advance a fundamental feature of the author's approach to the general problems of social ethics.

There are a great many persons who are by nature lacking in drive and energy, or who suffer from acquired inhibitions in their approach to their fellowmen for the pursuit of justified goals. In such a person the cultivation of unselfish ideals may accentuate the undesirable inhibitions. More accurately, the existent inhibitions may facilitate a too ready acceptance by their mind of restrictive ideals, making thus for general passivity. If a person—and in particular such a type of person—relies too much on absolute justice and the fair sense of his fellowmen, he may very easily neglect practical action and remain behind average people in mundane success. Disappointment may be followed by deep embitterment and an unreasonable fear of society; and this may drive the individual into unnecessary isolation.

The tragic element in this case is that ethical principles fetter a human type who at any rate would be comparatively harmless to the elementary interests of his fellow-beings. The real significance of ethical restrictions lies where natural ambition and drive would not allow for a spontaneous tendency to self-limitation in the interest of social harmony.

Is it quite responsible to educate youth in principles that are not going to rule the world in their lifetime? Is it justifiable to make susceptible people believe that decency and self-limitation are elementary rules of general behaviour, whereas we know that nothing but disappointment will be their share? It is as if we made unexperienced children believe that all animals of the earth are as tame and friendly as the dog at home, and then send them out into nature's wilderness. After a number of pleasant experiences with colourful birds, and timid hares, harmless goats and sheep, and perhaps on rare occasions with attractive fawns, the dramatic meeting with the fox and wolf is inevitable. Many would fall a prey to the beast before ever having had some of the pleasant experiences.

Indeed, the writer thinks it irresponsible to persuade kind-hearted but basically naïve people that, by the foundation of ethical and educational circles the affairs of human society are really safeguarded. Unfortunately, it is not even certain whether these fellowships and their publications have an influence at all on the socially important persons who do not belong to them. The creation of pleasant illusions for a large number of people is a goal important enough to justify the literature and organization in the service of such groups. It is also likely that some of the members may, on rare occasions, convert a cool and unimaginative person in office for a measure of mildness and modernism in a particular case. They may also on occasions decide by their numerical vote a relatively minor matter. All this in itself is important. But to rely entirely on these ethical-æsthetical movements in a world in which we are living implies a risk of surrendering the management of human society again to those who are archaic and reactionary even though their slogans may be modern.

The writer feels that the discussions relating to Co-operation, Tolerance, and Prejudice might prove to be stimulating; that both his novel formulations and his individual description of what has been in essence stated already by other authors will be found useful. He wishes to admit in advance that he has not been able to discover a solution in sight for the large scale difficulties prevailing in international spheres; on this point his book is likely to be felt disappointing to many readers. The writer, however, feels that unwarranted optimism, as contained in works of some authors, are out of tune with his efforts to contribute to a feasible social programme. There is enough wishful thinking in all plans and systems referring to improvements of social and individual life.

In discussing the phenomenon of *prejudice* the writer has in mind first of all the organized mass phenomena of this kind; and only in the second instance manifestations of a minor scale that have, nevertheless, a similar psychological background. The anti-Jewish attitude is referred to in several contexts; though, naturally, it may be said that it is of no immediate significance for the overwhelming majority of people. Yet if the instances quoted are true and the component problems associated with the phenomenon are capable of a psychological discussion, then the illustrative value of this material cannot be less through the limited practical significance of this particular social anomaly.[1] The reader, if interested, is referred to *Appendix I*, where a genetic survey of the problem in the light of social psychology is attempted. The writer thinks that the value of the concluding paragraphs might be generally acknowledged.

No doubt, the phenomenon called in this work "ethnic prejudice" is of a paramount significance. Its forces are observable particularly in recent events. The writer has had to content himself with referring, in various contexts, to this factor, without being able to hold out any hope for a substantial decrease of this anomalous element in the life of nations. It not only makes for unsatisfactory international relationships, but, what is of greater importance, it makes it well-nigh impossible for individual nations to create a peaceful atmosphere at home. It appears that mankind will have to put up with this factor—to some extent at least—as one of the many inevitable phenomena of life.

## III

Lastly a few words ought to be said as to the mode in which the writer discusses social problems. Statistics and experiments are in the main to-day's methods for drawing conclusions and making suggestions. The advisability of such a procedure needs no particular affirmation. It is also intelligible if some expert sociologists, and reviewers of publications, look with a measure of suspicion on works that do not comply with this pattern of

[1] It is perhaps even a dictate of scientific objectivity to take cognizance of and try to understand a sentiment that has been strongly characteristic in recent years of at least 100 millions of people in and outside of Germany.

research. Nevertheless, there is something to be said also in favour of discussion of the kind represented by this volume.

Statistics presenting phenomena in terms of quantity prove no more than the phenomena themselves. They do not decide whether a phenomenon is frequent or rare by dint of a natural law, or whether causes account for the existing frequency that are not unchangeable themselves. A statistical relationship states the frequency of a phenomenon provided that various factors associated with it continue to operate. Should one or more of the associated factors become different, the phenomenon in question is likely to change qualitatively or quantitatively.

A simple instance is the increase in the number of young men fit for strenuous exercises after they have been for some time in the army. Through the particular mode of life and training in the army the proportion of the very fit to the rest who are only average has changed.

Another instance of a changeable proportion is supplied when we compare children who live at home with those who are educated in boarding schools. Several children develop a better ability for mutual adjustment in the boarding school, though they were rather deficient in this respect whilst at home. It can easily occur that, whereas the percentage of pupils of a well-adjusted behaviour may be 75 per cent at a boarding school, the corresponding proportion amongst pupils of day schools will be hardly more than 50 per cent. It is, of course, assumed that the two materials compared come from similar sources; that is to say, that the boarding schools have not admitted a larger proportion of pupils who are by nature very adjustable.

Should we be able to point to a new measure in any field that promises better results than so far known, a large amount of previous statistical knowledge must recede into the background. A few cases of favourable results attained by one experimenting person have at least as much illustrative value as negative results of a larger number of workers with less enthusiasm. Should a scientific worker, whether he be a physicist, chemist, a medical man, or an educationalist, attain only once a result the possibility of which was unknown to the large majority of the others, he deserves as much hearing as the vast number of sceptics and those who refer only to negative results and the intrinsic difficulties encountered in all creative endeavours.

The knowledge of psychological processes is a foundation safe enough from which to look at the social process, provided one is ready to modify his psychology for the sake of a broader outlook. Statistical results inform on what is in existence ; but this photograph of social life does not necessarily show sufficiently the deeper forces behind the phenomena or the clear outlines of the phenomena themselves divorced from accessory features peculiar to changeable conditions. Our interest is, in the main, devoted to the question of what might be done and attained, and is not merely concerned with the knowledge of what does exist and why it does so. There is, of course, no guarantee that an author's psychology is the best one to serve as a basis for examination. There is no more risk in presenting what we deem worthy of publication than to fail in receiving attention. Even then, at a later period, suggestions of an author who was not successful at first may be reviewed and utilized within the frame-work of a new approach.

It is likely that the implications of competitiveness will remain the object of extensive study, and the psychology of prejudice, in particular of the ethnic type, have an interest at least for a number of distinguished research workers. The extent to which deeper mental automatisms can be influenced by the impact of environmental events may be capable of assessment only from large-scale social experiments. The factuality of such a causal relationship will hardly be doubted by any psychologist and sociologist with an outlook sufficiently broadened by available knowledge.

The discussions on the moral process might not at first attract a similar interest. Since the advent of Freud, psychology has been a matter of more passion than is desirable ; and for this reason, it is not easy for a relatively independent author to draw sufficient attention to a novel conception. But it is possible that before long, and clad in a new terminology, other authors will try a similar approach ; and this ought to be enough for the benefit of our cause.

## IV

To some readers it might appear that works dealing with the economic and strictly political difficulties, besetting the world after the last war, contribute much more to the task of immediate consolidation than a treatise on social psychology of the type this book represents. This may be the case. It may also be believed by some that it is out of proportion to write—and to read—so much on prejudice and about past events, in view of the urgent and apparently novel problems of world security and atomic warfare. The writer's answer is that the problems dealt with in this work are, and will remain, acute under all modern circumstances, even after the picture of the world might have regained some of its pre-war features. Moreover, social psychologists think that political and economic difficulties are but the manifest result of what could be termed briefly ideological and ethnical prejudices (cf. Ch. IIIc). It might prove a great mistake to go on in thinking, planning, and acting whilst ignoring most of the phenomena that have characterized European history in the last fifteen years. It is intelligible for people in general to want to forget these events in the attempt to settle down to a life of peace and comfort. This is the unalienable right of the masses. It is nevertheless indispensable that a selected group of people who feel impelled to search, teach, and suggest on behalf of their fellowmen should not lose sight of anything that has happened. One of the important lessons is that it is not difficult to transform individuals, groups, and even whole nations into deliberate torturers and murderers. This fact, in turn, ought to stimulate further research on the aggressive tendency of man ; we have to admit that since Freud and Adler nothing really new has been suggested.[1] Another important realization refers to the fact that the traditional concept of the state is archaic. It would be difficult to say that varieties of the present epoch are much less so. The third thing we must not ignore is that moral pacifism in the form known to us appears to be incapable of becoming a sufficiently effective and attractive factor. But the reader should judge for himself, stimulated by the suggestions of this work. All this is not a matter applying to a certain race or nation, but to human beings in general. The reader who wishes to study this book has, for a while, to shelve any sensitiveness or disinclination to face a realistic picture of human nature.

There is another point about which the writer has to say a few words. It is natural that a reader, wherever he lives, might feel that the expositions of the author refer to conditions in a particular country. The fact is that the author does not describe and even less attack the individual reader or his country, whichever it may be. The present work is *not* the result of recent thoughts evoked in the writer during his stay in Great Britain. The truth is that the psychology of tolerance and prejudice has occupied his interest for at least twenty years. Having lived, and worked, as a psychoanalyst, in four different countries—each

[1] Perhaps the present author *has* made a slight contribution. Cf. Ch. XI, XII.

of them representing a distinct social and cultural pattern—the author of this book has had ample opportunity of seeing a large variety of individuals and learning about several aspects of group life. In addition to his living amidst the peoples of these countries, he has had the opportunity there[1] of analysing consular officials, as well as refugees of two other countries of which much has been heard recently. All analysands inadvertently tell about a variety of things in the course of their free associations ; and if an analyst has an ear and a receptive memory for sociological data, he is in a position to accumulate a large amount of material, and later to correlate the details. Unfortunately, the writer has no acquaintance of Soviet Russia at all. The very few of his patients who stayed there for a period have given too incomplete a picture of the mass psychological conditions there.

## V

There is a notice in public vehicles advising : " Do not alight while the train is in motion." For years the writer's mind has " obsessively " transformed this warning into an advice of practical wisdom with a wider application. The idea put into words is : " Do not think that impressions or explanations are the essential truth ; do not believe that the temporary picture of social phenomena is final and unchangeable. A constant metamorphosis is in process, and disappointing surprises are the lot of those who mistake a phase for the permanent shape of things. Do not alight whilst the train of events is in motion ; but actually it will keep on moving."

For the life of the individual it is inevitable to assume that certain essential circumstances are permanent. A fair adjustment to life, and a fair measure of enjoyment of it, would be impossible were there not such a belief in the constancy of most things pertaining to life—whether fundamental ideas and principles or concrete circumstances in society. But it is not good to forget entirely that this constancy is only apparent, and is adopted by the mind as a working hypothesis. Those particularly who search and suggest ought not to be too credulous. For practical achievements in the immediate future, a somewhat blind belief in certain conceptions is necessary for one's efforts. Moreover, a leader's doubts may spread to numerous others and paralyse their dynamic contribution. Things are different—ought

[1] This refers to the period 1927–1938.

to be different—with a social psychologist. The relativity of phenomena is one of the paramount principles he has to keep in mind. His interpretations and explanations must be as careful and fitting as possible, so as to be borne out by other facts and later events indirectly connected with the original objects of his observation. This must not, however, mislead him into believing that he has found the comprehensive formula of human life and has discovered the full structure of the mechanism producing social and individual phenomena.

Thus, the writer is convinced that all he suggests is true in a certain sense, and capable of being applied to certain circumstances and problems. But he would deservedly raise strong doubts in his own objectivity, in the minds of those acquainted with the vastness of the field covered in this book, were he not to say clearly : " We are all only groping in semi-darkness, and shall never be able to find the ideal formula of human life ; and our ideas will always remain subjective, and valid only within certain limits."

It may be, however, that this work as well as others of its kind has no practical significance at all. It is possible that the world of actualities already contains the dynamic elements of those further developments of which the authors, indulging in the rôle of prophetic callers, speak in terms of hope and future. In this case the creative rôle of such works is insignificant or only imagined. Moreover, it is not so much the content of ideas as the form given to them by an author for which he may claim originality. It would be difficult to suggest something brand new, never thought of previously, and entirely novel to the contemporaries. And were it true that an idea is entirely new and peculiar only to its author, we ought to approach it with a measure of suspicion as something that has, perhaps, not sprung from genuine human nature.

Nevertheless, even mere thoughts on human life might be considered as having a significance. Should the actualities of life prove incapable of substantial amelioration, and consequently the proportion of positive life and frustration is to remain unaltered, in spite of new forms in the external aspect of society, then at least the pattern of ideas in which humanity conceives of its affairs and hopes might become increasingly attractive and mature. Progress in thought, even if objective realities remain unaffected, may ease the psycho-affective aspect of life. All attempts, therefore, to enrich our concepts on, and insight into, life merit a place among the multiform phenomena of the human world.

An author may consider himself fortunate if his contemporaries condescend to accept his work at least as a stimulation to their thought devoted to the deeper aspects of life.

I dedicate this small volume and any future research in the field of human psychology I am contemplating to those authors and students who have grasped the actual line of development, invisible as it is to the majority, but obvious to all of independent mind.

Dr. R. H. Thouless, of Cambridge University, author of *General and Social Psychology*, has written the Introduction after reading and criticizing the MS. I owe him a debt of gratitude for this as well as for the encouragement implied by his expert opinion.

A particularly valuable contribution has been made by my friend, Dr. D. S. Fairweather, M.A., M.D., M.R.C.P., D.P.M., Deputy Medical Superintendent at Stoke Park Colony. He undertook the arduous task of examining the MS. as to its intelligibility for the reader; it is to his credit if the style is improved in many places where the original version was not as clear and idiomatic as it is now. Very few are so well fitted for this task, both by their catholic knowledge and discerning personality, as he is. I am also very grateful to Dr. Herbert Read for his interest in my work and for the valuable suggestions he has made. Mr. E. W. Dickes and Mr. K. Murphy were also helpful in the preparation of the MS. for the press. The co-operation of all these persons has been limited to the formal aspect of the work; it does not suggest their personal attitude to the author's theories.

Finally, I wish to thank my wife for her secretarial assistance as well as for her numerous suggestions as to the choice of a more popular way of rendering my thoughts. It has been my aim that every educated reader might be in the position to understand certain parts of the work; but it is written above all for the advanced students of social and medical psychology.

## PREFATORY NOTE

Terminology is a matter of general agreement; but in some cases a writer has to use a certain expression in a somewhat original or limited sense. It is, then, necessary to define in advance its exact meaning, as it is to be understood in the course of discussion. In this work *prejudice* signifies a bias coupled with an aggressive attitude for which an inadequate reason is given. Bias alone, without the element of aggressive resentment, and without a quasi-delusional stereotyped concept, is something different. Obviously, there is no exact dividing line between sentiments, beliefs, and preferences on the one hand, and gross bias on the other. In general, people apply the word " prejudice " to all these phenomena, that is, when they do *not* agree with them and the person professing or showing such attitudes appears to be uncompromising about it. The writer, however, wishes to restrict the notion " prejudice " in this work to the resentful, quasi-delusional stereotyped mass-phenomena, as well as to comparable particular attitudes of individuals. Clearly, there can be no mental life without preferences and biased sentiments. A constant weeding out of one's mind of such elements may greatly interfere with mental ease and with the feeling of happiness. Very few people have a large capacity for this type of sobriety. Concrete life in general, and one's fellowmen in particular, give frequent reasons for disappointment; consequently, people cannot help seeking uplift and consolation in a number of beliefs, as well as psycho-affective compensation through what we may call *bias*. It is a fact that the display of such attitudes may strike the observer of a different make-up unpleasantly; but this does not alter the human as well as indispensable character of these sentiments. The less capable such a bias is of leading to irrational resentment the more remote it is from what the writer prefers to call prejudice. It is natural for people to resent an attack on, or interference with, their biases and sentiments of the aforementioned type; but this again is not identical with resentful prejudice. In the opinion of the writer it is unpsychological to attack—whether in writing or by political measures—such sentiments where there is no real social necessity for such a step; and what is an unpsychological and unnecessary measure, might amount to mental cruelty, practised for its own sake. Cf. the discussion in Appendix III.

## CHAPTER IA

## FELLOW-FEELING, CO-OPERATION, AND COMPETITION

*There is a natural positive interest in the fellowman; small children display this inborn social sense clearly.—Other factors are bound to interfere with this basic sentiment.—The limiting significance of fellow-men.—The realization of this fact is not equally clear with respect to all fellow-beings.—The competitive factor.—The inner circle.—The impression the subject has of the "small neighbour and friend".—Human inadequacy and the limitations associated with it.—Identification and its implications.—Why is sympathy with the manifestly ill greater than with those labouring under social difficulties and poverty in happiness?—Where identification is destroyed by propaganda, inhuman attitudes are likely to become natural.—The social backing of the individual and the loss of this support.—Contemporary events illustrate the discussions.*

1. THERE is in the human being a natural, elementary interest in his fellow-beings. Healthy infants smile happily at each other; they smile similarly when faced with their own image in a mirror. Children of all ages display clearly this elementary social sentiment, and their keenness to play with each other is, in essence, based on this elementary social attitude. As we know, they easily forget quite recent differences and soon approach each other with a view to restarting the common play, as if nothing had happened that could stand between them. Adults, too, frequently enough display the same elementary interest, particularly on journeys or at any time when the individual is allowed to relax. But in the adult this elementary reaction toward his fellowmen is no longer present in its original purity; it is greatly modified through additional factors. The vast number of experiences during life results in a variety of ideas regarding the significance of fellow-beings for the individual.

It is obvious that an environmental person may be a friend or rather indifferent, or may be a competitor in the enjoyment of the good things of life, and even a definite adversary. There is naturally an uncertainty as to these possibilities where a stranger is concerned. But, obviously, one cannot be quite sure even with regard to an acquaintance or relative, since new situations may evoke in him an attitude different from the previous one. A degree of caution and suspicion arising from this uncertainty necessarily modifies the elementary attraction felt by an individual toward his fellowmen. Vaguely—but to some extent even explicitly—there arises the question : How far can the other individual satisfy or interfere with my present needs, and further, or hinder, my future as I would have it ?

2. The significance of fellow-beings for the individual embraces a great variety of aspects. The maintenance and protection of his physical life, the satisfaction of his pleasures and mental needs in the broader sense, and amongst these his craving for friendship and appreciation as well as for a certain personal position in his environment—all these spheres of individual life are obviously dependent on the fellowmen. Co-operation, indifference, or manifest antagonism are three possible rôles assumed by environmental persons towards the subject.

No doubt, relatively few in number are those who appear immediately necessary for the individual's needs, or with whom personal relationship is desired. But the number of those who are joint claimants and competitors for practically everything is large. There is no unlimited freedom in space for the individual ; he has to share it with others and frequently to give up his preferences. In the choice and use of various facilities, objects, tools, institutions of all kinds, food, clothing, etc., there can be no autocratic freedom for a person. In his striving for friendship and love, social significance and prestige, he is not alone, he is only one of many. Of necessity, there constantly occur frustrations and disappointments in the course of various attempts ; and the automatism of wishing and striving can never remain smooth, but undergoes continual modification. Simultaneously the mind tries to find an interpretation of these experiences, whether right or wrong. At any rate, there must ensue a realization of the fact that environmental persons are intrinsically connected with the limitations of life's spontaneity. The result is the awareness of the *competitive factor* which modifies the original autonomy of human life.

3. This awareness is vague only in so far as the extent of this interference by the fellowmen is concerned. But the concept

about this unavoidable factor in social life is clear-cut in the mind. With respect to particular persons and occasions, the subject knows distinctly that frustration is due to the antagonism toward his own aims manifested by fellow-beings. Moreover, the tendency to such antagonism felt by the subject toward the aims and claims of his fellowmen must also illustrate for him the existence of the *competitive factor*. Self-observation thus confirms the competitive significance of others. What is recognized as a constant tendency within the self, is bound to suggest that the concrete experiences of being opposed and limited by others are not incidents but spring from universal human characteristics.

4. The interpretation by the mind of the customary difficulties in life, and of their causal relationship to the behaviour of environmental persons, is not in every respect accurate. For the sake of adjustment to one's closer environment it is imperative to ignore, as much as possible, the knowledge of the competitive significance of a selected number of people, and to retain this knowledge only with respect to the more distant outside world. There is an obvious necessity to consider the members of one's closer environment as friends, and thus legitimate claimants for all the good things of life. Members of the family and a few friends are, as a rule, parts of this *inner circle*; all those outside this circle constitute the world of competitors and potential adversaries, toward whom it is found natural to feel and to act accordingly. Whereas one is prompted to develop a certain degree of friendliness toward the members of the inner circle, it is considered enough to view the members of the outer environment with a fair measure of toleration.

5. Owing to the human desire for emotional attachments, there also exists genuine warmth and love towards a limited number of persons of the inner circle; and this sentiment substantially screens the obvious fact that these selected members of society are actually just as much limiting factors as are the others. The tangible signs of goodwill, co-operation, and requited love displayed by these members of the closer environment stimulate and intensify in the subject the further growth of his own friendliness toward them. To a large extent they can be perceived as part of one's own personality; their share in the good things of life can thus be easily acknowledged as natural. Within such

a limited circle the elementary interest of men in each other comes more frequently and manifestly to the fore than toward strangers. And the character of being competitive and ruthless in the pursuit of goals is attributed in the main to the " outsiders ". In brief, in the course of social adjustment the knowledge about the competitive attitude of people is associated with those who are in the periphery of the individual's environment. Close and distant are, of course, notions not necessarily congruent with spatial proximity or distance ; the phenomenon is governed by the degree of emotional interest extended by the subject to his various fellowmen. We should rather speak about a centre and periphery of the individual's social interest.

6. This presentation sounds logical ; or, rather, it appeals to our desire for a clear-cut system. But soon we have to realize that just the opposite is also the case. Not infrequently, the individual finds the members of his closer circle burdensome, and he is only too ready to shift his interest to persons of the outside world. In essence, however, this is again the same phenomenon. In such cases the individual wishes to carry out an exchange ; he wishes to make the new object of his elementary interest a member of his inner circle, on whom to pour the rays of his friendliness instead of on one or more members who happen, through circumstances beyond his control, to be his relatives or friends. It is no secret that antagonism and resentment amounting to hatred frequently exist toward the closest members of the inner circle, whereas the outside world is imagined as consisting of nicer, more decent, and worthier people.

7. The fact that this paradoxical behaviour does occur, is not simply a sort of failure of the mind to comply with the desirable rule. We have to bear in mind that the division of the environment into an intimate inner and a strange outer circle is, to a large extent, an artifice of the psyche. In point of fact, the members of the inner circle are no less competitors and limiting factors than are the multitude of others. In many respects they are even more so. The spatial proximity, and the sentimental obligation toward them, result in substantial limitations for the subject. In addition, it is human nature to expect from friends more than from strangers, and to resent strongly the smallest degree of thoughtlessness or opposition if it comes from members

of the inner circle.[1] This human propensity constitutes, in essence, a limitation for the self. The psychological effect of disappointments amounts to a restriction of subjective ease; and the very idea that with relatives and friends the depth, significance, and frequency of such incidents is larger than average implies a limitation of personal expansion in the psychological sense.

Nevertheless, these facts have largely to be ignored (annulled). The individual cannot bear the clear knowledge that all the world around him consists of actual or potential competitors. He *has* to create for himself a division of the world into close friends and strangers, associating the idea of competition and limitation with the outer environment, and ridding a number of people, largely or entirely, of this unpleasant characteristic. This division, carried out from a subjective need, is not entirely without confirmation in the world of concrete realities. Friends and relatives *are* in fact more frequently helpful and considerate than the others; they behave so from the same motive as that which prompts the subject to include them in his inner circle. Consequently, the subject is enabled to feel a measure of confidence, to view at least his inner circle with trust, to allow himself to love a number of them, and to expect from these few individuals similar attitudes and behaviour towards himself. All this enhances the subject's belief in the *significance of his own personality*, and reduces to a certain extent his fear of the outside world.

8. We are thus entitled to state that the idea of an intimate circle consists of two components. One is based on real experience, that is on the measure of kindness manifested by friends and relatives toward the subject; the other is an intra-mental element created by the mind for the sake of subjective security. No wonder that an artifice of the mind cannot always function smoothly. There are too many manifest signs of the competitive

[1] The explanation of this phenomenon in accurate terms does not appear an easy matter. Clearly, disappointments in connection with relatives upset the libidinal balance in the subject to a larger extent than in the case of strangers. It is possible that this occurs because the subject ties, as it were, himself to the relative or friend, and limits his own potential capacity for transferring emotional attitudes on to a number of other people; by experiencing disappointment he feels cheated of the recompense for his self-limitation. All ties imply, to a degree, fetters (Cf. Ch. V); and the bitter feeling of disappointment in the instances under discussion is an indicator of the fact that there is, indeed, repressed resentment behind emotional ties. The writer, however, feels that more might be said in explanation of the phenomenon referred to.

and limiting significance of the closer environment, which it is impossible to overlook. Thus, even the amount of repressed resentment against them that is due to the sentimental ties is constantly revitalized. It cannot be expected that a repressed element so frequently stimulated by unpleasant incidents should remain in dormancy all the time ; it is intelligible that it does come, with various frequencies, into the fore.

9. We can also describe the problem of the burdensome inner circle in a somewhat different way. Those with whom one has to share space, materials, and opportunities are competitors *whose reality is felt immediately* ; whereas it is only at exceptional moments that the limiting significance of the broader environment, and also of national and international events, is visualized and resented by the majority of people. In the case of relatives and friends who do not live in local proximity to the subject, there exists the element of emotional proximity felt by the subject toward them ; and this may make the opposition or limitation coming from them, however small objectively, a significant event because experienced as " immediate ".

10. This leads to the discussion of a peculiar phenomenon that is of particular importance for the life of small communities such as, for instance, a group of neighbours.

It appears that people in general are more readily envious of the share of their close acquaintances and of neighbours in their district, than of that of the world at large. This may be the case though the persons envied have nothing extraordinary in their possession, and have merely had some small incidental stroke of luck. Less notice is taken of the millions of others who are strangers, and amongst whom not a few are wealthy or powerful people. Their share—at times a disproportionately large share—remains simply an object of knowledge, but is hardly ever the cause of passionate resentment. Naturally, one is more concerned with what occurs near by than at a distance. Moreover, from the point of view of envy and begrudging each other, the small man, even if living far away, may be nearer to the critical eye of another small man than is the powerful and wealthy person who dwells spatially in his immediate neighbourhood. The extra-territorial social position of the latter is to the small man frequently quite acceptable, though he cannot help resenting any temporary progress in the life of another person who—in his opinion—belongs to his own level of existence.

11. We can easily recognize the mechanism at work here. It is the process of *identification*, which operates more readily in one case, and less in the other. In his friends, relatives, and neighbours, the small man can see his own picture ; and about himself, his own value, and significance, he has no very high opinion. He is well aware of his own smallness in various respects, since human beings in general are undoubtedly far from perfect, never even approximating to the ideal they themselves desire. Beneath the surface of contentedness with oneself—which is necessary for life—there is some realization of one's deficiencies. The external circumstances of the individual, being always short of his wishes, his original plans, and actual necessities, underline the feeling of smallness. And somehow, one is more easily aware of the similar smallness in a friend, neighbour, or relative ; in all probability, because one identifies oneself more readily with these than with the other members of society.

Thus, since the close acquaintance or the relative is just a small creature, conceived with his faults and limitations in gift and power, he is not felt to be worthy of a little addition in luck or of an opportunity not given to the subject. In this phenomenon the human being appears to subscribe to the principle of exploitation ; as if holding that weakness deserves nothing else than further weakening, and only the strong and efficient—though he be a total stranger, and one who is reckless in his principles—is entitled to luck and a substantial share in social position, rights, and worldly possessions.

Thus, the root of this attitude toward the neighbour and relative is essentially a depreciation of the self, projected on to those who are felt to belong to a similar low category of existence.

12. The subject is always aware, to some extent, of human insufficiency in general, and of some of his individual limitations in particular. And this very awareness implies dissatisfaction with the existing position. One natural consequence of this dissatisfaction is the tendency to create compensatory facts. The urge to produce and to attain, the desire for appreciation by others, the wish for protection and security, are logically direct results of the realization by the individual of his insufficiency.

Since weakness of the self is recognized as a potential source of disappointments and pains, physical and mental, fear of one's own weakness develops. But frequently—perhaps in everybody—there is, besides, a definite hatred of weakness ; and with regard to fellowmen, it is combined with contempt of all manifestations of personal limitation, physical and social, and an adoration for power and success wherever and however it shows itself.[1]

There is admittedly a sympathy toward the sick and injured ; and the readiness to help in such cases manifests itself with promptness. But it has always been surmised by some—and even firmly stated by wise cynics—that the subject's vague fear of becoming ill or injured himself and stricken with pain largely accounts for this sympathy. There is a kind of superstitious motive in this helpfulness, with the secret aim of averting misfortune of the same type from oneself. In the ultimate result it is good that such an irrational but emotionally potent factor exists ; however primitive, it provides driving power for the sense of duty and reinforces the ethical element of the mind.

13. There is, in general, no such prompt sympathy for people who are weak in initiative, in competitiveness and in cunning ; even though all these minuses have led manifestly to a poverty-stricken atmosphere in family life, and to a pitiable absence of self-confidence and healthy vitality in millions of people, the onlookers feel hardly any sympathy comparable with that manifested toward the sick and pain-stricken.

I suggest that this is so because of the absence in this case of the superstitious fear referred to. Social and emotional poverty, from which the millions suffer, does not strike people as sufficiently appalling ; they also hardly realize the agony due to these conditions. Consequently, their mind does not apply such a possibility to their own life, with the same penetrating intensity, as in the case of illnesses proper. True, each person, knowing about human weakness in general, is aware of potential risks to his own social and economic position, however well established at the moment. But the very fact that their circumstances *are* satisfactory, does not allow for a full identification with those

[1] The tyrannical person takes pleasure in subduing and exploiting the able-bodied fellowmen ; to prove superior to others who are potentially capable of attack and self-defence is a source of satisfaction. But there is hardly any attraction in dominating the cripple and the slow-witted.

who are in so much worse a position. And thus there cannot occur that panicky fear through identification, which is a potent stimulus of sympathy and helpfulness.

14. It is possible to describe in other terms, too, the difference in reaction to the economic distress of fellowmen on the one hand, and to their serious illness on the other. It is more or less clear to everyone that nothing can fully guarantee for the individual the uninterrupted enjoyment of his economic or positional superiority. These things are too much dependent on others, and in various circumstances quite beyond the control of the individual [cf. (2) ]. At all times, a certain number of people have had to give up their power and position and to come down in the scale of material possessions. But the confidence in one's skill and ambition, coupled with a desire for enjoyment, sufficiently counteracts the realization that a come-down is not excluded. The mental process of wishing the fulfilment of goals, together with the realization of one's practical faculties, results in what we may call confident hopefulness ; and this amounts as it were to a promise of restoration should a temporary loss ever occur. Consequently, the superstitious identification with the poor and miserable is rarely ever felt.

On the other hand, illness is conceived as a threat to life, as a messenger of death, in fact, as death in the making. No one can escape illness through his own efforts, and thus no one can whole-heartedly hope to avoid setting his foot on the path that may lead toward death. Thus, the superstitious fear emerging in face of serious physical conditions in a fellowman unavoidably enforces identification and sympathy. There is no direct danger to the foundations of life in intellectual slowness, lack of success, and social inferiority. Hence, a process of identification and resulting sympathy as in the former case hardly ever occurs in most people through witnessing poverty and social misery.

15. At any other period during recent centuries—considered the modern epoch of history—the above presentation, like all discussions by psychoanalytical authors on aggressive tendencies might have been regarded as rather academic. The writings by contemporary psychological authors, particularly if members of definite " schools ", have indeed created the impression of a selective bias in favour of the exceptional and pathological.

To-day, however, we have witnessed and will experience even more, social phenomena that more than confirm the various statements made in the past by psychoanalysts.

Exact reports coming from various parts of Europe, for several years dominated by organized brutality, throw a light on human nature that is indeed startling. A vast number of people in possession of businesses and flats, whose original owner suffered the tortures of concentration camps and are amongst the few to return, are refusing to give them up or even to share them with these rightful owners. If our customary concept of human sympathy had been factual, these unfortunates would have been received with open arms and would have returned into homes prepared for them.[1] Undoubtedly, also, events of this latter kind are occurring, in a minority of cases; but a substantial number of people are manifesting no factual sympathy or even sense of justice at all in these circumstances; so much so that Governments think that they cannot afford to enforce the elementary principles of human right and are delaying decisions or compromising, in order to avoid political troubles at home.[2] This has been the case even in countries where previously democracy, tolerance, and modernism in all human affairs was the professed programme of social science and government.

16. We psychoanalysts always thought that the tendencies to

[1] Desire for scientific objectivity requires the following statement by the writer. Reference is made in this work to contemporary events associated with the political regime in Germany in the recent past. The sole aim of discussing these events has been the utilization of these phenomena in social research, for the future good of society. What the cultural position of the German nation is going to be in the future, is at present difficult to predict. Even though concluding from the past is the favourite reaction by the searching mind, this procedure may not be entirely free from mistake and bias. There is no doubt that a substantial number of individuals there are genuinely fond of humanity and freedom.

The writer has tried to gather data of people's spontaneous reactions to the horrors of the past regime, after they were rid of its tyranny. Unfortunately, he did not succeed in finding unequivocal instances of such an indignation on the part of large German groups. Maybe that hungry and beaten people are not quite capable of such a moral indignation; or, maybe that the writer is not in possession of sufficient information. We must not ignore that in countries other than Germany large sections of the population readily collaborated with the criminal German regime; and here, too, the manifestation of regret and indignation has been far below what might be expected. Apparently, it is not easy to become fully humane after having been used to the fact that crime may be the essence of law; this confirms the assumption that cruel aggression is not a strange element in human nature, and its becoming dynamic is easier than its full suppression.

[2] This paragraph was written in June, 1945. In March, 1946, such conditions still prevail to a considerable extent. In a certain part of Europe propaganda has created the belief that more Jews returned from the concentration camps than there had been in that region previously. In fact, only 10 per cent have remained (1947).

aggression and gross brutality revealed in dreams, and disguised in psychoneurotic symptoms, were merely intra-mental elements, with no aim at realization, and no dynamic charge suitable for manifest action. All this has proved to some extent a mistake. Where social conditions allow or even encourage aggressiveness, all the tendencies of the savage may be actually manifested in behaviour. From now on we shall know better. Now we can better grasp why the psychoneurotic suffers so much from his anxiety attacks. Though there is not the slightest question of his ever committing an act of aggression,[1] the energetic charge of these intra-mental tendencies is indeed great. There is reason enough for the psychoneurotic to feel uneasy, and to try to rid himself of such processes, directed against his self.

17. The contemporary phenomena referred to above illustrate more than the bare facts. They demonstrate how shaky the foundation of a just social order is if it be based on intellectual insight and voluntary fairness alone. These events also show the peculiarly firm grip which possession or economic superiority can have on people, up to the point of eliminating from their minds the elementary sense of justice and every trace of sympathy with sufferers. The facts prove also a point to be discussed later in detail, the great significance of social backing for the development of a more, or less, satisfactory ethical behaviour. It depends very much on the spirit of the broader social environment and the administration, whether *a*-social or criminal tendencies in the individual are recognized as wrong, or alternatively are allowed to assume a rôle in the mind unopposed by moral rejection. These masses under recent German domination were systematically taught that a society and a government can legally be based on criminality ; and consequently a vast number of individuals are now void of the requisite minimum of self-criticism and self-restraint.

These people were encouraged to consider themselves different from those singled out for persecution ; to think that the victims belong to a different category of human existence. Consequently, the process of *identification* with the suffering fellowmen ceased to operate, and the fear, the vague superstitious fear, of a similar fate did not prompt humane reactions. I think, indeed, that the astonishing conduct of these people demonstrates that, *where the*

[1] In the psychoneurotic the element of moral self-restraint is considerable ; his psyche cannot tolerate the *mere idea of a-moral tendencies*.

*fear of a similar threat (jus talionis) does not operate, there may be an absence of spontaneous sympathy.*

It is obvious in this case that the material gain, made possible through the elimination of a group of fellow-beings, was the decisive temptation. In the competition between such temptation and the dictates of justice and sympathy, under average "normal" circumstances the latter do appear, to a varying extent, to be victorious. But in the absence of sufficient identification—and the implied fear—there seems to be merely a conceptual knowledge of the victim's claim, but no emotional understanding of its absolute justification. In other words, there is no emotional element strong enough to help in combating the crude competitive tendency, and therefore no real sympathy develops. Clearly, to give up a possession to a fellow-being means, in essence, readily to suffer a limitation through the existence of others. In "normal" circumstances, likewise, the competitive principle interferes with the elementary inter-human attitude; but its influence is greatly reduced towards a fellow-being in distress, through the process of identification. In the sad phenomenon of our times a potent factor of the social attitude has been eliminated; and through this fact the competitive tendency, the resentment at unavoidable limitation by others, has become dynamically strong, sweeping away the application of elementary justice in the cases mentioned.

The reader will do well to recall to his mind once more the discussion in the last paragraph, with the view of noting the interrelationship of various factors in the creation of a manifest attitude. The individual factors here referred to are: the fundamental social sense; the competitive attitude (resentment against limitation); the approval by Government and organized society or body of just or criminal attitudes; and the phenomenon of identification, with the implied fear of misfortune, or the apparent absence of such repercussion, as the case may be.

*Note.* A close analysis of the social sense is attempted in Appendix II 11, 12.

# CHAPTER IB

## HUMAN INADEQUACY AND FEAR OF THE ENVIRONMENT

*Human behaviour is the result of an interplay of motives.—Primary and secondary causal factors.—Secondary elements are not necessarily of a secondary rôle.—Which is more important, the fear of the environment or the feeling of human inadequacy?—The nucleus and development of the feeling of inadequacy.—The feeling of moral insufficiency in the child and adult.—The environmental factor in this element of the mind.—The environment's attitude forces the individual to hide features of inadequacy.—Fear of the environment is a potent factor.*

1. IN the analysis of human behaviour it is not always expedient to ask which is the primary factor among the several motives jointly operative behind a particular phenomenon. Human feeling and conduct is the outcome of compound processes. It is like an orchestral piece in which the musical impression on the perceptive mind results from a combination of accords and the tones of various instruments.

Besides, a mental motive can be actually the product of an earlier process or tendency, but nevertheless it may prove ultimately of a greater functional significance than its creator element. An incidental defeat suffered by a youth at a moment when a friend of his was enjoying a minor success, proved to be a stimulus for the revision on his part of his earlier life-plan; at first over-idealistic, he later did his best to become a practical success. It is obvious that there was no intrinsic relationship between the irritating incident and the later attitude of this young man in repressing most of his idealistic inclinations for the sake of demonstrable material successes. Clearly, the resulting attitude was of a far greater significance than the incident, which in itself might have implied no more than a brief spell of uneasiness.

If a child breaks a window in a house, the owners of which are away on holiday, and torrential rain entering through the window damages valuable furniture and clothing beyond repair, the significance of the secondary event for the owner far exceeds the annoyance about the broken panel. If, further, the little boy who was the initiator of these events is afraid to pass the scene of his past misdeed, and avoids, perhaps for years to come, the street in question, this case would be an even apter illustration of the point mentioned. The broken pane may soon be replaced by a new one ; whereas the fear leading to the avoidance of the street may influence the boy's life to a substantial degree and for a considerable period. This example may at first appear to have no adequate parallel in the sphere of intra-mental processes. It is nevertheless a fact based on indubitable experiences that secondary processes closely dependent on a still current primary one are not infrequently of superior content and dynamic significance as compared with the primary factor.

2. In the case of our main theme, dealing with the function of co-operation and the factors interfering with it, it appears nevertheless profitable to inquire into the relationship of the two disturbing factors mentioned, the fear of the environment on the one hand and the realization of self-insufficiency on the other. It is undoubtedly of practical consequence to see clearly here, since the possibility of remedy is not equal with regard to the two factors. We can try to encourage a person and persuade him into believing that he is not less in the eyes of his fellowmen than are average people. It is possible to remove some of the doubt felt by an individual with regard to the personal values and significance he possesses. But in this our endeavour we must be prepared for a substantial limitation. Admittedly, not a few sensitive individuals will readily listen to encouragement, and will avail themselves of the opportunity to create a somewhat optimistic conception about themselves. But in this process they will soon be opposed by their more exact knowledge of the factual circumstances. Their sense of realities will not cease to reveal to them how small are the chances of a fair deal throughout life, even where deserved. And even more must it be realized that only comparatively few persons are attractive or impressive enough to feel sure of some success and appreciation, in almost all walks of their life. All the others must constantly live in some fear of being ignored and consequently denied even their fair share in the good things of life, if its acquisition depends mainly on the goodwill of others.

From these few remarks it can already be guessed that for the problem of co-operation the environmental factor plays possibly a greater rôle, if practical considerations of remedy are in question. It will not be difficult to ascertain the probable relationship between the two sources of disturbance running counter to the elementary desire for friendly co-operation, if the genetical development of both " complexes " is kept in mind.

3. In the infant, and the small child, there must be a feeling of absolute dependence on others, particularly when biological needs require satisfaction, or circumstances of an uneasy character arise making for the child the presence of the adults acutely desirable. This experience is, probably, the nucleus of the later feeling of self-insufficiency, though not quite the same as that feeling. Soon the child learns that the " kind " persons of his environment are at the same time the sources of limitations imposed upon him by them for educational reasons. The fact, moreover, that adults enjoy more freedom of décision, and more direct access to desirable goals, becomes very early an obvious experience, and the desire to grow up soon largely dominates the feeling of all children. Thus the *feeling* of *self-insufficiency* is introduced into the child's mind from two aspects. One is the positive, more pleasant experience that the adults are the source of subsistence and protection for himself. This, however, implicitly informs the child of his own smallness. The other type of experience consists of the repeated instances in which adults impose their will and guidance on children against their spontaneous wishes. Acquaintance with the *competitive element* in life, together with the knowledge that the weaker suffers limitation, thus becomes the unavoidable experience of all human beings.

4. But, as we know, the adults support their claim to superiority by pointing to the inferior intellectual and moral standard of the child. Not only does the young individual learn about his concrete weakness and his need of external help, but the awareness of his mental inferiority is instilled into him. He is not clean enough, not clever enough, not obedient enough, not nice enough, etc. This is obviously the real foundation, and the first instalment, of the feeling of insufficiency ; in the adult it becomes, to a great extent, a moral one. One has only to take this notion of *moral insufficiency* in a sense broader than that in general use.

In the course of mental growth there develops an intramental picture of what may be called the average human dignity, an image of the ideal in various respects for the person's character and behaviour. This desirable picture not only includes aspects of morality in the customary sense, but is composed of all the features of a man or woman that together contribute to the formation of an appreciable and pleasant personality. Skill, intellect, gestures, voice, and external appearance as well as moral character in the narrower sense, are the individual items relevant to the functional picture of the personality. And, as suggested, there exists within the subject's mind an image of ideal composition which appears desirable to him and also applicable as a plan of manifest life to his particular make-up.[1] All tendencies, decisions, and actions are measured by this subconscious ideal picture ; and the realization of self-insufficiency has reference to this moral character (general quality) in the broader sense suggested here.

5. It is undeniable that the sentiment of self-regard and feeling of responsibility in a broader sense owe their development to the explicit wishes of the adults, who encourage and discourage, advise and check as well as praise or disapprove the individual actions of the maturing child, and, in essence, its personality as a whole. This external pressure constantly moulds the personality in the making, and similarly later, the adult individual. It is easy to realize that the natural tendency of the individual to consider the environment is stimulated in an equal measure by the desire to please others and by the fear of others. Both factors are highly emotional in charge, and this genesis is probably responsible for the strong emotional urge of what appears as one's autonomous conscience.[2]

The hypothetical idea of what people might think and do *if* they knew about various individual tendencies of the subject constitutes a force constantly influencing the mind. By such a fear the subject seems to assume that a great number of others

[1] In the spontaneous choice of ideologies and ideal pattern of personality there is always a tendency to please the particular make-up of the subject. Even though practically the attainment of a certain ideal-ego is impossible for the subject, there may be deep down a feeling of a psychic ability for its development. Otherwise, there would ensue a tension beyond endurance between the ideal and actual personality. This seems manifestly to be the case in obsessive personalities ; their psyche appears to be particularly intolerant towards their sexual and aggressive tendencies. The difference between the ideal and the actual personality can be ignored only where there is a general capacity for dividing between the spheres of wishful imagination and those of actual manifestation. In the obsessive type the tabooed idea becomes equal to action, and this prevents the subject from recognizing sufficiently the separateness of wishing and acting in general. Thus he is also unable to tolerate the gap between his ideal and his feasible ego.

[2] Cf. Chs. VI, XIV.

are different from himself both in character and value, and that many of these others are in fact better, more clever, and more dignified on the whole. But there is mainly a vague fear that other people may easily overlook their own moral and intellectual deficiencies and yet expect from their fellowmen—the subject included—an entire absence of such weaknesses.

6. The individual is doubtlessly dependent on others for very many things. He needs their physical help, their advice, their appreciation, and their very company. But these others, so much needed and craved for by the subject, are often unfair; they allow themselves to be guided in their social attitude by the appearance and the externals of behaviour of their fellow-beings. They wish him to be pleasant and virtuous before they are ready to let him have his due share in life, however morally deficient and unpleasant they themselves may be. In this respect people behave in general just as employers in particular; they themselves may be unable to carry out the smallest detail of the productive process, but they expect from the wage-earners skill, experience, and subservience. In the case of the employee, things cannot be different; the expectations put on his efficiency are justified. But the average human attitude in expecting from others more perfection in general human values than one possesses oneself is in its effect cruel. People wish to make up, as it were, through the perfection, grace, and goodness of others what is lacking in themselves. It appears, indeed, in many instances that the less perfect a human being is, the less he is able to forgive deficiencies in his fellowmen.

Skill and efficiency in general are appreciated and admired; on the other hand, weakness, lack of driving power, and even incidental mishaps suffered by another person, evoke, besides some pity, a measure of disregard. Thus the subject has to be careful to hide, as far as possible, his average human deficiencies, and has to bring, as much as possible, into the limelight any signs of his efficiency and attainments.

7. The feeling of inadequacy in average human beings refers to a large extent to the realization that it is, in fact, impossible always to impress others to the degree that is desirable in various situations. Thus, the fear of the environment results in an intensification of the feeling of insufficiency that exists owing to

a more primary cause. In other words, not the realization by the subject of his objective inadequacy is the chief disturber of self-confidence, but the associated fear of unjust reaction on the part of fellowmen to the discovery of this insufficiency in the individual.

Why people react so unfairly to the average deficiencies of their fellowmen is a less simple question than might be inferred from the few words devoted above to the phenomenon. It has to do with the function of tolerating oneself, and the association of this self-toleration with the tolerance of others. This process will be discussed in a later chapter.[1] Here we wish only to note that the very existence of defects in the subject's personality makes for a desire to meet other fellowmen who give pleasure in their appearance and outward behaviour.[2] Yet, as already indicated, this fact spurs people to the display of advantageous aspects, and to the hiding of all their faults and weaknesses, to an excessive degree that implies a strain for them and becomes the source of an undercurrent of anxiety lest they fail.

[1] Cf. Ch. IV.

[2] Cf. Ch. IV (2, 3) about the mixing within the mind of the " subject " and the " object ".

# CHAPTER Ic

## REACTIVE TRAITS SECONDARY TO THE FEELING OF INADEQUACY

*The realization of human inadequacy.—This realization is a variable factor of the mind.—Compensatory traits.—The instinct of self-preservation lends its dynamic force to some of these secondary elements.—The rôle of general intra-mental weakness in the perception of complexes and the realization of inadequacy.—The prospect of improvement in social attitudes follows from the socially conditioned character of some undesirable attitudes.*

1. THERE is in everybody a certain realization of his human insufficiency. The claims made on the human being by various situations in life cannot be met fully. Only too often one has to resign oneself in advance to the prospect of partial or total failure. In all respects—in strength, skill, endurance, and in goodwill and morals—there is a gap between the imagined ideal pattern of perfection and the actual attainment. There is, in fact, a considerable gap even between what appears to be the minimal requirement of personal accomplishment for practical life and the manifest ability of the individual to cope with things.

A certain measure of realization of human deficiency is obviously normal. It would be a delusional state if the mind took no notice at all of the real position. The shock of disappointments unavoidable in life would be beyond endurance. But the realization of human weakness varies greatly in various persons. There is also no proportion between the limitations of the personality and the feeling relating to this relative weakness. People who suffer greatly from what we call a feeling of inferiority are, as a rule, not below the average in human accomplishment ; they are not rarely above the average in ethical orientation and even in practical ability. In the life of the same person, there are moments when the awareness of insufficiency interferes with the dynamics of the mind more than at other times, though the general structure of the personality may be to all intents the same.

There is a similarity to the dynamic effect of what we call subconscious complexes in the psychoanalytical sense. I hold that the influence of these on the mind is dependent not only on their absolute intensity, but also to a great extent on the measure of their realization by the rest of the self.

The significance of the realization related to human inadequacy lies in *secondary processes* which it stimulates. It is not surprising that not a few of these secondary elements are clear attempts at compensation. They reveal themselves as derivatives of the complex to which in our opinion they owe their existence.

2. It is hard to assume that the urge for unreasonable power, or the tendency to deny full esteem to the weak, are elementary forces, comparable to what we call fundamental instincts. Such anti-social tendencies, one has to admit, can be of no vital significance; they are never needed for the maintenance of the individual's life or of his race. It is, therefore, justifiable to consider them, and similar manifestations of the personality, as *reactive* in nature; that is, as stimulated by environmental events, and coming into being in a quasi-logical sequence to such events.

This may be surprising, in view of the universality and dynamic force of such tendencies as lust for domination or possession *per se*, or the sentiment of envy where the subject does not lack in essentials. If the amount and intensity of the educational measures required for checking such tendencies are taken into consideration, they can hardly be thought of otherwise than in terms of elementary, instinct-like forces of the human race.

But it is nevertheless true that we are dealing with phenomena of a secondary order, though of supreme social significance. One has only to rid oneself of the notion that powerful tendencies, of widespread manifestation, must be elementary and autonomous in the same sense as the vital instincts of human life, which latter need no independent mental process to create them. Character traits, even if not innate but obviously reactive, can be endowed with a force that makes it almost impossible for the subject to resist their urge voluntarily.

3. The instances referred to above are secondary products reactive to the realization of self-insufficiency. They have been recognized by the Adlerian school as compensatory attempts.

We should, perhaps, more accurately say that they are meant to compensate for the loss in psycho-affective equilibrium incurred through the realization of human imperfection. They are not only secondary in order to a primary force stimulating them, but also logically associated with it. And the primary force through its continued existence plays the part of a conditioning factor in the constant creation and maintenance of the secondary element. The analogy to primary and "induced" electrical currents presents itself obviously.

In essence, the above-mentioned instances of reactive tendency spring thus in the wake of a genuinely primary element of the mind; it is the actual insufficiency of the human being, and its realization, that stimulate the attempts at compensation. Perhaps, this origin accounts for the intense force and universality of such phenomena as lust for domination or possession, or envy, which latter is only another mode of expressing a desire for unlimited and unnecessary possession. In other words, the elementary fact of insufficiency, with its realization, possesses a dynamic force comparable to that of fundamental instincts; and some of this force can be transferred to reactive elements ensuing from this primary one. It is very likely that the subconscious realization of human insufficiency has a dormant but strong affective potential; this mirrors, even though only partially, the actual significance for life of various deficiencies. Much potential disappointment, pain, and even danger is implied in imperfections of the human being; it is only natural that the subjective realization of this should create reactive products of a powerful drive and resistance.

4. Returning to the primary factor under discussion here, which is the realization of human insufficiency, we should bear in mind that its painfulness exists only because of a side glance at the social environment. The comparison of the individual's self with the others, and even more the fear of their opinion, with all possible consequences of this opinion to himself, are the obvious sources from which the painfulness of self-insufficiency springs. This has been clearly explained above. We can now add that, from this genetic angle, secondary traits associated with the feeling of insufficiency are *reactive* even in the narrower sense of the word, in so far that they are really stimulated by the environment and are not merely results of an intra-personal difficulty.

One must also recognize that this influence of the broader social environment is different from that of particular persons who determine or interfere with the subject's private affairs. However great these persons' actual significance, in either sense, may be for the subject, he might get rid of them. The subject is logically allowed to imagine at least the possibility of freeing himself from them through leaving them, or seeing them dead. But there is no escape from the broader human environment, and its materialization cannot be even imagined as long as the subject is sane. Individual members or even groups of this hostile environment may go, or may have to surrender their relative power and influence ; but this makes no more change in the impact of the broader environment on individual life than the removal of a bucket of water makes in the level of the sea. Consequently, reactive sentiments stimulated by the broader environment are very potent mental elements ; and attitudes that are attempts at compensation springing from a fear of the environment may assume a deep-rootedness such as is familiar in vital instincts.

5. This conception of reactive trends link up with the theoretical problem of deflection of mental energy and sublimation. I assume that once a tendency emerges in the wake of a particular mental process, the energy and drive manifested in the secondary attitude springs from the supply of energy of the personality as a whole, because it is the balance of the integrated personality that is to be restored through the deflection. It is, therefore, perhaps too narrow a concept to think of " sublimation ",[1] that is, of a real transformation of a particular instinct and tendency.

Thus it can be said that compensatory traits may display the elementary force of a quasi-inborn factor, because they are measures in defence of the feeling of the *self*, and thus aptly comparable to attempts at defending physical life. In a broader sense they are thus manifestations of the self-preservation instinct, though somewhat " derailed " from attaining its genuine goal, which is peace of body and mind. The psychiatrist will be reminded of the explanation offered by psychoanalysis on the general significance of delusional systems in the psychotic process. These formations are recognized as attempts of the mind at the restoration of contact with reality, which has been largely destroyed by the pathological process.

[1] Cf. *Man and his Fellowmen*, Ch. VIII (6), (8).

6. If the mind brings into operation tendencies of anti-social character, because the sense of a loss stimulates the creation of reactive substitutes, then there is always much in those tendencies that goes beyond the mark. It is true that with selfishness and aggressiveness there is something—whether much or little—to be gained. In this respect there is in these reactive tendencies no character of unreality comparable to the delusions of the psychotic. It is a fact that attainments, whether they be objects, or power, or even merely harmful interference with the life of others, may to a degree buttress up the feeling of the self, if it is somewhat "shaky". But on the whole, such a reactive tendency, being anti-social in its goals and scope, can never contribute to a harmonious balance within the mind. There is bound to emerge in the mind the simultaneous knowledge that a programme of aggression can arouse in the personality of others, the intended victims, only resentment and the wish for revenge. This intra-mental conclusion, it may be thought, should in fact increase the tension of disharmony; whereas the very stimulus for the creation of a compensatory element was the desire to relieve an uneasiness ensuing from the realization of insufficiency.

Nevertheless, the increased tension, as a rule, does not prompt the person to the abandonment of his reactive aggressiveness. The satisfaction from the aggressive plan and its actual results seem to thrill the mind to a too great extent to admit of such a process of self-regulation. The general spirit immanent in the affairs of the world unequivocally admires success and envies the pluck for aggression. This environmental approval does not allow the subject to give up a surplus of his exaggerated reactions. In other words, it is ultimately the environment, through its presumable spirit, that decides whether a certain type of reactive tendency is adhered to and increasingly developed, even though the increase of the intra-mental tension, which the subject originally meant to reduce, should warn against its continuance.

7. From the practical viewpoint of the sociologist and reformer, the reactive, that is, the *secondary* character of anti-social traits implies, as a matter of fact, a measure of hope for the future. It does not matter that envy or lust for unreasonable possession and power are so universal and so strongly at work, if only there should remain the prospect of partial remedy, effected through measures on a larger scale than the mere ethical appeal to the individual. There may logically be expected a decrease in such

tendencies, if the realities in the social environment should not unduly stimulate the feeling of self-insufficiency.

8. But it is well to extend our examination to a more accurate analysis of the feeling of insufficiency. If our expectations of a possible improvement are not to disappoint us, it is imperative to look for weak points in our explanatory concepts. It has been suggested that the reactive attitudes of an anti-social character spring from a concrete fact, that is the subject's actual lack of perfection. Yet it has been pointed out previously that, in essence, it is the *realization of this imperfection* that is the immediate stimulus of secondary products. It has been assumed that it is not so much the actual insufficiency of the human being as the degree of its realization by the self that causes the uneasiness and all its reactive consequences. It has also been pointed out that there is no proportion between the actual degree of imperfection and the feelings related to it. Thus, from intrinsic psychoneurotic sources the feeling of insufficiency may be increased unduly, and then its undesirable products may come into the fore more forcefully.

If this is so, then the extrinsic conditioning of the reactive traits cannot play the decisive part ascribed to it, and the hope of remedying them through alterations of the social factor may be much smaller than has been assumed. It cannot, and should not, be doubted that the feeling of insufficiency plays a greater part in the production of reactive traits than does the objective fact of human imperfection *per se*. The more critically we approach the problem, the more it must appear probable that *the undesirable direction which the attempts at compensation take, results from the psychoneurotic uneasiness developing in view of human weakness, rather than being the adequate consequence of the objective fact*. Excess of realization of the implications bound up with human weakness is very probably based on an innate lack of the psychic process as a whole, peculiar to a large number of people. Optimistic concepts to the effect that an encouraging tone of early and later education may in itself prevent such feelings of " inferiority ", seems to me, indeed, unwarranted.

Similarly, however, unjustified it may seem to deny that extrinsic influences *are* capable of increasing or decreasing the difficulties arising in the course of intra-mental processes. But as suggested, it is of no avail to overlook the fact that the intramental complications themselves are largely intrinsic, i.e. expressive of a faulty development. Just as there exists a scale of variants in efficiency of all physiological functions in various persons, so there are in the spheres of mental functioning weaknesses of various degrees, on account of obstructions in development. If an infantile trauma can substantially interfere with mental development and render the individual prone to fixations and regressions, this in itself is due to innate lack of resistance. The same is the case if the impact of a single trauma appears to have interfered with the " naturalness " and spontaneity of the subject. A surplus of self-criticism, shyness, and intense awareness of self-insufficiency, are due to a constitutional excess in realizing all that is deficient and disturbing, whilst taking insufficient note of what are the assets of the personality. Psychoanalysis proper can, nevertheless, improve such conditions, through bringing relief on other points and thus altering the intra-mental balance as a whole.

9. Nevertheless, there is no cogent reason for relinquishing our fundamental concept in its application to social improvement. Though the immediate stimulus leading to unfavourable reactive formations is, admittedly, the feeling of insufficiency—in essence largely of a psychoneurotic causation—the resulting attitudes are but defences of the *self*. As suggested above, it is the maintenance of an integrated personality that is the original goal of all compensatory formations, however ethically wrong these may be. *In the creation of certain social attitudes as attempts at compensation for the feeling of weakness, the central aim is not the presence of these attitudes but the restoration of balance within the personality.*

If this latter assumption is true, then we need not be unduly concerned about the prospects of improvement in the social sense of individuals. They will be only too ready to give up compensatory traits of an *a*-social and ludicrous type, if the deep-seated uneasiness which gives birth to these reaction types should be eased by suitable reforms. Cf. XI (2). The lust for unreasonable power or possession, and the like, are deep-rooted, if once created, not for their own sake but for the sake of the personality desirous of a psycho-affective balance.

The second point to be borne in mind is the fact that uneasiness and the urge toward the creation of compensatory attitudes does not necessarily mean the direct and exclusive desire to assume *a*-social attitudes. As long as power can be used to exploit others, as long as a conspicuous " more " possessed by a few gives them extraordinary opportunities of attaining elementary human happiness, we must understand that the compensatory attempts will tend in these directions. But if exploitation and undue power should come to be regarded as in opposition to cultured life, if envy and the contempt of the fellowman because of his physical or positional weakness should come to be looked upon as archaic tendencies [1] disqualifying a person from retaining public esteem, people's minds would choose differently.

10. Every law and regulation has to force itself upon society, and the assumption that everybody genuinely agrees with legal and ethical principles is but a working hypothesis, admittedly a hypothesis that really does work. A vast number of individuals assume these desirable principles from, we may say, opportunism. And this is good, because it is in fact the only way of educating the average masses. Why should it be impossible for all the authorized representatives of administration and public education to assume a kind of pretence that absolute decency within society is the *natural standard*, as if another serious alternative did not exist in the mind of an average human being! Such assumed attitudes on the part of influential bodies and persons could not fail to have far-reaching social effects. Cf. Ch. XI (13) (14).

It is clear that there is at present no justification for hoping that an essential change of principle in handling society is round the corner. In proportion to the degree to which such a working hypothesis will permeate administration and society, there is bound to ensue an appropriate improvement within the minds of many individuals. The frequency of compensatory traits that are undesirable are likely to decrease. Public disapproval, with the threat of loss in esteem, is a powerful regulator even of deeper mental spheres in the choice of the ultimate type of reactive traits. Cf. Chs. VI, XII, XVI.

[1] Cf. Ch. XI (15).

## CHAPTER IIA

## TOLERANCE AND THE FACTORS OPPOSING IT

*Tolerance is a function, operating constantly.—Resistance to new suggestions.—A new idea or an impression may be perceived as a threat to mental stability.—The rôle of competitive resentment in intolerance.—The dynamic rôle of symbolic associations.—An instance.—The moral conflict.—The internal aggressor may cause more uneasiness than the potential or real competitor.—The relationship between the competitive complex and the amoral tendency in the psyche.*

1. For reasons discussed above (Ch. I), the elementary friendly interest in the fellowman cannot remain an unadulterated sentiment ; it is modified through the interference of other tendencies and processes. The resulting attitude toward the fellowman is rather that of toleration. This is clearly the case with regard to the vast majority of fellow-beings, that is, to those who do not evoke our affection, or, through some of their characteristics, our interest or admiration. More accurately, the average attitude towards a fellow-being is a compound sentiment, consisting of friendly interest, antagonism from the competitive complex, and a measure of acceptance of the unavoidable ; the proportion of these components being variable.

2. This acceptance, or tolerance, is a *function* and not merely a passively receptive attitude. Let us think, for the sake of analogy, of two bricks with a larger or smaller interval between them. If the space between the two is large enough to receive a third brick without being touched on either side by the two others, then there is no mechanical interaction between the three. But if the middle brick has to be forced into the space, it exerts a certain pressure on the two, just as it receives such a pressure from both sides. This is comparable to what I call the active function of tolerance. The factors opposing the elementary interest have constantly to be dealt with by the mind ; that is to say, their influence diminished and adjusted according to existing needs

of the inter-human situation. There has to take place a constant process of toleration with respect to each person in the environment; the presence of a fellow-being keeps the function of tolerance constantly occupied, and not only at the moment of the first meeting with him.

3. Like every function in the human organism, that of tolerance may operate either smoothly or under a strain. It is only natural that those fellow-beings whose limiting significance to the subject's freedom is obvious, stimulate the function of tolerance to a great extent. The presence of such individuals in the field of the subject's existence implies an element somewhat difficult to "digest"; their toleration implies a measure of strain for the psyche. The difficulty for the subject's mind in this type of case is caused by the fact that the fellowman in question represents a limiting potential.

But there are individuals whose capacity for tolerance is intrinsically below the average; within them there is a habitual difficulty in coping with the presence of fellowmen, including even those who, by dint of their personality, would imply *no* exceptional task for an average mind. Moreover, to get on familiar terms with a new phenomenon, as for instance a point of view contrasting with one's previous belief, is not equally easy for everyone. More often than not the mere mention of such a novel suggestion, or opinion, different from the subject's own, makes people irritable.

4. One readily understands that an average person feels uneasy if a sacrifice be asked of him for the benefit of another man, for whom he cares very little; or, if someone makes a suggestion, even though only a theoretical one, the materialization of which would interfere with the subject's rights or expectations. We understand also that a person reacts negatively to a statement that might imply a disappointment of his hopes; thus, people do not like critical remarks on their religious conceptions, because they realize that if these statements were true—as they might be—the hopes they place in religion might prove without foundation.

But a similar irritability is, at times, aroused in people by statements that contain no such undesirable elements; by statements whose unpleasantness lies apparently in nothing else than in not being congruent with the listener's knowledge or opinion. The offensive character of such statements is obviously *the implicit disagreement with the subject.*

5. Since daily life provides such frequent illustrations of this type of reaction, we are inclined to consider it natural, with no further background worthy of analysis. But a little thought must reveal that this is not entirely the case. Just as frequently the receiving of news—unexpected news—or that of corrective information or entirely new knowledge, is rather a pleasant experience for people ; they show no signs of resentment at the implied alteration of their previous knowledge and opinion.

We may assume that much depends on what group of associations are being touched intra-mentally by the literal statement.[1] The emotional reaction to new information is irritability only if any association is stimulated that might imply an attack on the subject's wishes and expectations. Yet this answer, though psychologically correct, cannot be the end of our inquiry. The real question is why far-fetched unpleasant associations are too easily stirred up in some individuals, on certain occasions, though it is sure that the speaker cannot be suspected of any intention of aiming at such sore points in the subject's mind, and the manifest meaning of what has been said appears far from being irritating in character.

It seems not even logically necessary to feel resentment when one's opinions and theories are openly criticized. No one can really compel the subject to change his mind ; if his opinion is so precious to him, no one can take it away by merely disagreeing or criticizing it, unless the subject himself chooses to give it up for the sake of an improved concept. In this case he is in fact a gainer, a fortunate fellow who has got rid of something useless in exchange for something valuable. The resentment follows apparently from the fact that people associate their *personality* too closely with any of their particular opinions, and feel the rejection of their statements as a wholesale denial of appreciation, a denial of their personal significance. This personal attack *may be* the aim in particular instances of criticism ; but, as a rule, even a simpleton or an ignoramus enjoys a measure of friendliness and personal appreciation by his fellowmen, so long as he does not wish to appear more than he actually is.

[1] Cf. Appendix II.

6. Observation shows, indeed, that many of those who are over-sensitive to discussion and criticism, are, in other respects, too, somewhat unstable in emotional balance. An opposing statement always challenges the mind to deal with it, to compare it with one's own opinion ; and this process implies, however remotely, a consideration of the possibility of abandoning one's belief. This small " storm " within the psyche seems to be a good deal of a burden to personality types of emotionally unstable composition.

We may also assume that deep down in their mind these people have not a firm enough conviction about their chosen opinion ; probably they even have some doubts with regard to their general intelligence and faculty of judgment. There is, as it were, a constant though dormant opposition in their own mind to the very ideas for which they profess preference or even claim exclusive validity. If then an extrinsic opposition to their belief has to be received into their mind, examined, and dealt with in the afore-mentioned way, this foreign idea greatly intensifies the existing intra-mental doubt about themselves, and this constitutes a threat to the precarious stability of their chosen belief, and also to their ease of mind as a whole.

7. But I feel that the type of intolerance here under discussion has in numerous cases a different and greater significance. A large number of those suffering from instability and defective tolerance seem to be on the whole lacking in elementary interest in their fellow-beings. They are deficient in the capacity to *accept their fellowman as an independent personality*. For them, all the others in their environment count only so far as they confirm their own opinion ; or at least so far as they do not conspicuously manifest their independent personality. Subject to that, these others can at least be imagined to be in agreement with the subject. But as distinct, manifestly independent personalities, with their own rights and claims, they are undesirable, intolerable, and quasi-non-existent.

8. An opinion or attitude differing from that of the hypotolerant subject activates in the latter's mind *competitive resentment*. This is one of the probable reasons why a novel statement with no element of personal attack, or with only a remotely implied one, can cause in a great number of listeners marked irritability.

It is the aggressive element associated with competitive resentment that supplies this emotional over-reaction. It may also be said that the two differing ideas, that of the speaker and that of the sensitive listener, vie with each other, and this process stimulates the elementary and more significant competitive complex, which we have outlined in Chapter I.

The foreignness to the subject's mind of an opinion advanced by another person evokes in response the elementary *competitive complex*, which makes the mind realize that all fellowmen are strangers and potential limiting factors in life. The new, differing idea becomes representative of the person who utters it ; and thus, for the mind of the listener, the distinct and competitive significance of that person, of all other persons, indeed, is brought home.

9. We are faced in this psychological process with the phenomenon of *symbolic association*. This consists in the stimulation of a particular sphere of ideas (complexes) by a different category of mental elements, if there is an emotional link and a symbolic relationship between the elements of both spheres. Whether such a link exists or is possible between two logically disparate spheres depends largely on individual psychic factors, which themselves may undergo a change in significance in various phases of the individual's life. The dynamic significance of a certain memory, for instance, may change with time. At one period one aspect of that event may be more dominant within the mind, and another aspect at other periods.

10. A woman who was friendly with a man and almost engaged to him severed this friendship because she discovered that her would-be mother-in-law was not a trustworthy person. First, the feeling of great regret for having been obliged to give up the man was prevalent in her. As time went on she discovered in herself some annoyance with the man for his reluctance to admit his mother's fault. She now felt quite glad to have been spared all the trouble that would have been unavoidably her share had she married him. The thing, however, that she did not know—it was only realized much later—was that the would-be mother-in-law reminded her, in one particular feature, of her own grandmother, who had caused much irritation to her own daughter, the mother of the woman in question. On a later occasion she

recognized the similarity—a reminder of the grandmother—and she was again glad, but now from a different point of view, that she had not married her friend.

11. It is easy to see that a memory always has various aspects. And it is also easy to understand that not every aspect can be equally prominent in the mind at all phases of life. Certainly the whole question of the grandmother was bound to lose much in significance in a few years—she could not live for ever; whereas the untrustworthiness of the friend's mother was a problem of much greater practical significance for anyone who married him.

Let us now assume that this woman in certain situations proved to be weak. On one occasion she had, in fact, lacked the courage to tell her employer that his attitude towards a customer was rude. She then regretted her own weakness and the necessity to be in the employment of such a man; and suddenly the friend of the past came into her mind amid her solitude in life. His weakness in not seeing his mother's faults might have been the element that was stirred up subconsciously by her own weakness in the present. If one may be allowed to venture on a reconstruction of the whole reasoning deep down in her mind, perhaps she thought that, had her friend proved stronger and less blind to his mother's faults, she would have married him in spite of all, and would so have been spared now from being in the employment of a man of whom she disapproved.

The sole purpose of this instance is, however, to show how a particular element of a complex memory may be more capable at a certain time of being stirred up at the cost of other aspects of the case. It may be assumed that, if this woman's employer had been a liar, this fact would have been more likely to conjure up deep down in her mind her past friend's mother. Instead of her regret at not being married there would have been, possibly, the comforting idea that "it is better to have a liar as a boss than as a mother-in-law". It is hoped that this instance sufficiently illustrates the individual and variable conditioning of stimulation by an associative element.

12. But there are symbolic associations within the psyche that are of a more universal character. Though each individual is unique, and in details the workings of his mind are peculiar to

him alone, there is so much that is common to all of us. The impact of social life, in its deeper influence, does much to account for this. It results in elements of the mind common to many. Consequently, there are also symbolic associations that are of more or less universal occurrence, or at least are common to individuals of a similar personality type.

Returning to our original problem, we wish to state that the *strangeness* to the subject's principles of an idea expressed by a fellowman is able, by way of symbolic association, to stir up the competitive complex ; the idea of the intrusive and limiting character of fellowmen in general being associatively related to the foreign idea intruding, as it were, into the mind of the subject. Both ideas have obviously a common abstract denominator ; and this for the mental mechanism of perhaps all people, but particularly for those lacking in tolerance toward what is new or different.

13. But all this is not yet the deepest root of the phenomenon, and certainly not the only one. I think there is an obvious pointer to the fact that this symbolic stimulation is, in its turn, made possible by a yet deeper underlying factor. I suggest that difficulties in the *moral function* are important contributors to this type of intolerance. The tendencies that are kept dormant for the sake of morality are nevertheless not void of dynamic charge. Their impact on the integrated personality is felt in various ways. It is possible more or less to protect from them the freedom of moral choice ; but not to eliminate them. Similarly we can protect a child from the attack of a dangerous dog without in the least diminishing the animal's aggressive potential.

This constant struggle within the mind against tendencies and concepts that are in opposition to the aims of the moral function, can create amongst other results a sensitiveness against *strange ideas* in a broader sense. That is to say, any statement in opposition to one's existing knowledge, opinion, or belief, may become a symbol of the strange anti-moral world within the mind. As suggested, the different opinion of a fellowman throws into relief the distinct individuality of persons other than the subject. But at the same time, the foreign idea can become a symbolic reminder that the homogeneity of the moral spheres within the subject is only a working hypothesis ; that the moral composition of the personality is not free from volcanic elements menacing the whole structure. It is not difficult to understand the symbolic relationship between a strange idea coming from outside, and that part of the mental content which we would preferably throw out of our personality. In a functional sense, such symbolic relationship implies that stimulation of the one complex can be transmitted to the other.

14. I wish to suggest that it is this difficulty in the deep moral process that lends so much irrational passion to intolerance towards the opinions and tastes of others. Admittedly, the competitive complex alone possesses emotional charge enough to evoke resentment and antagonism. A superficial view of a materialistic orientation might suggest as sufficient the assumption that a strange idea evokes the realization of the fact that all fellowmen are intruders and limiting factors in concrete spheres. The moral element, so this superficial explanation might assert, is at best an equal contributor to the intolerant reaction. But, I feel, this view would be a mistaken one ; and any conclusion drawn from it might lead to practical failures.

Admittedly, the competitive element, with all the fear and resentment implied by it, is undoubtedly a fundamental force. It is so, because it links up with the tendency of elementary self-preservation and self-assertion. Competitive intolerance—if looked at closely—is largely of an unjust, superfluous nature, since there is in fact room and opportunity in plenty for others.[1] Thus, in essence, the competitive complex aims at *unlimited opportunities* for the individual. But since the elementary needs of life and of the mental personality do require a certain struggle and purposiveness, it is easy for the unjustified part of the competitive tendency to buttress itself with the principle of elementary rights. In simple words, the person can persuade himself that all his resentment and suspicion and intolerance come only from elementary self-defence and not from the tendency to seek unrestricted power in the choice of vast opportunities. Thus, the emotional charge of this factor—so may it be argued—is great enough to account for various manifestations of intolerance, if it is unduly stimulated.

15. Against this trend of thought we have to realize the following facts : As we have pointed out above, generalized competitive resentment (with all its implications) cannot really be accounted for by actual conditions. It *is* certainly justified in face of those

[1] Cf. Ch. XI, p. 176.

fellowmen who concretely interfere with the fair claims of the subject; and also towards those who manifest anti-social tendencies in general, even if not against the particular subject. But its generalized operation is not warranted by objective facts. If, as we assume, the competitive phenomenon in all its aspects is an object of implicit knowledge for all of us, then this corrective realization must also be included in the concept relating to it. Indeed, I assume that it is partly responsible for lessening the fear and suspicion ensuing from the elementary crude complex. There must also be a knowledge, based on personal experience, that many situations of the individual do allow of an improvement in his favour, through some change of the external conditions; that there is, as it were, a possibility of partial escape from the factual inconveniences due to social restrictions. This means in essence that as long as the adversary is an outside factor, there appears a possibility—whether immediate or remote—of the subject escaping from its proximity.

16. But if the aggressor is an internal factor, the prospects of escape are almost non-existent. Without an intra-mental rearrangement, as brought about by psychoanalysis or other rare types of emotional experience, there prevails a constancy within the mind as to its basic composition; and the realization of this allows no real hope of escaping from the impact of unpleasant inner processes. Admittedly, one creates incessantly for oneself a hypothesis that the "bad" tendencies opposing the desired programme of life may one day cease to exist. It is even a fact that for the conscious awareness there is a fluctuation of their intensity. But deep down within the psyche there must be a realization of the full truth about the component elements of the mind; and the fact is that the group of "dangerous" tendencies remain alive as long as the life process in general shows no decline. The manifest influence of the disapproved tendencies *is* largely checked, to various degrees in various circumstances; but they still continue to exist. It is assumed throughout this work that the moral process has constantly to take place in order to maintain fundamental morality; just as there is a process continually concerned with preserving health and replacing used-up energies.

17. The vague or subconscious realization of the fact that the moral enemy is always in existence must be a potent mental

element. The great variety of anxiety neuroses ensuing from moral conflicts illustrate the dynamic significance of the amoral tendencies. And the psychoanalysis of all persons, however free they may be from manifest neuroses, suggests likewise the existence of the amoral category of tendencies in everybody. All this needs no particular mention. What *is* intended to be pointed out, is something else, related to these phenomena. If you fight against somebody or something, and the limitations of your fight become apparent, there ensues an element of disappointment, and even fear, that is not directly congruent with the actual harm done by the person or thing fought against. The partial futility of the fight, and the necessity to remain on the alert, and the very fact of the continued presence of the undesirable factor within the spheres of life, are a source of particular tension. This discussion will perhaps convey better the significance of the part played by the " inner enemy ".

18. In view of the differences in the nature of the two objects of fear—*the host of competitive fellowmen* on the one hand, and *the inner enemy to morality and mental peace* on the other—the latter is obviously the more discomforting. There is no element of genuine hope of ridding oneself of its impacts, still less of its presence.

19. In the discussion of the competitive complex we must remind the reader that it consists naturally of an active and a passive component. There is a wish for autocratic freedom of the subject, but also a fear relating to the same tendency in others. Clearly, from realizing one's own tendency to autocracy, one can also experience fear through visualizing the same and even stronger desire in others.

This centrifugal result of the subject's own aggressive tendencies has been recognized by modern trends in psychoanalysis.[1] It has even been suggested that the aggressive significance of persons in the subject's environment may be imagined by the mind to an exaggerated degree, through magnifying one's own annoyance about various smaller or larger obstacles in life, and projecting the associated subjective resentment on to others. I think that this may really be the case ; but it occurs only because what I call the competitive complex lends its

[1] Cf. M. Klein's theory on the infantile origin of aggression, discussed by Flugel in *Man, Morals and Society*.

dynamic charge to such exaggeration and projection. This complex is very strong because it is largely based on facts. There can be no explaining away of the modifying influence of society on the individual's physical and mental life. And this influence is in many ways of a competitive nature.

20. Thus, it might still be argued that an irrational fear of the *new* or *strange* is stimulated mainly by the competitive complex; that the intolerance comes in the first instance from this element and only in the second instance from the fear relating to intra-psychic immorality.

Yet, it has to be admitted that the overcoming of the competitive tendency—and also the fear of other people's competitiveness—is closely related to the moral process and its difficulties. Self-limitation is demanded by society and its moral system. Transgression of laws, and disapproved conduct in general, may be followed by retributive measures. If an individual is being restricted in his freedom of life and earning, whether by a court of law or merely social disfavour, his place and share will be transferred to others and satisfy their desire for more, that is, satisfy their competitive tendencies. It is thus obvious that a fear ensuing from intra-mental moral difficulties connects up on some points with the fear attached to the competitive complex. The writer, therefore, prefers the concept that marked intolerance of the *new* and *strange* originates mainly in the fear of immoral elements within the self.[1]

21. It is true that the competitive complex in both its aspects is something more elementary than the moral fear in a comprehensive sense. From the viewpoint of mental dynamics, however, the difficulties in the moral process are of a superior significance. Certainly, processes in this sphere are more apt to be the object of *symbolic stimulation*.

Training in moral restriction—this taken in the broader sense (as described in Ch. I)—starts very early in life, whereas the full realization of the competitive complex begins only later. Training in cleanliness and regularity in feeding is a moral education. The significance of the competitive factor, on the other hand, requires much experience in the course of life for its full realization. Though the related complex is based on an

[1] Cf. Appendix II.

archaic tendency [Ch. XI (15)], the individual's particular experiences mobilize its dynamic charge. Thus, it is conceivable that the moral process possesses a stronger dynamic significance than the competitive complex.

It will be seen in the next chapter that fully blown prejudice, which is a systematized form of intolerance, cannot sufficiently be understood without reference to the difficulties in the moral process. The contribution of the competitive complex in prejudice is duly recognized in the course of the discussions (Chs. III and VI). But the central rôle of the moral factor in the development of prejudice is difficult to overlook.

# CHAPTER IIB

## INTOLERANCE TO REFORMS

*Individual opinion is based on intrinsic and extrinsic factors.—The tendencies of conservatism and revolutionism.—Flugel explains them by the bipolar attitude to parental authority.—Additional factors are the variable capacity for responding to new suggestions, and the degree of mental harmony.—Public discussion, even if not logical, is an advantage.—General conservatism in the service of moral stability.—Adherence to mere externals diminishes the capacity for essentials and progress.*

1. THE reader who has carefully followed the discussion so far—and especially if he is already acquainted with the fundamental assumptions about subconscious determination of thinking—will realize that the psychological background of any individual opinion must be complex. The reason for individual differences with regard to the same event or problem can only be looked for in the deeper psychological-affective world, which is peculiar to each individual. What is common to various minds, and even universal, is partly racial inheritance, but to a large extent the result of environmental influences.[1] It is one of the fundamental concepts of this work that the environmental factors very substantially mould the subconscious spheres, in addition to their obvious influence on consciousness.

2. It is clear to every student of psychology that experiences during early development determine not only the general structure of the personality and decide not only on the future stability of the psycho-nervous system, but must in some degree pave the way for the main trend of thinking and judging, characteristic of the adult individual. But it is comparatively new knowledge that people's social attitudes and opinions are dominated—amongst other elements—by two antipodal factors, the tendency to conservatism and the urge for changes even of

[1] Cf. Ch. IIA (12).

a revolutionary extent. Obviously, there is always a mixture of both tendencies present ; and what accounts for the variety in people is the proportion between the two polar elements. It has been suggested by Flugel [1] that the obedience to and admiration of parental authority constitute the nucleus of the conservative attitude, whereas the tendency to revolt originates from sentiments of antagonism towards parents and persons in authority in the life of the child.

3. This explanation is so self-evident that it cannot be disregarded. The fact that individual analyses of various persons do *not* show in a clear-cut way the validity of this rule, is due to the contributory influence of other mental factors of no less impact. One is the constitutional slowness or quickness respectively in responding to new suggestions and new situations. Another operative factor is the measure of relative stability within the emotional spheres of the individual. An urge for change, for attack on existing conditions and principles, is often expressive of a stormy atmosphere in the psyche, and not necessarily of a genuinely progressive outlook.

4. He who does not realize this fact, who does not wish to open his mind to this phenomenon, which is so manifest with regard to quite a number of " leftish " individuals, is himself deprived of that measure of wisdom necessary for evaluating things, and of that calmness so valuable in attaining individual peace and happiness. By this statement the human value of any " leftish " progressive principle is not questioned ; just as the social value of any " conservative " principle is not dependent on the quality of the motives that might prompt a person to adhere to it. There is thus no absolute parallelism between the social significance of a principle or an institution, and the degree to which the intellect of the person who advocates it is free of emotional complexes.

5. Fortunately, the opportunity for public discussions, even if not conducted in a logical manner by all taking part in it, may contribute to a clarification of issues in the course of time ; people attending such meetings go there in most cases with the idea of having their own point of view confirmed and seeing the

[1] *Man, Morals and Society.*

defeat of other opinions. They cannot consciously realize that another course within their mind may be possible. Nevertheless, this does take place frequently enough, by dint of the fact that human thought is complex. However great the subjective, even psychoneurotic, factor may be in the preference shown by an individual for particular social principles, the environmental influence ensuing from public discussion, and even from violent criticism of each other's opinion, can and does, in some degree, correct the subjective bias. Violent outbursts in the course of discussion may appear unpleasant and undignified ; but I am inclined to see the potential advantage of such manifestations. They exert a corrective influence on the power of chiefly subjective motives. As suggested in another context, the reception of a new suggestion is always a challenge to the mind to consider its value ; this process implies a greater or lesser possibility of revising and even abandoning one's existing opinion. It is to this weighing-up process occurring in hazy subconscious spheres, that I am referring here in assuming the purifying influence of public discussion.

6. The corrective influence does not mature at once, or for each individual in equally manifest degrees. It is rather a wholesale influence that I have in mind, imparting to society, to the public mind, some elements of the objective truth. For, the conscious realization of these corrective elements may remain obscure, or absent, for a considerable time ; but they hover, unrealized, above all passions and partisanships. For the social psychologist with knowledge of these facts it is impossible to wish that public discussion, even if at times irrational and passionate in manifestation, should cease to exist. This does not conflict with the firm conviction of the present author, and of others, too, that the decency, humanity, and justice of public life and of public feeling should be decisively supported, and even enforced, by those in possession of administrative and academic authority.

7. The comprehension of conservative tendencies in a substantial number of individuals is possible through a closer understanding of the concern of men for the maintenance of their moral stability. As pointed out several times in different contexts, the apparent stability of morals is the result of a process going on constantly, though with little conscious awareness. This process as well as the very necessity for it imply the existence of a constant current

of amoral and anti-moral tendencies. Beneath the surface of outward adherence to morals, there is a fluctuating process in which a variety of " viewpoints " with regard to morality take part. It is enough for average mental health and emotional balance if the subject is unaware, or almost unaware, of this state of affairs in the deeper layers. There is a natural wish to retain the hard-won peace of the conscious mind, and no desire to experience the deeper events.

In some people the customs of life, private and social, become closely interlinked with their conscious morality. And thus, the tendency to retain the apparent solidity of the latter leads to the simultaneous tendency to adhere strictly in general to all that is deemed right and normal. Any suggestion of change in the traditional customs of private life, and particularly in those of society, is intolerable to them, because it is conceived by them subconsciously as a threat to their moral stability.

8. This psycho-sociological phenomenon, though so evidently widespread, has remained apparently unrecognized by authors. If there should ever exist an antidote to this source of conversatism, it can only be a different attitude of people toward what are merely the formalities of life. At all times formalities have been considered as something essential,[1] and, as it were, of eternal validity. Children have been taught to consider them as quasi-moral laws, and adults have adhered to them often more than to genuinely indispensable principles. As long as the study of history and ethnography, and modern psychological and sociological research did not sufficiently open men's minds to the limited and temporary value of so many phenomena, it was justifiable to overlook the difference between the really eternal or essential and the only temporary or formal. But it appears that a change of attitude in this respect ought to develop in future generations, in order to free men's minds for devotion to principles that offer greater promise for the maintenance of an enjoyable society.

9. Admittedly, the life-span of a generation seems an eternity to its members ; and the externals customary in the course of their life-period are part and parcel of life to them. But the circumstances of civilized life and the multiform claims on the personality

[1] Cf. Forma dat esse rei.

have become complex almost beyond endurance. The first thing that loses ground in this competition for attention is the genuineness of social morality. The available mental energy cannot be concentrated satisfactorily on too many interests and obligations. If there are to be too many things with which the personality has seriously to concern itself, priority will be given to those tendencies that serve selfishness, prestige, vanity, and other fictitious social values with appeal to primitive desires ; then there cannot remain nervous energy, sentiment, and genuine interest for self-restriction, friendliness, and co-operation. For this reason, mankind needs to be relieved of having to take too seriously formal aspects and temporary customs in private and social life. Then, so many people who are now afraid even to consider reforms, will become keen on probing into various possibilities of human progress. But as long as they are trained to make the forms of life the essentials of their existence, there will be an unjustified degree of close association between these forms and the moral essentials. The result of this undue unity in men's minds of the two elements will be an adherence to unhealthy conservatism, which is more an inhibition than a principle.

10. From the previous discussions it must be intelligible that there are in fact two types of tolerance. The one is the fair capacity of the mind to perceive impressions that are new, or in opposition to what the subject's mind spontaneously prefers. Such a psychic structure to varying degrees enjoys the new or strange type of impression, or remains more or less indifferent. Clearly, this tolerance is difficult to reconcile with deep *religious belief of a distinct traditional kind*, or with enthusiastic nationalism. In these cases the mind is, on principle, biased ; full tolerance is impossible. Individuals who *are* capable of it may belong in the category of the wisest, shrewdest, and most pleasant people ; but they can never constitute the masses of those who make up devotion-filled congregations, militant political parties, or the host of faithful lovers of certain newspapers or authors. From the viewpoint of social welfare in the broadest sense, it may be said, however, that without these broad-minded " sages " the world would be rather backward and stale.

The other phenomenon, not less deserving to be called tolerance, is a different mode of coping with the *new* or *strange*. The psyche of these people tries to ignore, as much as possible for each individual, the impact of the impression that contradicts preferences and beliefs. Morally, this type of tolerance must be considered a high achievement in so far as it implies sacrifice and is not actually the result of a smooth functioning of the mind. It is, however, inconceivable that the psyche of this group could really accomplish what it does, without some degree of *tolerance* in the genuine sense. Perhaps, the mind of the individual of this second category is less prone to "externalize" than that of the less tolerant. Or, we may assume that their mental disposition is similar to that of the dogmatic believer and is, in fact, incapable of remaining unaffected by foreign impressions that are allowed to enter their mind; but their capacity for anulment, that is, for ignoring the stir caused by the foreign element, is of a sufficient degree to result in a fair measure of practical tolerance.

It would be unwise to tax the practical tolerance of these, in essence fair and even kind people, by our forgetting to consider the dynamic difference between the two types of tolerance. A note of warning the reader of unwarranted psychological optimism is necessary. All that is known or thought about the function of tolerance and the factors conducive to intolerance does not yet influence actual conditions. Much more is needed for this than the writing of a few books which are read by a few interested persons. It is unwise and "unpsychological" to approach people in various walks of life so as if their psyche worked according to rules of psychological objectivity. Consequently, the old advice still remains valid. If you wish co-operation and a working tolerance do not touch people's sensitiveness too much. In questions of scientific discussion this rule of prudence cannot hold, and must not hold, if some progress in insight is to be attained.

# CHAPTER IIIA

## THE PSYCHOPATHOLOGY OF THE MORAL PROCESS. PREJUDICE IS A TYPE OF PARANOIA

*Moral decision is an* ad hoc *function of the mind.—There is besides a constant moral process; it refers to the general capacity for self-restriction and adaptation.—Its disturbances are frequent.—The question of inborn capacity for morals and the rôle of the intelligence factor in the process.—The cardinal point is the self-perception of a tabooed tendency, not its quantitative aspect.—Repression and elimination.—Removal from the conscious may amount to practical elimination.—Two different instances.—The rôle of the unsatisfactory moral process in the genesis of obsessional neurosis.—Preoccupation with morals is a symptom.—The prejudiced type of social reformer and purifier.—The harmless paranoias.—An advocate of natural methods of healing.—Religion and paranoia; similarities and differences.—A simple instance of prejudice—Prejudice is the paranoia of the " normal ".—Both prejudice and paranoia are indicative of an unsatisfactory moral process; paranoia is a breakdown of the social faculty.—Psychoanalysis is not always capable of laying bare the fundamental etiological factor.—The homosexual complex in paranoia is not the root of the disturbance, even though often manifestly in the foreground.*

1. THE moral character of judgment and conduct at any moment is an *ad hoc* attainment of the personality. On each occasion it results from the rejection of the exact opposite of the chosen alternative, and from the overcoming at the same time of all other tendencies which may stand in the way of that alternative.

If, for instance, the predicament of a fellow-being calls for a substantial financial sacrifice to help him, this implies for the subject something more than the simple giving up of part of his possessions. The subject may be one of the types for whom love of money is a substitute for a specific libidinal satisfaction; or he may be a person whose intense feeling of inferiority has culminated in an unreasonable fear of losing any part of his possessions. In addition, a relative of the person in need may have aroused in the past the resentment of the subject, who is now called upon to help, and there may still be sufficient antagonism left to make the sacrifice no easy one. A further obstacle may be the idea that a helping gesture in the present might later induce the beneficiary to rely once more on the giver. The person who is thus faced with the alternative whether to give or not may, in addition, look into a more or less distant future in which he himself will need all the money he can get together in order to launch an enterprise he already has under consideration.

2. The element directly opposed to *giving* is the tendency to *hold on* to one's possessions. All the other reasons enumerated, relating partly to the would-be beneficiary and partly to the person approached for help, are contributory factors that might militate against the positive alternative. This instance may serve to illustrate how a variety of tendencies have to be dealt with in the course of moral decisions.

Since the components of any problem are always different even from those of a similar one, the moral decision cannot simply be based on the employment of a ready-made pattern of behaviour (the ideal-ego). However automatic and spontaneous a moral choice may appear, it is suggested that it is a fresh decision and not a routine one ; and it implies the neutralizing in a unique situation of all but one of a set of divergent tendencies.

3. It may also be suggested that there is a constant moral process that maintains the general ability and readiness to make a moral decision. This intra-mental process is not solely concerned with particular decisions regarding each individual action or inaction, but with the maintenance of a satisfactory moral standard and functioning. The individual judgments and decisions are only possible because of the presence of this general function. The promptness and the quality of individual decisions must be dependent on the quality and the stability of this fundamental moral process. In the case of each new decision there is an analogy with incidental attitudes and reactions of the personality to various emergencies. If there habitually exists a fair degree of optimism and desire to live, actions taken by the person in defence of his physical or mental interests will in each successive instance be more appropriate than if there is less fundamental vitality and general self-confidence.

4. Thus it is not enough to agree on the uniqueness of each moral decision, whilst believing that the general moral standard in the adult is a static element, instead of a constantly operating function. Morality itself, as a principle and a dynamic factor, is never unopposed within the mind ; and it has to be safeguarded and " overhauled " in a way analogous to the maintenance of health in general.

Morality means self-restriction through regulation of the spheres of feeling and action ; but this restriction of the self by the self is certainly not a claim accepted once and for all. There is at all times a revolt against the very principle of self-restriction, particularly if its working is not required for securing the satisfaction of immediate needs of the person concerned, or for protecting him from pain. The idea of morality as a dynamic mental element requires a constant process maintaining it as a functionally fit factor.

If an appetite for a certain food is not satisfied, this means not only the denial of that particular enjoyment, but more generally a restriction of the personality as a whole. If adults interfere with a particular game played by a child, they not only deprive the child of that enjoyment but evoke in him resentment against their control in general. Even more is this the case when adults are interfered with in the attainment of their aims. The element of resentment at being interfered with is quite consciously and distinctly present, apart from the regret at not having reached a certain objective. In most cases the feeling of resentment on the general ground is definitely more prominent in the mind than the sense of frustration with respect to the particular wish.

5. These instances will be helpful in illustrating the fact that in the case of moral self-limitation, too, there are two aspects to be considered. One is the principle of moral readiness in general, and the other is the particular case in which the moral function is called upon to operate in the forming of a decision.

In another context [1] a similar division was suggested by the present author between a general emotionality of the self and the particular emotional reactions. It was there pointed out that there is a fundamental feeling referring to the self as a whole, which is the basis of the incidental changes in feeling that are the particular emotions. For the sake of analogy it was also

[1] Cf. *Man and his Fellowmen*, Ch. V.

mentioned that the muscular contractions required for definite tasks are only possible because there exists continuously in the muscle a tone, which is in essence a constant readiness to get into action. The same analogy may apply, of course, to the phenomenon under discussion.

6. It is, indeed, inconceivable why such a thing as a disturbance in the moral process, in a broader sense, should not exist. There is no functional domain within the human organism in which there is not a gradual scale extending from prac ically perfect efficiency, through various degrees of weakness, to manifest inefficiency. The phenomenon called moral deficiency (moral insanity) is the peak of unsatisfactory moral functioning. In these cases there is an innate deficiency of the capacity to feel and behave in accordance with moral precepts. The close relationship between such conditions on the one hand and intellectual feeble-mindedness on the other, illustrates the part played by strictly organic factors in the moral function, since genuine feeble-mindedness is undoubtedly due to an under-development or functional deficiency of the brain. The lack of efficiency in regard to morals, and to self-limiting adaptation in general, in these mentally deficient people speaks in itself for the existence of a *general moral process* which is not the same as the *ad hoc* decision in favour of a particular line of conduct.

7. It is not suggested that the moral process, or the moral sense, is something innate ; though we may feel sure that it is for the individual largely a matter of developing a disposition inherited through generations. It is probable that the nucleus of the moral sense is the realization of the necessity to adapt oneself to others and to please others. If this realization is coupled with a measure of satisfaction relating to the individual's acceptance of such necessities,[1] then, perhaps, this combination constitutes the foundation of the moral sense ; the maintenance and continuous elaboration of this intra-psychic element *is* the moral process.

We must agree with *Burt* that the inborn quality of general intelligence plays a part in deciding the quality of the moral sense. The ability to understand the social significance of morals and the implications for the individual of approval and dis-

[1] Cf. p. 273 ; also Flugel, Man, Moral & Society p. 201.

approval by society, is obviously part of the intellectual function. Yet it appears that after the moral function has been established within the mind it exists as an independent sentimental factor. It is concerned with imparting to the personality the indispensability of self-limitation and the actual capacity to practise it. Clearly, the acknowledgment of the necessity for all this is just as much an intellectual operation as it is an emotional process. Thus, it is possible that some defects of the intellectual (*g*) factor may, from the outset, interfere with the development of the moral function.

8. It is also obvious that there are individuals in whom the instinctual tendencies aiming at personal gratification are stronger than in others. And on the other hand, the proneness to react with fear, disgust, or submission is not equally developed in all individuals; some react more readily in this way, some less. Since, however, training in morals and adaptation is largely dependent on the fear of parents or society, as well as the fear of "sin", a minus in such reactions of "surrendering" and "refraining" may well account for a deficiency in the moral sense. There are also a variety of experiences in youth, such as the right proportion of love, acknowledgment, and encouragement received on the one hand, and discipline applied on the other, that are directly responsible for the development of the moral sense.

9. All these details throw a light on factors whose interaction in the course of maturation in youth decides the ultimate quality of the moral process which is the main subject of the present discussion. It has not been for the mere avoidance of verbal repetition when I have spoken now about the *moral sense* and now about the *moral process*. The former notion refers to the degree and readiness of recognition of the moral aspect in various situations. The moral sense is thus equivalent to the notion of the superego or ego-ideal of psychoanalytical terminology. The moral process is, as the expression suggests, a comprehensive function. Doubtless, there is a short though complex moral process in every decision, as the instance above (pp. 61–2) illustrates. But the expression was introduced to refer to a more comprehensive and continuous process maintaining the principle of self-regulation in general.

10. In the morally deficient the unsatisfactory social conduct results from a fundamental weakness of the moral sense and therefore of the moral process, and not simply from the excessively strong impact of the individual tendencies. Where this latter phenomenon does make its appearance, it is the consequence of the fact that one or more of the tabooed tendencies act in comparative isolation, that is to say, without being subject to countertendencies within a well organized psychic system. Thus they manifest themselves with insistence. (See pages 67–8.)

That which in a simplified mode of description is referred to as a moral inhibition, curbing in the average person the impact of amoral tendencies, does not function merely after the fashion of a brake or of reins. This mode of interference could change the *quality* of a tendency merely through changing its *quantitative* aspect. But the great variety of cases in which moral conflicts in the narrower sense, and difficulties in the moral sphere in the broader sense, reveal themselves to the eyes of an unbiased psychologist suggest a rather more complex process.

11. Indeed, the process of deflection and sublimation cannot but be comprehensive functions. Unfortunately the basic concepts of psychoanalysis have been allowed to be influenced too much by a psychopathological bias. Normal, necessary functions of the mind have been frequently overlooked, or their manifestations conceived as quasi-psychopathological occurrences. It is true that what has been so much discussed as *repression* and *sublimation* are already secondary processes stimulated by a conflict ; and, admittedly, such conflicts are constant incidents in the life of all human beings. But we may feel sure that there operates a broad and fundamental moral process as defined above, which is independent of the particular moral conflicts.

It is fundamental, not incidental. It refers to the personality as a whole, and not to individual problems, emotions, and tendencies. It is as fundamental as is the physiological process that constantly maintains energy and the desirable chemical composition of the cells and body fluids (homeostasis). The processes of repression and deflection, on the other hand, are comparable to the activity of leucocytes in destroying and removing agents that are dangerous intruders into the organism. Deflection and repression operate, of course, also with respect to tendencies cropping up from within and not manifestly in response to particular events outside the self. A surplus of hatred or of sexual urge may be the result of difficulties in the hormonal or affective metabolism, with no primary reference to particular events or to impressions received from the environment. The repressive function called forth by these latter difficulties may be compared with the various biochemical processes that render innocuous the poisonous products created within the organism in the course of assimilation. But all these physiological functions are distinct from the general vital process that supplies food to the cells, restoring energy and maintaining the homeostasis within the organism. In an analogous way, the broad and fundamental moral process is concerned with the personality as a whole, imparting to it the characteristic of and the capacity for moral self-restriction in general.

In essence, admittedly, both the maintenance of morality in general and the individual decisions arrived at, alike imply self-regulation and self-restriction. I have nevertheless introduced the above distinction because it does not seem to me feasible to explain various phenomena simply by assuming that the moral function consists in the suppression of individual tendencies.

12. It has been customary in psychopathology to assume that definite tendencies or emotionally charged complexes of a tabooed type may become too intense to remain in repression ; then the manifestation of psychoneurosis may occur. Various considerations and observations have led me to believe that in most cases it is in fact only the degree of *perception* by the self of such tendencies or complexes, and not necessarily their quantitative dynamic potential, that has grown stronger than can be endured. Cf. Chs. IV (6), VI (6).

I have suggested that, under average circumstances, there is within the psychic structure a working balance between the different components, but that pathological processes of emotional or hormonal nature may interfere with this harmony, and, in some degree *isolate* a particular component from the integrated sum-total of the others. Through being isolated, this element becomes a disturbing factor for the mind. I think that the increased dynamic power of such an isolated element may be due in some cases to the absence of a counter influence exerted on it by other elements after the fashion of anti-hormones. But in other cases the *isolation* mainly brings about an intensified perception by the self of that element, and then it is this latter fact that becomes the cause of the trouble.

I assume a similar possibility with regard to the moral process. The most frequent difficulties of the psyche are probably those of the moral function in the broader sense defined above. The disturbance of this function may then lead to a difficulty in coping with one or other of the individual tendencies which are always present within the psyche. This means that the tabooed tendency in question—be it of a sexual, anti-religious, aggressive, or otherwise anti-social nature—can no longer be sufficiently repressed, and consequently it appears subjectively to be extraordinarily strong. For subjective awareness the emergence of this particular tendency or temptation is the only apparent trouble, and the mind tries to fight it. Since, however, there is a deeper trouble, a difficulty in the fundamental moral process, this attempt at remedy can hardly have a full measure of success.

13. There must obviously be a difference between an *a*-moral tendency that has obtruded itself upon consciousness, through a process of isolation in the above sense, and a case in which external stimulation is chiefly responsible for the tendency. In the latter case, the issue of the struggle for the suppression of the tabooed wish will be dependent on the relative strength of the repressive faculty and of the emotional charge of the incidental reactive tendency in question. But in the case of an obtrusive element that itself owes its dynamic power to a yet deeper-lying disturbance of the moral process in the broader sense, in point of fact a third factor also participates in the struggle. What has been called the capacity to repress, or to sublimate, needs to be more accurately brought into relationship with what has been defined as the fundamental moral process.

14. The concept generally held on this point has been that the moral factor, or the superego (Freud), sets into motion a process for the elimination from consciousness of the wish or idea in question. Accordingly, the repressing function acts in the interest of the superego. This concept can safely be retained. It should not be forgotten, however, that elimination of conceptual contents or of incidental tendencies from consciousness occurs also for another reason. So many elements have to disappear, not for

the sake of morality, but with a view to clearing away what has become useless ballast. There are not only conceptual elements that have to be " forgotten ", discarded, but also the pattern of a number of emotional reactions that are still existent even though no longer actually justified by the presence of external circumstances that stimulated them. There are also a number of habits that came into being as reactive formations, but after a time are no more than strange features. In all these instances a process of elimination, similar to repression, has to operate.

15. In the case of moral repression proper it is necessary to look more closely at the factors that may be assumed to take part in, or to be associated with, this repressive process. Repression implies, first of all, elimination from consciousness; and then, the transference of the impulse into new channels. This latter phase is, in my opinion, not always necessary. The very elimination of a tendency from conscious spheres may lead to its gradual but absolute dissolution. There are mental elements where it is the conscious concept, and not the emotional component, that accounts for their vitality and significance; in its absence the associated impulse or emotion quickly wears off. If, for instance, a person introduces himself to another as a relative, and describes his precarious situation with a view to receiving considerable financial support, there will emerge in many cases a distinct emotion of sympathy in the person addressed. But if, subsequently, it should be discovered in the course of conversation that the two persons are not relatives, then, even though the assumption made by the applicant was a genuine mistake, and this person in need was a likeable fellow, the feeling of sympathy might greatly diminish and even disappear entirely. Apart from such special cases, it may be said in general that in many instances the elimination from conscious spheres may be enough for a total dissolution of a tendency when external stimulation was the chief factor in giving birth to it. Thus in a number of cases repression has to concern itself merely with the removal of the reactive tendency from the spheres of conscious striving.

16. A person may have been insulted by his wife in the presence of another woman, who, incidentally, may have more of what is called sex appeal than his own wife possesses. Through having his vanity hurt in such circumstances, he may for a time feel no

attraction toward his wife, whilst his phantasy may occupy itself with desires concerning the other woman. These desires, together with the coolness toward his wife, are *reactive elements*. Both may wear off in a comparatively short time, without leaving behind in the memory any trace that might prove of practical significance.

17. In other cases the reactive tendency may become more firmly rooted. A woman had consented to marry one of her suitors out of financial considerations. Her parents had given her little chance of going out to dances and attending shows, and she had hoped that being the wife of a wealthy man she would be able to follow her inclinations. At the time of her marriage she even felt genuine love for her husband, and everything started well. Later the husband insisted on what he called a sober rational life. He himself was insensitive to dramatic or musical art, and consequently he felt that money spent on it was wasted. In quick succession two children were born. The first pregnancy and birth went off smoothly. With the second pregnancy some dizziness and vomiting appeared. These symptoms are not exceptional with expectant mothers ; but this woman took them somewhat seriously. Destiny willed it that childbirth should also prove difficult in the second case ; and in addition the young mother had to spend some weeks under treatment for eczema, which had developed owing to the use of a certain chemical material used during the process of the confinement. Eczema makes most people irritable. And excessively matter-of-fact men have not much tolerance for irritable wives who, apart from this sort of minor complaint, are physically well. Moreover, the difficulties of pregnancy and childbirth are more easily forgotten by husbands than by their wives. These experiences were clearly remembered by this woman, who felt disappointed in general with her life, past and present, though she never admitted the extent of this feeling to herself. All the resentment had now been shifted on to the inconveniences of pregnancy, childbirth, and subsequent eczema. She felt that it was not worth while being a woman, a wife, and a mother. Of course, only disappointed women have such a philosophy ; or women who are by nature incapable of enjoying family happiness. In this case, the incidents associated with the second childbirth had lent a dynamic charge to the disillusionment about the " sober " make-up of the husband.

A strong desire emerged to leave husband and children and to free herself, perhaps for other men. The woman felt that she was by nature unfitted to live the life of a wife and mother, in the narrow bounds of a household. If we recollect the motive that made her consent to her husband's proposal of marriage, we must recognize that from the very first she was, to some extent, lacking in the qualities required for a fairly contented marriage. The later events—her husband's soberness and the various minor mishaps associated with the second childbirth—powerfully developed this small anti-marital complex.

The reactive element in this case was one with a much greater dynamic charge than in the former instance; it was grafted on an older characteristic of the personality. A "forgetting", that is, a simple process of repression, was here not enough. A sublimation of a complex, or its transference into different channels, could hardly be expected in this case. It is difficult to imagine another reactive psychological process as an alternative to this wholesale resentment that would have coped satisfactorily with the intra-mental storm. An obsessional neurosis with strong depression followed.

The analysis suggested, throughout its course, a *deficient moral process* in the broader sense. Not only was this woman by dint of her personality-type unsuitable to be a happy wife and mother; but clearly, she was able only with difficulty to adjust herself to almost all the existing limitations imposed on the individual by customs and law. There was no question of transgressing in conduct the bounds of legality. The practical spheres of morality and social decency were in her case—just as in many similar ones—unaffected by the psychic deficiency. It was just an instance where the moral process in general worked under constant strain. The almost obsessive ideas of leaving her family and becoming a semi-prostitute were, in my opinion, results of the intra-mental process of isolation described above. We know that almost every woman has a subconscious prostitute complex; and certainly every married woman may dream at times of freedom and romance. In the case of its "isolation" in the sense described, such an idea may become strong in dynamic force and may contribute to obsessive formations.

18. The case illustrates the following. Incidental repression with an alternative utilization of the impulse or tendency depends on the quality of the moral process. A pure impulse of hatred

can be transformed into some useful antagonism in politics or social activities. A distinct sexual tendency may be " sublimated " to some extent into various interests. But where the problem is concerned with a resentment against the obligations and duties imposed by marriage, and against family life in general, a repression in the full sense can occur only if the fundamental moral process works well. In the absence of this prerequisite there is no other mental mechanism at hand to create a tolerance of duties and obligations in cases where the compensation through pleasure is too small to counterbalance the awareness of the burden. An unsatisfactory moral process implies ultimately a deficient capacity for self-restriction. Yet in cases where the weight of the burdens implied by duties enters too much into consciousness, the only process suitable to cope with the condition would be a well functioning moral process which makes self-limitation a natural and even a satisfying act for the personality.

19. We know that in cases of psychoneurosis in which the hatred factor dominates—as in the obsessive-compulsive form—treatment is difficult and the prognosis not as frequently favourable as in other forms. I feel that this is the case because of a particular difficulty which such people have in submitting to obligations in general. What appears to the psychoanalyst as hatred is, indeed, in the social psychologist's view fundamentally a resentment against duty and moral restriction. This is, however, not the place to discuss psychopathology proper.

But it seems certain to me that a constitutional difficulty in the basic moral process leads, in a vast number of individuals, to the formation of prejudice. This is the case, perhaps, when the basic disturbance is not complicated by the " isolation " of a particular tabooed tendency. To express it in other words—there are individuals who consciously and manifestly subscribe to average moral conceptions, but whose moral process actually operates under stress. This may be compared with the condition of some persons whose function of digestion is never free from some difficulty, though their appetite and their weight remain virtually normal.

20. There are a great number of persons who in principle readily subscribe to the necessity of ethical conduct, without, however, being much concerned with the problem of actual morals in

society. In an analogous way, a person may be kind and helpful to children whom he meets by chance, though he may have no desire whatever to have children of his own. He finds it right that other people should have a family, and should feel this to be an essential part of their life. He also recognizes clearly that society as a whole can only be based on family life, and that the continuous propagation of the human race is a logical phenomenon. But he himself has not the slightest urge to participate in this social process, and he also finds it natural that there should be many people like himself. On the other hand, there are fanatics of family life who miss no opportunity of advocating it and giving their active support to the cause of children and mothers.

The purpose of this analogy is to bring home that two individuals may equally subscribe to an important principle, but their minds may be dominated by the problem involved to quite different degrees. Regarding the question of morals, there are, as we know, people who cannot encounter any event of private or social life without thinking at the same time of some moral question raised by it. If these are individuals of a pleasant and tolerant type, they earn much appreciation from congenial fellowmen for their efforts in spreading and protecting higher morals. But another group of people, in a way similar to those just mentioned, appear so obsessed about the " immorality of the world " that they cannot avoid being unattractive in their fighting attitude towards the evils in society.

21. Let us now think of a particular type of person resembling but at the same time conspicuously differing from the two just described. There are individuals who emphatically subscribe to the supremacy of morals, but who at the same time have a subconscious moral process that works under constant strain. The non-initiated may be puzzled by the simultaneity of two such phenomena, as a great concern for ethics and justice in society, on the one hand, and on the other a disturbance in what we call the subconscious moral process. The first answer I can offer for easing the logical difficulty is that the psyche of these persons have been unable to adopt sufficiently the extrinsic claims of education and social convention as their own quasi-autochthonous principle. Cf. Ch. XI (12). In other words, for their subconsciousness the claims of morality are still too much of an enforced element, supported too much by the fear of

society. A deficiency in the deep moral process has not permitted a proper digestion of the education they have imbibed in the art of self-restriction, though this education has instilled into them a deep-rooted appreciation of the significance of morals. It may also be that their respect for morals is due to their egoistic desire to gain appreciation from society, an aim that necessitates compliance with the avowed ethical principles of society. The interaction of such divergent forces produces a disharmony of the personality, and a resulting psychoneurotic " complex " is seeking conscious manifestation.

Such a person may feel a restless urge to concern himself with the task of purifying society, he will display a marked interest in social morals, but one that is interlinked with gross aggressiveness and with the tendency to wreak painful retribution on those suspected by him. He is apparently not concerned with the improvement of those whose conduct is, in his opinion, improper and dangerous. Their punishment and elimination from society is the problem for him. In other words, aggression in the service of morality is his manifest aim. Every observant reader must have met more than one example of this type. It is also noticeable that such persons easily find a following in their hatred and their attacks. It is not difficult to stimulate hatred and aggression in a large number of persons who can hardly suppress the manifestation of resentment about grievances of their own and who welcome any legal or approved occasion for giving vent to this resentment of theirs.

22. The type just described is, as a rule, not concerned with such social problems as, for instance, criminality, the unscrupulous dissemination of venereal diseases, or the ubiquitous economic exploitation of the weak by the strong. These offences against society are obvious, are generally disapproved, and, each in a different way, are prosecuted by law or attacked by certain social groups. The objects of attacks for individuals of the type under discussion are different—the " hypocrites ", or the " undiscovered offenders ", people accused of being inferior and dangerous in general. The less clearly specified the alleged crimes are, and the more hazy the elements that can be introduced into the accusations, the more passionate is the interest in social purification shown by this type. " Lustfulness," " badness " of mind and heart in general, " destructiveness," " anti-social character " and similar charges are preferred ; and in most

cases whole groups, religious, political, or racial, have been the objects of such accusations.

The psychoneurotic colouring of the whole phenomenon is obvious to the comparatively few who are free from this type of neurosis. The passion, the exaggeration, the wild generalization, the preference for what is in the main unprovable, for what can be alleged but is difficult either to prove or refute, these features are for the psychiatrist reminiscent of the delusions and the behaviour of a paranoiac patient.

23. It is more than an analogy, or the assumption of a distant relationship, when we regard the social attitude of prejudice as closely comparable with the psychosis called *paranoia*. No approach to this problem of social prejudice can be satisfactory without a reference to that type of mental disease. Paranoia is one of the psychotic manifestations in which it is still justifiable to assume the absence of a material, organic process in the etiology, and to conceive the mental process as a faulty reactive attitude toward the environment. Paranoia is a logical, systematized delusion which leaves the integrity of the mind otherwise fairly intact. Measured by reality the delusion is, in its literal sense, of a more or less absurd character, an invention of the phantasy that has become a firm belief. Taken in itself, the delusional system seems to possess a logical coherence and meaning. In many cases fellow-beings are even inclined to listen earnestly to the statements and complaints of a paranoiac and to sympathize with them, and they only later realize the presence of a psychosis. The conversation and reasoning of these patients on subjects other than those that touch on the delusion may be entirely rational.

24. There are, for instance, persons who gather people round them in order to preach to them a new religious revelation. In the opinion of one of these prophets, everything so far taught and proclaimed is out of date, and only his particular concept is the real and full truth. He himself, naturally, is a chosen, exceptional personality. There is nothing really unpleasant about such a person, nothing dangerous. But his talk and his persistence soon become boring and seem sterile to the ordinary man, whether educated or only in possession of ordinary common sense. This type of prophet is a paranoiac. It must be admitted that any

individual " conviction " differing from what a group of others believe resembles paranoiac delusions of the kind just described. What reveals a person as a paranoiac is the degree of his preoccupation with his belief, to which he would sacrifice other normal aspects of people's life.

25. I once met an elderly gentleman in a spa where I was then in practice. He was an advocate of " natural " methods of cure, to the exclusion of all drugs and chemicals. He tried to convert all his new acquaintances, and me as a doctor even more so. I should not like to have any exaggerated bias in favour of contemporary medical methods—my psychoanalytical experience is enough to prevent that. I am also ready to believe that it would be better to avoid chemical methods of treatment if cure could be effected solely by fresh air, warm water, and specific diets. Consequently, it was not difficult for me to remain polite and attentive when my new friend explained his theories. But I felt sure that he was a paranoiac. I asked him whether he thought a person suffering acute pain from an incurable cancer should not receive morphia. His answer was : " Certainly not. Morphia is not natural. Warmth is capable of reducing pain." This adherent of natural curative methods gave as the only reason for his preference for natural methods that drugs are unnatural and thus harmful to health and subjective well-being. But his answer with respect to relieving the pains of a sufferer from an incurable cancer showed that he was prepared to persevere in a principle at the cost of real helpfulness. This is delusion.

26. There are large communities in the world, such as orthodox Jews or Hindus, that have their traditional dietetic laws, to which they strictly adhere as long as no medical consideration demands a change. They accept many restrictions in life for the sake of religious happiness that for them ensues from the compliance with these regulations. Freud went out of his way to argue against all religions, as they were in his opinion mass-paranoias. Clearly, in so far as assumptions of religion do not conform with actuality—as the atheist supposes—beliefs are comparable to delusions. But who could deny that the social attitude of a religious person—so long as he is not incidentally a psychoneurotic—is satisfactory? And his frame of mind is more frequently one of happiness than is that of many doubters and atheists. Here, there is no similarity to paranoia, and therefore

the two types of belief cannot be based on an identical underlying mental process.

In addition, the various ritualistic restrictions adhered to by members of traditional denominations do not purport to be individual inventions. The belief in their obligatory character is for them secondary, following from obedience to God. The "naturalistic" restrictions of the type mentioned above are admittedly based on an individual original belief. Such a person is proud of his exceptional cleverness, and he does not cite an external command. Therefore his adherence to a principle at any cost, even when manifestly nonsensical and cruel, is a sign of delusion.

Now there are paranoiacs who do refer their peculiar attitude to some revelation, just as religious communities profess to adhere to the commands of their Heavenly Father. But the difference is obvious. In the case of a member of an established denomination, his fellowmen's declaration and persuasion is the decisive factor; whereas in the case of the delusional paranoiac the whole system of his belief is based on an alleged individual revelation. That is to say, on an intra-mental experience of individual character. Admittedly, the concept of a divinity and the fear of God may be capable of a psychoanalytical explanation (cf. Freud, *The Future of an Illusion*). But the beneficial results of religious beliefs in general with respect to the feeling, conduct, and social attitude of people invalidates the diagnosis of religion as paranoia proper.

In more serious forms of paranoia the patient regards himself as God, an Archangel, a second Jesus, the Messiah, King of the World, the Blessed Virgin, the Great Inventor, the supreme Wizard, etc. Or, alternatively, he complains of persecution by invisible or distant enemies, or by a gang of powerful people who possess "electro-radio" or "telepathic" devices with which to interfere with his life. These two types seem obviously different. In one group the patient is something great and exceptional, though not understood and acknowledged by the world. In the other group he is a mere sufferer, but his adversaries and his sufferings are of an exceptional type. However, in this fundamental feature of the *exceptional* or *mystical* the two kinds of paranoia are similar.

A third and distinct type is the querulous. He troubles the courts and authorities with complaints about personal injustice, or with memoranda on public affairs which, in his opinion, are "scandalously" dealt with by the authorities. He is never satisfied. Even if a judge were formally to declare that he was right, he would start another campaign on the same matter or another one.

There are various " fanatics " both of the aggressive and of the mild type [1]; believers in eccentric ideas, and advocates of and fighters for " certain systems ". Some of them attract followers, others remain alone in their belief. I consider their dominant ideas comparable with the delusions of paranoia in the clinical sense, even though clinical psychiatry may assume that the underlying processes are different.[2] Clinical psychiatry has not yet approached the problem from the angle suggested in this work; though there *is* a link between the theory of the writer and modern trends in psychiatry. Cf. Appendix II.

27. It is well to define the phenomenon that is to occupy our attention in the following discussions. Prejudice is not a mere conceptual opinion, but a sentiment. There are, in fact, only two possible types of such a sentiment: a bias in favour of somebody and a bias against somebody. This sentimental bias is the essence of the phenomenon called prejudice, and the judgment included in it is, in fact, of a secondary order and of secondary significance. The reasons given by the subject for such a sentimental bias may be demonstrable facts, though they are more frequently inventions; yet even where they do conform with actuality, they are not the primary source of the sentimental attitude. They serve as an explanation; they are meant to vindicate the attitude in question, though actually they can never do so fully. There is, first of all, always a disproportion between the intensity of the emotion aroused by the prejudice and the fact to which the subject points in explaining his attitude. And if, alternatively, the reasons given for a prejudice *are* of a serious nature, they prove in the vast majority of cases to be invented or exaggerated. But however factual may be the reason advanced in support of a prejudice, it is secondary in origin to the sentiment and, as will be shown, it stands in no causal relationship to it. This phenomenon is actually the main characteristic of the external aspect of prejudiced attitudes.

[1] *Matte Fanatiker* in German psychiatry.

[2] As long as a psychopath or psychotic person remains fit enough for living in a community and is considered, by a smaller or larger number of people, as worthy of being listened to, his delusions or eccentric ideas are a factor of significance. The problem of the composition of the deeper psychological structure in such a personality alters this fact very little. It is not always right to disregard the manifest aspect of psychopathological phenomena in favour of the deeper processes. Cf. Ch. VII.

28. It will be useful to introduce at the outset a simple instance, and to continue the description of the phenomenon by referring to this instance. A man who for years had been reluctant to marry, suddenly discovered a particular woman for whose sake he felt inclined to change his view. This woman was superior to him in many respects; she was steady, experienced, and popular. It *was* more or less intelligible that her company should stimulate in him the desire to marry her, despite his habitual disinclination to make any woman his wife. But the very fact of her superiority made it impossible for the woman to consent. The man was not only hurt, but his references to the woman—whom he had so much admired—showed blind resentment and prejudice. Suddenly she became in his opinion a person "only good enough to be a receptionist at a hotel, a woman with no particular intelligence or personal dignity". We cannot fail to recognize the formation of prejudice. It is true that in this simple case there was a concrete reason for the annoyance. But there was no logical justification for the new concept about the woman. At first she was so exceptional as to be the only person whom he would like to marry; later she was in his eyes a woman whom hardly any person of social standing would choose as his partner in life.

If this man had merely harboured resentment against the woman, however strong, and had unduly criticized her actual human deficiencies (as for instance her conceit or sarcasm, or her educational shortcomings), we should have been unable to speak of pure (unreasonable) prejudice, and only of a rational resentment exaggerated by some prejudice. But as the case was, the deficiencies alleged against the woman by the disappointed man were sheer inventions, and in flagrant contradiction to his previous conception of her.

In point of fact, the man in question was manifestly feminine in many of his ways and he had a strong mother fixation. The psychoanalyst could well understand his bachelor attitude. But the content of his critical references to the woman of his previous choice needed a psychological interpretation. I thought at that time that he was shifting his own complex on to the person who had disappointed him. He himself was sexually fixated on his mother, and for this reason, and also from fear of having to adapt himself to a strange woman, he had developed an antimarital attitude. This disinclination to put up with a wife and her individuality was expressly admitted by him. Thus in effect he tolerated only incidental girl friends; that is to say, *he* himself was like a receptionist pretending friendliness to all strangers who pay for their room. I admit that the whole phenomenon would also allow of a somewhat different interpretation. The point to be illustrated is the unjustified blame thrown upon another person in response to an embarrassing situation. A man who had developed for years an affectation of disregard for all women, considering them unworthy even to be in the same room with him (he never invited his girl friends to his home), was bound to be greatly shocked by a refusal from the only woman who had impressed him. There must have dawned upon him the realization that he was not so superior to women as he liked to think ; that there might be others besides this particular woman who would reject his approaches. This realization stimulated some vague awareness of his being burdened by a definite psychopathological complex (see above). And the intolerance towards his own complex was somehow instrumental in creating the prejudiced concept about the friend he had so admired.

29. It should be pointed out that in all cases of genuine prejudice the alleged reason for condemning the object is a second thought, a secondary invention. There may actually be much or little for which the object could justly be blamed. He may be an average individual, or a person marked by definite faults or even vices. The prejudice, if directed against him, may refer to such demonstrable defects. But the sentiment of prejudice itself is not the consequence of these faults and vices. And since this is so, we shall not be surprised to find that the accusations levelled against people from prejudice so frequently contain, among some facts, a large proportion of invented, even fantastically untrue, elements.

30. People do not as a rule waste much passion on condemning the thief, the burglar, or the murderer. On the occasion when they first learn about the crime there is—though not always—genuine indignation. But soon this passionate interest wears off, and what remains is only an intellectual disapproval of the anti-social deed, coupled with the idea that some legal proceeding is necessary. This rather lukewarm attitude of the average person holds no comparison with the passionate manifestations of prejudice. Consequently, if people habitually have a prejudice against any group, such as the Jews or Roman Catholics, the

Negroes or the British (among the Irish, and conversely), Capitalists or Communists, etc., then any human weakness or vice displayed by one member of this group will be condemned by two sorts of sentiment. One is the general disapproval of the deed in question, and the other—far more passionate—is the emotional reaction associated with the pre-existent prejudice.

There are cases where it might require a great deal of detachment to recognize the admixture of prejudice in a hostile reaction that in itself is natural. A policeman or soldier might have been killed by a member of a group that is an habitual object of prejudice ; it is understandable if the grief of the family is coloured (though not necessarily intensified) by a measure of this prejudice. Should fellow-nationals who are not close friends of the victim display a similar degree of indignation, it ought to be easy to see the substantial rôle of the irrational prejudice. As we know, the reaction in strangers to murder is, as a rule, short-lived and lukewarm ; even more so in the case of a death in the battle. There will be a large number of people who object to a condemnation of all contemporary Germans, even though their own relatives died through maltreatment in prisoner-of-war or concentration camps. The numbers of those able to think with a similar fairness will be much smaller if, for instance, Negro or Jewish persons are connected with their bereavement or any harm they might have suffered. There is on the whole no prejudice against Germans comparable in deep-rootedness and irrational character with the anti-Negro or anti-Jewish sentiment.

31. Prejudice—whether dominating the subject to a greater or only to a lesser extent—is a paranoia of the non-psychotic. It is a passionate belief preferably in something not proven or even unprovable. It consists in an accusation and disqualification of others and a lifting of oneself above those others. It is unassailable by objective argument ; the very nature of prejudice includes an a priori rejection of any objective truth incompatible with the belief it implies. The prejudice answers, as it were, an intrinsic desire of the subject, just as does the paranoiac delusion ; and the correction of the delusional belief would run counter to this pathological need of the mind. (See p. 88 and Ch. VI.)

There are apparent exceptions to this description. A limited number of persons have undoubtedly abandoned a prejudiced belief they had held earlier in life. In the writer's experience this occurs only within a more general maturation of the personality, resulting in a better balance of the psyche. In a few cases the change-over is manifestly connected with a mental crisis. But, whilst in full flourish, a prejudice is unassailable by logical arguments or friendly persuasion, because it has assumed a certain function within the psychic processes.

Prejudice based in the main on wrong information is a different phenomenon. Its correction is almost as easy as that of any other mistake. That is to say, if the subject is not too much dependent on projective condemnation for his self-confidence, he will more or less readily accept the truth. (Cf. Ch. II.)

It need hardly be mentioned that, just as in paranoia, the source of discomfort in prejudice is the subject's own mind and not the external circumstances stimulating the complex (cf. however pages 84, 95) ; likewise, the assumed enemies of the subject, and of society in general, the base and inferior people against whom the prejudice is directed, are primarily inner enemies, intolerable elements of the subject's psyche. In prejudice there is also, as in paranoia, a mixture of what appears to be to a certain degree logical and sensible with what is absurd and exaggerated. Just as the paranoiac delusion contains novel concepts and references to things and persons remote from the subject's concrete experience, so prejudice prefers as its object strangers and whole groups of whom any close personal knowledge is unlikely and impossible.

32. A person dominated by prejudice is never really happy, and only on comparatively rare occasions is he capable of mental relaxation. Where, as in the prejudiced person, an outburst of indignation can so easily be stimulated, below the surface of apparent calm there is a volcano. What we know and assume about this psychological background of prejudice can indeed suggest the existence of such eruptive elements.

The preoccupation of the prejudiced person with the morals of others betrays the essential character of his own mental conflict. It is, indeed, peculiar that psychology and sociology of the past have not clearly recognized this fact. Perhaps, the scientist's own unrecognized bias, the subliminal prejudice present in so many persons, may account for this blindness. If anything can be gathered from the manifestations of prejudice in an individual, from the content of his delusional beliefs, and from his passionate and aggressive demeanour, it is the existence of an intense disturbance in the moral spheres.

Here is a difference between the obsessive ideas of paranoia and those of prejudice. In the psychosis the literal delusion is entirely symbolic, entirely phantastic. Only the expert in dreams and neuroses can to some extent understand the reference to the original elements. In prejudice, on the other hand, as just noted, the moral conflict suggests itself unmistakably. This difference exists because of the very fact that in the prejudiced the integrity of mental functioning in general is not affected by symbolism to such a degree as in the paranoiac patient. (See also Ch. III (2).)

For this reason the prejudiced person is a far greater potential danger to his fellowmen than is the psychotic. Some paranoiacs do commit acts of aggression, if their delusion prompts them to self-defence against imagined attacks. But on the whole the faulty functioning of their mind incapacitates them for more comprehensive plans, and naturally they can persuade only a very few weakminded people to place trust in them and give them support. The prejudiced person, on the other hand, is practically in full possession of his mental abilities, and his passionate attitude, aiming at the elimination of the " bad ", even renders him impressive to many of his fellow-beings. He is suggestive and may prove efficient. If given power and opportunity, he becomes an unscrupulous torturer of the bodies and minds and even the killer of his chosen victims.

33. Full-blown paranoia is thus able to throw light on the phenomenon of prejudice. There cannot be the slightest doubt that prejudice is a type of paranoia. But the writer thinks that the phenomenon of prejudice can in turn suggest something about the essential character of paranoia. In the interpretation of paranoia by Freud and his fellow workers the chief interest is focussed on the manifested persecutory delusion. These analysts have stated that an excessive disturbance of psychic structure by the homosexual tendencies of the subconscious may cause paranoia. The enemy is, in this concept, a symbol of the subconscious homosexual tendency. Other theories, too, have been advanced by various authors who have observed, analysed, and even improved paranoiac patients.

I find myself forced to the conclusion that both paranoia and prejudice are signs that the sense of social responsibility does not function too well in the individual affected. It is so obvious in the prejudiced person that he has difficulties in his attitude to his fellowmen, and also that he is too much concerned with the question of social morals. In short, the subject is beset with a deep-seated difficulty in imposing on himself the restrictions of morality for the sake of society. I think that fully-blown paranoia is a *psychotic breakdown* of the social-moral function in the sense just mentioned. In my opinion the paranoiac feels too acutely that the claims of the social order are beyond endurance for his mental structure.

34. If homosexual tendencies or other infantile elements show a predominance in the analysis of such patients, this is only the case because of the disintegration and isolation of intra-mental factors referred to on p. 67. It is one of the great mistakes of psychoanalysts to consider that which comes into prominence under observation as the main root of the trouble. What remains intangible may be more truly the primary etiological factor, and what obtrudes itself plainly may be only a secondary product. If a stone has wounded a person and soiled the wound, and pus develops, which hurts, as we know, it is right to remove the pus ; on removal the pain will be relieved. But no surgeon will forget that the accumulation of pus is secondary to the original injury by a dirty stone.

It is, of course, impossible to discover during analysis tangible evidence of the deep-seated difficulty in social and moral adjustment. This latter is a comprehensive function of the personality as a whole, with deep and ramified roots, and hardly recognized by the average subject either in its positive working or in its difficulties. The individual moral problems which *are* the immediate object of self-observation are, in fact, particular applications of this wholesale function. Whether the competitive attitude or the fear of it, whether sexuality or chastity, free aggression or yielding are the manifest problems, the social analyst must not forget that all these are but phases in the general process of moral and social adjustment.

## CHAPTER IIIB

## CONTINUATION

*The rôle of facts in the genesis of prejudice.—The intellectual function in the prejudiced person.—The man who contradicts himself on the same principle.—A paranoiac theory on the discovery of Salvarsan.—A prejudiced medical man.—Past sexual experiences in the development of later prejudice.*

1. IT is in the very nature of prejudice—being a kind of paranoiac delusion—that the subject cannot realize its unobjective character. He may recognize prejudice in another person ; though it is exceptional for one person to recognize in another person his own peculiar type of prejudice.

The reason with which a person justifies his passionate hostility towards another person, group, ideology, or project, may be partly or entirely factual. What makes his objection a prejudice is the passionate intensity of it, which interferes with his logical function. A theft or exploitation whether committed by a friend or business-competitor is objectively the same ; but, as we know, the observer's attitude towards the act may be markedly different in the two instances. It would be difficult to prove that a person's lacking efficiency, reliability, or pleasantness has anything to do with his being of a certain religious denomination or political adherence. Nevertheless, it is a matter of routine, all over the world, for people to assume such causal relationships. Even people who are educated, and otherwise logical in thought, have to make an effort in order to prevent the full development of such an idea that begins to emerge when they are annoyed about a person's conduct.

2. A distinct prejudice does not always equally interfere with the subject's judgments. In this, too, there is a similarity to ordinary paranoia. Such a patient may be intelligent, and appear logical in his reasoning, when he does not feel that his particular delusion is touched by the discussion or any statement.

A lawyer who thought himself the " incarnation of the heavenly kingdom and the sole ruler of Hungary " spent his life from the age of 32 in the psychiatric wing of the University Hospital at B. He applied himself there to the study of languages and sociology, and the professor of psychiatry—himself a well-read man—used to enjoy the conversation with this man. There was in his conversation no trace of a psychosis for as much as half an hour on certain occasions, until by some association he found himself involved in a sphere where he could not help referring to his delusions.

3. The intellectual faculty of a prejudiced person is intact to a much greater degree. A fierce anti-Semite may on one occasion be able quite calmly to discuss with the chairman of a synagogue the internal affairs of the Jewish congregation and advise him in a friendly way, and on other occasions, however, deny with conviction the right of all Jews to equal citizenship. It is well-nigh unpredictable where delusion steps in to interfere with ideation and attitude; but, undoubtedly, prejudice prevents the subject, at times, from seeing a most obvious point under discussion. I had a schoolmate, son of an aristocratic family, whose parents wished him to become a priest. He was on the whole a well-behaved and intelligent boy. On many occasions he lectured to the boys about "the beauties of the Jewish religion". This, however, did not prevent him on other occasions from speaking passionately about "the secret custom of the Jews of using children's blood for the Passover". He stated that their religion prohibits the Jews from eating blood of animals "only for the disguise of the criminal ritual mentioned".

People of average intelligence and logical ability usually find it practicable to discuss problems of common interest. Though on certain points divergence of outlook or liking becomes apparent, it does not cloud the trend of discussion. The partners understand that, given a certain view on one matter, a number of associated conceptions must be influenced from the outset.

There are, however, occasions when it is impossible to see why a person becomes adamant about a certain point without being able to clarify the fundamental difference between himself and others. It appears that he recognizes all that the others say, and still, as if without any particular reason, he cannot reach the same conclusions as his partners in the discussion. This strikes one as an absence of logic; yet, it is hard to imagine that a person with otherwise unimpaired logical faculties should be unable to apply it to one particular point.

4. This phenomenon is the clearest illustration of how an element of prejudice may obstruct the trend of logical ideation. In most cases it is hard even to guess the kind of element in the mind of a certain individual which interferes with his intellectual intercourse. On rare occasions it is, however, possible to see more deeply into the phenomenon. I shall attempt to reconstruct a simple instance, more accurately, to simplify one such a case. The person in question, a man of academic education, was at a party where the question of corporal punishment at schools was discussed. He declared himself in favour of this measure, whereas the other members of the party were against it. This might be merely a difference in opinion of a fairly objective character. It is not illogical to doubt whether gentleness alone is really capable of replacing stronger, deterrent measures. It is even admissible to think that the occasional employment of force cannot do much harm to a child, and, therefore, it is justifiable for teachers to make their task easier ; unquestionably, education through infinite tolerance and refined psychology might require the expenditure of too much nervous energy.

In the further course of conversation the same man stated that corporal punishment by parents "is definitely wrong". He related that he himself received a thrashing at home only on rare occasions, but he thought that it ought never to have happened. For his differentiation between school and home he tried to adduce a few reasons, all interesting enough, but certainly not convincing. He himself admitted that the difference he made was for him a matter of firm conviction rather than something for which he could clearly account.

An explanation of his peculiar attitude became possible when in the heat of further discussion he mentioned the misery of a distant relative, a teacher who was dismissed because of repeated brutality towards children. "It was wrong to ruin a person for such a small cause," he added. On the face of it, the instance of the teacher was meant to serve as an illustration of the subsequent remark that it was wrong to punish him by dismissal. But actually, I suggest, the disturbing complex in the mind of this man was the idea that one might jeopardize one's career through being impulsive. He himself was of a rather impulsive disposition, and the instance of his relative was a frequent topic of conversation in his family.

5. This instance is different from the type of prejudice dealt with

in Part I in so far that the accusation of others is no component of the abnormality. Implicitly, however, there is a wholesale rejection of the logic of all those who *are* able to reason against corporal punishment. The inclusion of this type of irrational judgment in the broader group of prejudice is reasonable because of the obstructive character the particular idea has on the general thinking of the subject. However, only the fact that these judgments concern inter-human relationships—in this case in the educational sphere—makes them fully comparable to prejudices in the ordinary sense.[1] In all cases of prejudice its deeper psychological function is an imaginery defence against an anticipated discovery that the subject bears in himself condemnable elements. We can also say that prejudice formation in the broader sense is an attempt to deal with anxiety referring to the subject's moral insufficiencies. The function of prejudice and comparable obstructive ideas is a psychoneurotic vindication of the self. Here we may also refer to the instance described in the first part of Ch. III (page 79).

6. In the year 1922 I saw in a general students' reading room at Prague a small book which was left there by its owner. It was, I realize now, a kind of ideological compendium for the use of German aryan student unions in which, amongst other things, it was stated : " The Jew Ehrlich has discovered his Salvarsan with a view to enabling Jewish men and women to be immoral without fear of venereal diseases." " . . . likewise the modern custom of wearing light weight or conveniently cut dresses in the summer has been introduced by Jewish women from motives of sexual immorality."

At that time I did not realize the implication of this booklet and thought it to be a piece of pornographic literature. In the majority of " Burschenschaften "[2] the student members vied with each other in the art of duelling and in heavy drinking. Owing to this latter fact, the incidence of venereal diseases was—so far as I remember—not small amongst them. At the commencement of the University terms leaflets were given to each student by the Bursar's office at the German University pointing out the rôle of alcoholism in the acquisition of venereal diseases. This instance is adduced merely for the illustration of organized prejudice and its background.

[1] Cf. Appendix II.

[2] Students' Unions.

7. The following episode provides an instance of some interest. Many years ago I treated by psychoanalysis a young woman who soon after her marriage had developed an obsessive neurosis. Amongst other details of her life she told me about a comparatively recent period in which she had suffered from "abdominal tension"; an experienced medical man treated her, for several months, by intra-vaginal massage. This recollection occurred to her repeatedly in the course of free associations, and on one occasion I asked her to remember the full facts. She related then that after the first few treatments she observed that the doctor intentionally masturbated her, to which she readily responded. There was never a word spoken between him and her about this fact, but she knew clearly that this prolonged treatment was not called for by her condition.

The story so far does not merit our attention. Incidentally I knew that the wife of the doctor suffered from an incurable illness; and the other party, the patient, was never contented with her marriage. The circumstances were obviously conducive to what had taken place.

It was still during the time this patient was in my analysis that another woman consulted me with a different complaint. Several weeks earlier she had received a blow in the course of a dispute with a neighbour and stated that since this time she suffered from headaches and was incapable of working. She wanted, in fact, a certificate for a court proceeding in which she was to claim compensation for the loss of her working capacity. I was unable to diagnose the presence of a neurological illness; moreover, it was obvious that her complaints were due to the loss of prestige in the neighbourhood. Thus, I had to refuse her request. She came once more and repeated stubbornly her wish for a certificate. In the course of conversation I pointed out that actually the doctor who had seen her soon after the alleged injury had occurred was best fitted to testify on her behalf. To this she rushed to answer: "Of course, I asked him for a doctor's note, but he ironically said that I should go to a Jewish specialist who might be ready to make a good business out of the case. Isn't he an anti-Semite?" When I asked her for the name of the doctor she mentioned the practitioner referred to in the afore-mentioned analysis.

The problem here is not one of a person who, though himself not without blame, utters wholesale slander of a prejudiced character. One might calmly say that whatever intimacy takes place between two adult persons is their own business, whereas the issuing of an untrue medical certificate is a serious matter; undoubtedly the doctor in question had refused to commit this offence. What it is intended to demonstrate is the probable connection between difficulties in the moral sphere and resentful prejudice. In other words, people who in a prejudiced way accuse whole groups of being morally deficient are themselves under the pressure of a specific difficulty in their moral process. In most cases this difficulty leads only to occasional manifest offences; on the whole, such people present to the world an impression of being correct gentlemen, and at times even altruistic idealists.

8. Here is the place to discuss the influence of past sexual experiences in the development of biased attitudes later in life. Let us assume the case of a young man who, for whatever reason, had a passionate love relationship somewhere abroad, where political ideology and concepts on inter-human relationships are different from those prevailing in his native country. This man marries later at home in ordinary circumstances, and as time goes on his psyche has to cope with the difficulties ensuing from obligations and limitations of his conjugal status. In such moments there takes place in deeper layers a comparison of the present with past periods of life, infantile and later; imagination also conjures up a course of events that might have occurred were the subject not married to his present wife. It is obvious that in such a process the memory of past love scenes cannot fail to emerge, and in various degrees to disturb the work of intramental adjustment. Should there be a strong repression in the mind preventing some realization of this process, and at the same time the memory in question, at that period, be strongly dynamic, there has to take place a process of compromise. The person beset with such difficulties may surprise his friends by favouring a political or cultural programme strange to them, from no intelligible reason at all.

It is possible that such a dissension is an expression of the subconscious desire for the revival of the past relationship with the foreign girl. The objection by the sense of realities to this obsessive element may evoke some tendency to externalization, prejudice formation, or it may simply block at certain points of ideation the integrity of logical thought.

Similar mechanisms interfere with thinking and sentiment in general to a very substantial extent. It is obvious that owing to the complex nature of mental life these events are not avoidable at all. There is always some element, or the interplay of numerous factors, to account for a certain trend imposed by the emotional spheres on thinking and judging. A general resistance of the mind towards irrational tendencies can limit the frequency of processes of this kind ; another kind of psychic resistance decides the degree to which recent difficulties enforce *regression* and various psychoneurotic manifestations.[1]

[1] *Note.*—The writer's attention has been drawn to the case of Wordsworth and the book by Herbert Read devoted to the poet. This author attempts a psychological explanation of the fact that Wordsworth turned from an enthusiast of French revolutionary ideas into a determined adversary of the same creed. Read suggests that this metamorphosis might have been a subconscious reaction to the poet's severance of his relationship with the French girl, Annette, and their child, and to his subsequent marriage to an English wife. Read seems to assume that beneath apparent indifference there was in Wordsworth a sense of guilt which resulted in militant conservatism.

It is true that a turn towards conservatism, traditional dogmatism, and even reactionary hostility to new concepts is a frequent phenomenon. One might refer it to growing maturity in general, if it were not obvious in many instances, that this metamorphosis has been stubbornly irrational and not associated noticeably with other signs of improvement in the personality.

On the other hand, an emotional change-over such as that of Wordsworth, never occurs without giving rise to some new element within the mind. A love-relationship, deep as his was, cannot simply disappear and give place to a legal marriage with another person. This is even more improbable if the relationship implies serious obligations or the abandoned partner has been left in unhappiness.

We do not know how the large number of people who are not cool psychopaths achieve their readjustment if faced by a similar problem. It remains nevertheless probable that some form of reactive formation is bound to manifest itself, immediately, or at a later period of life. Memories are either easily assimilated into the subsequent psychoaffective structures of the subject, or they constitute foreign bodies requiring particular mental processes to cope with them. This does not apply, of course, to the equally large number of impressions that fade out of the psyche because they lose subjective significance in the light of later attitudes and interests of the personality.

Admittedly, a number of attitudes and beliefs in early man- and womanhood are stimulated to a substantial extent by the impact of neuro-hormonal processes that are not yet as steady as later in life. After this phase has been passed, several of the subject's beliefs and aims appear less dynamic and may gradually be abandoned. This alone, however, cannot account for the emergence of new attitudes diametrically opposed to the previous ones and held passionately or stubbornly. Read is right in recognizing the rôle of remorse and the ensuing tendency to develop new attitudes. There is always a number of memories—relating to facts or tendencies—that are felt by the psyche burdensome and in need of some new element or process capable of neutralizing them.

Changes in ideology or habits in the forties–fifties may have another, additional root. The inevitable realization by the individual of being no longer young is bound to create some envy and resentment of those who enjoy the privileges and hopes of youth. This, in its turn, may be displaced to ideas representative of contemporary youth, or to attitudes that are characteristic of daring, venturesome people.

It is obvious that the merits or demerits of any ideology or tendency are not affected by the character of deep psychic forces contributing to their development. This has been pointed out above (Ch. II, B (4).[2]

The writer thinks that there is one instance where we may take a change in ideology later in life as a probable sign of growing maturity. It does occur that a person of much experience and unfettered intellect is able to recognize in the middle period of his life that some traditional concepts are in fact dispensable and had to give way to newer ones. If the reformed outlook implies for the subject a lessening of his social power, then maturity as a source of the metamorphosis is even more probable. Persons with religious-ascetic tendencies displaying similar self-denial are, of course, dominated by different mental motives. But as a rule they are not in favour of modern sociological concepts, and thus there is no difficulty in distinguishing them from the former type.

[2] Page 56.

## CHAPTER IIIc

## THE COLLECTIVE (ETHNICAL) ELEMENT IN PREJUDICE[1]

*Proneness to prejudiced reactions is a variable factor in various ethnic groups.—The same type of religious belief common to different groups acquires a somewhat different colouring.—The collective factor.—There may be in the collective spirit (psyche) an element intolerable to the group; this prompts externalization as well as passionate hatred of others.—The rôle of external, international pressure in qualifying this process.—The environmental factor in paranoia.—The positive and negative aspects of religion.—The particular character of religions in moulding social atitudes.*

1. Experience shows that the proneness to prejudice and the susceptibility to passionate group hatred may be prominent within certain sections of humanity. The cultural pattern in accordance with which groups and nations live, the concepts of religion and nationality prevailing among them, always contain specific additional elements that give in each instance a distinctive character to sentiments and reactions universal among mankind. The ideas of national pride and patriotism are not only universal but, on the face of it, identical in all countries. But the actual composition of these sentiments as they exist in the minds of individuals belonging to a particular country, is seen by the psychologist to differ from group to group. The same is the case, for instance, with religious concepts. It is not only a matter of historical chance that the religious concepts and customs of various people develop so differently. It is the collective mentality of each group that gives the local colouring to its religious ideology, however great the similarities, and however extensive the identities, that may undoubtedly exist between the religious atmosphere of any two countries.

2. Two different groups may equally subscribe to a belief that all men are brothers, all being children of God the Father. Yet the actual conduct towards fellow-beings manifested on the two

[1] Cf. Appendix p. 259.

social soils proves unequivocally that deep down there cannot be a psychological equality between the apparently identical concepts. I am assuming that the prevailing economic conditions in the two instances are not widely different, and therefore it is not the different intensity of the competitive element that is responsible for the two types of social atmosphere. There are specific mental elements, collective features, that colour the thinking and feeling of most members of an ethnic group ; though we are hardly able to define these obscure though potent factors. These are responsible for the fact that, for instance, the monotheism of some groups is more intellectual, and that of others more primitive. These obscure mental components are also responsible for the phenomenon that one group of people extends human recognition to broad masses, whereas other groups are only able to do so within a limited circle. Logic would require that two groups, equally believing in universal human brotherhood, should make at least no fundamental difference between those nearer to them and those more distant from them. But experience shows that this is not the case. Instances to the contrary are too numerous. There are groups who passionately subscribe to the principle of human equality, and with the same passion exclude larger or smaller groups from this recognition, without realizing the ethical inconsistency manifested in their social behaviour. Some mental element makes them insensitive towards an inconsistency that would hurt the sense of justice and the very intellect in others belonging to a different mental type.

To put it in other words, the intra-mental conditions for the creation of prejudice are substantially dependent on a collective factor (ethnic psyche). It is also certain that various religious concepts and national ideologies constitute a different soil for prejudice. But, on the other hand, it is obvious that it is the collective particular element operative in men's minds, that is largely responsible for the preference of the particular religious or national ideology by that group.

3. It is not overlooked that all that is peculiar to an ethnic group is the consequence of historical events—political and economic—and of the geophysical characteristics of the piece of earth it inhabits. Hardships from natural causes, and lack of stability in life owing to wars and political pressure, satisfactorily account for the unpleasant colouring in the deeper psychological

make-up of groups and nations. But the devices of science and progress in general civilization have for some time now reduced the natural differences in the life of various nations; and the basic principles of social administration are no longer so widely different in various countries as in the past; accordingly, a great deal of the unpleasant features in the psychological atmosphere of groups continues to exist only by virtue of tradition or inheritance. Undoubtedly, an individual member of such an ethnic group may change even in the deeper structures of his psyche if transplanted into a markedly different environment.

4. By assuming that certain mental elements, peculiar to the spiritual make-up of a group, may increase the proneness to prejudice, we have actually assumed that these people have in their subconsciousness a surplus of complexes that are a menace to the harmony of their own minds. Or, viewing it from another aspect, the individuals of such a group find it more difficult to remain tolerant because they are burdened by the collective element peculiar to them, that is because the toleration of the *self* is not easy for them.

Tolerance towards others, it has been explained, is largely the reflection of the subject's tolerance towards his individual *self*. It should be added that intolerance is more frequent and intense among members of a group if there is something in the spirit of the group that is a burden to the individual mind. Intolerance and open hatred prominent amidst a religious, national, or political group is, in the writer's opinion, a manifestation of its self-condemnation. It is unfortunate that in the practical sphere the only victims of this self-condemnation are the chosen or chance objects of intolerance.

The condemnation of the pathological elements in the spiritual atmosphere of their group by its members remains a subconscious process; it may be as little realized as the background of a paranoiac delusion is by psychotic patients themselves.

There appears to be little hope of easily eradicating from ethnic groups the excessive readiness to yield to prejudice. Traditional concepts and the whole spiritual and sentimental atmosphere of the group keep the "complex" alive. Much external pressure, political and cultural influence on the part of other nations, exerted for considerable periods, can alone do the work. But so long as there are such frequent upheavals in the world, armed conflicts and economic struggles, it is impossible for attention to be paid by such a peculiar group to criticism coming from other nations or groups. Their disapproval is reacted to by a simple psychopathological "trick". They are declared base enemies of the country or group in question, and of human decency and progress in general; and thus their criticism ceases to be a force capable of a moulding influence.

5. It cannot be repeated too often that potent motives, perhaps the paramount ones, leading to prejudice and consequent attitudes spring from environmental sources. There is something in the public spirit of a prejudiced nation or group that is intolerable to the minds of the individuals amongst them, an element that is incompatible with their mental stability. At the same time there is in such societies a more or less explicit encouragement and manifest approval of prejudiced attitudes.

Incidentally, in the genesis of paranoia proper, which the writer considers to be related to prejudice and unmotivated hatred, there is similarly at work an environmental factor. It has been noted by Freud that it seems as if the patient suffering from persecutory delusions has sensed the subconscious hatred (we should say, the "competitive complex") existing in his fellow-beings. I should like to add that in the ultimate analysis it is the environment, animate and inanimate, that has made the paranoiac, and also the neurotic, ill. The claims made on the human personality by various situations, and by the co-existence of fellowmen, are not easy to satisfy, even to an average degree, for every individual. If then, owing to an innate weakness the mind breaks down under the burdens of daily life, there may be a vague realization by the subconscious of the part played in the difficulties by the broader environment. This element of deep knowledge may be personified in a delusion of being persecuted or interfered with by people in a mysterious way. There are other forms of delusion in which the sufferer's own weakness is expressed in the delusion following a psychotic breakdown. If, for instance, the patient feels that "everything in him is rotten" or is "dark" or "numb as though without any feeling", this may be interpreted as delusional realization of the very weakness that could no longer cope with individual and social life. These latter forms of delusion are, however, not characteristic of paranoia proper but of melancholia and schizophrenia.[1]

[1] See Appendix II.

6. Allusion has already been briefly made to the rôle which particular religious ideologies can play in paving the way for prejudice and associated aggressiveness. Indeed, those with knowledge of history need no further proof for this causal relationship. Our examination of possible prospects of social improvement nevertheless justifies an accurate analysis of the phenomenon. Let us start first with a statement in defence of religion. To a very great extent, all the horrors committed throughout history against heretics were associated with religious zeal because the cultural poverty in the civilization of previous centuries (as that of some ethnic groups to this day) knew of no other " sacred " pretext for giving vent to general aggressiveness. Thus, for centuries the logical and ethical contradiction between the religion of all-forgiving love and the unscrupulous exploitation and destruction of Jews and heretics was not even recognized by the masses.

But there can be in religion itself an element of potential prejudice ; or, more accurately, a specific colouring of religious concepts and teachings may increase, and has at all times increased, in the believers that psychoneurotic disharmony that makes for prejudice. The tendency to eradicate " sin " in its various forms clashes so frequently with the weakness of the moral process defined above. The more superhuman the idea preached the less can the individual's mind forgive itself the operation within it of anti-religious and anti-moral tendencies. The more general, consequently, must be the pressure of the tendency towards externalization, that is of prejudiced accusation of others. The traditional idea of an external *devil* who tempts weak mortals introduces a ready pattern for the process of externalization (projection). The idea of the devil in contributing particularly to Jew-hatred in Christian countries has been clearly recognized by recent authors.

7. On the other hand, I agree with those who state that a deep religious conviction is a certain antidote to psychoneuroses. I agree that psychoneuroses may be the outcome of a moral conflict particularly where it is fed by an intellectual doubt about the absoluteness of moral precepts. Simpletons in religious feeling are less prone to develop, let us say, an obsessional neurosis ; but they are very apt to react to mental difficulties with prejudice-formation.

To clarify this statement it should be added that a deep, uncomplicated religious belief does not exclude difficulties in the moral process as defined above. Consequently, a person may be very religious in a primitive sense, and relatively free from common neuroses; but, owing to an insufficient moral process, very prone to the most stupid and unassailable prejudice. His simplicity and lack of general intellect is but a further factor permitting the development and maintenance of his prejudice.

The difficulty of the moral process has reference essentially to the necessity for self-restriction in various fields. At the same time primitive religion is based on expectations of blessings in reward to faith, and primitive religiosity is associated with the subject's conviction of being better than others and therefore entitled to more than others. The revolt against morals can thus easily be projected on to those who are deemed condemnable on religious ground. Cf. Ch. XIV (10), (14).

*Note.* The large-scale massacre in India illustrates the coming to the fore of "ethnic complexes" in the wake of paramount changes; cf. Ch. VIII. (Sept. 1947.)

## CHAPTER IV

## PERCEPTION OF THE SELF AND OVER-SENSITIVENESS TOWARDS ELEMENTS IN THE " INNER ENVIRONMENT "

*We understand our fellowman through self-perception.—The I and the Thou, and their complementary rôle in the process of identification.—The perception of the self in the course of moral choice.—The mixing of " outside " and " inside ".—The dream.—The perceptive agent is the integrated personality; theoretical difficulties.—The faculty of self-perception is dependent on outside influences.—Intolerance of the self may lead to concrete intolerance.—The discussion of atheism in various types.—The Jewish anti-Semite.—Intolerance is a defence mechanism.—Stimulation of intra-mental disharmony by impressions from the outside.—Intra-mental regulation.—A father concerned about the coolness of his child.—Emotional unresponsiveness may prevent irrational hatred.*

1. IT has always been recognized that we understand our fellowman through the medium of self-perception. We assume in others the operation of motives and feelings similar to those in ourselves. Though it is the other person's manifest behaviour—that is, his actions, the expression of his face and his gestures—that is the immediate source of our knowledge about him, the interpretation of these externals takes place largely through comparison with ourselves. We guess what similar behaviour on our part would indicate about our feelings and intentions, and project the resulting causal connection on to the other person. In brief, in the course of interpreting the behaviour of a fellowman, the subject introduces, as it were, the other man's personality-image into himself behaving as he does at that moment, and constructs a state of mind appropriate to this behaviour.

2. First an identification of the subject with the manifest behaviour of the other person takes place, and there immediately follows the identification of an imagined *ad hoc* frame of mind of the subject with the mind of this other person. But it is clear that

only the first phase is an instance of *identification* proper. The subject imagines himself behaving as the other person does at that moment; in the second phase the subject merely assumes that the type of feelings he himself has in response to this imagined imitative behaviour are elaborately present in the other person. This assumption is, more accurately, a process of projection (externalization). But taking the interpretative process as a whole—as the two phases are practically simultaneous—we realize that the *I* and the *Thou* are compounded into an *ad hoc* unity within the mind of the subject.

Something similar to this occurs in another process, different in essence and goal. I refer to the process of moral decision. In the course of this function, two opposite alternatives are conceived through the subject imagining himself definitely acting in each of both ways. There is also clearly present a third aspect of the ego, the real personality, *not yet* committed to any of the alternatives, and capable of observing the two imagined types of attitude or conduct. Here the subject views the image of himself—in two differing editions, as it were—just as one observes an external object. There is thus a mixture of the ego with a quasi-external (double) image of the ego. In fact, however, yet another image of the self participates in this process, Freud's ego-ideal, by which the two (or more) recent alternatives are measured. This representative of one's purest conscience is, in fact, the deposit of external education and intimidation. In point of fact, the possible judgment of the external environment explicitly enters, to a varying extent, into the conscious process of weighing up and choosing. What the world at large, and particularly certain members of this world, would say or do in the case of the right or the wrong choice respectively, is a consideration always present in the process. Thus, even the picture of the genuinely external world is introduced into the mind and mixed up with the two alternative pictures of the ego.

Only too often the ultimate decision is not in accordance with the ideal-ego or with the strictest claims of society (or religion). But, I think, the picture of the society does always enter the complex process of moral consideration. Not infrequently, the picture of another type of environment becomes involved, that part of society which it is believed would choose the less strict alternative, the subject thus encouraging himself in rejecting the ideal choice. Whatever the details and components of this complex process may be, one fact remains certain, that there takes place an *ad hoc* mixing of the environment and the self.

And this is actually the point which we should like now to discuss.

3. The phenomenon of prejudice-paranoia is obviously based on this fundamental mixing of the " outside " and " inside " within the psychic processes of the subject. In general, all misunderstanding between human beings results from the fact that the subject assumes the presence in his fellow-man of a certain trend of thought or a frame of mind ; it is inevitable that such assumptions spring from the wishes or fears of the subject.

On the other hand, there is much that is really common to the minds of various people, and through empathy a proper understanding of each other is very frequently possible. Only, there is no provision made by nature that the function of empathy should work accutately in all circumstances. The human psyche is an admirable and complex instrument, but certainly not one endowed with mathematical precision. Therefore, the fact that there is within the mind a mixture between concepts relating to environmental persons and those to the subject himself, leads at times to conclusions which are mistaken if measured by outside reality. The emotional emphasis put on the various intra-mental elements is not always in accordance with the requirements of orientation in the outside world ; the emotional processes in general are to a great extent beyond the control of the rational.

Spotlights projected on the stage may create a variety of unrealistic impressions, for instance, through artificially uniting the left and right half of two groups or pieces of scenery and putting into the shade the two lateral halves belonging to each concrete part of the scene. Analogously, the intrapsychic flashlight of affective emphasis can make two heterogeneous elements coalesce, resulting in an irrational mixing of the ego and the object.

A most interesting instance in this respect is the dream mechanism, ascribing the subject's tendencies to other persons and endowing the subject with characteristics of other individuals. Moreover, the dreamer's tendencies are symbolically expressed by persons, animals, objects, and localities having a specific significance. This phenomenon betrays some of the intra-mental processes in which the mixing of the " outside " and " inside " takes place. We may say that this propensity of the dream, as well as the underlying mode of mental functioning, indicates the deep-rootedness of the human being in his broader environment.

The dreaming psyche is able to express its components and processes only in terms of objective environment. This leads us to the discussion of a further point related to the main theme of this work.

4. Individual tendencies, and particularly those of an instinctual character, are as it were distinct objects for realization by the *integrated personality*. This is not only a fundamental thesis in psychoanalysis, but a phenomenon consciously clear in many moments to every individual. Tendencies of a sexual nature and phantasies of the similar group, aggressive impulses, envy and jealousy, critical sentiments toward relatives or revered authorities, may appear to the subject as though foreign to his genuine ego. Thus, the function of tolerance includes the particular aspect of self-tolerance. An inquiry into the relationship between centrifugal and centripetal tolerance seems inevitable.

It is difficult to suppress the question : What is the *integrated personality* if not a sum-total of psychological dispositions, particular tendencies, and the whole content of the mind, conscious and subconscious ? If this be the case, then the faculty of perceiving one's own component tendencies, however manifestly it operates, presents a difficult problem to logic. But, obviously, there is such a thing as a perception of the personality as a whole. Consequently, the perception of components of the personality need not present a problem of its own. We may, perhaps, say that each mental element (tendency, disposition, and definable content) has a double aspect—the element or tendency *per se* and its dynamic activity, its function. The former aspect, as may be imagined, is a component of the whole personality ; whereas the latter retains a certain measure of distinctness and is capable of being perceived by the integrated personality. This concept is open to question ; but the questions are not unanswerable, so the writer feels. Only this is not the place to enlarge upon the problem.

5. The question still to be answered is, how does the integrated personality perceive its *self* as a whole ? On the face of it the subject doing the observation and the object observed by it is the very same thing. An answer to this intricate question is possible when we realize that in observing our fellowman we

perceive actually his personality as a whole. This perception transferred to the self, is probably the fundamental element for self-perception.

It has been stated earlier that we understand our fellowman only through the medium of perceiving our self. But this thesis refers to component elements and processes, such as the images, feelings, tendencies, and overt actions associated with them. The subject perceives within himself these individual processes and the causal associations, and applies his knowledge in the course of understanding the environmental person. An answer to the question how the component elements of the self are perceived by the integrated personality of the subject has been attempted above (4).

But it is obvious that a picture of the subject's personality as a whole develops, first of all, through the experiences of perceiving his fellowmen. Even though an infant would never look into a mirror he would acquire a picture of his own personality through frequent observation of others. These others appear in a large variety of behaviour-forms, and the ensuing impressions on the mind of the infant—and adult—develop the function of perceiving the self as a dynamic whole.

Naturally through perceiving within the self continuously the large variety of sensory feelings, emotional currents, and tendencies, the image of the *self* is much richer in content, much more differentiated than the image referring to the environmental person.

6. Returning to the main theme of this part, we can take it as probable that a deficient self-tolerance may interfere with satisfactory tolerance towards outside objects. An environmental person is clearly a reminder of the self. Moreover, various impressions coming from the outside world can stimulate associatively intra-mental elements in the subject (see Appendix II). Thus, an outside impression, whether it is a person or a complex event, may become a symbol of the self or its components, and dissatisfaction with the self can be projected on to outside objects.

There may exist a selective intolerance toward specific elements of the self. In consequence of this, the manifestation of intolerance towards external objects may also be selective, in accordance with the association evoked within the subject by the external impression.

7. It has been recognized that a tendency or feature of which the subject himself would like to be rid, may irritate him to an exceptional degree if manifested by others. This may be so if the subject is conscious to some extent of the presence of the element in question within himself. More frequent are the cases of intolerance towards certain characteristics in others if the subject possesses the analogous tendency in repression. We cannot dismiss, for instance, the idea that moralists who concern themselves overmuch with a particular kind of vice in society, have some deep-seated difficulty with the same kind of temptation.

There is, however, no need to assume that a religious or moral leader who, for example, speaks constantly and in a stereotyped way about sexual chastity would in reality easily succumb to sexual temptation. In most cases of such selective "intolerance" the subject has rather a particular difficulty with the mere idea of sex. His psyche has, as it were, an allergic sensitiveness towards the realization of sexuality in himself, however average its dynamic power may be. Likewise, such a person may be hypersensitive towards the idea that a great number of people are indeed sexually licentious. In brief, it is the dynamic charge of an idea and not exactly a practical weakness in this instinctive sphere that may result in an intolerance towards a laxity of sexual morals in the outside world. (We consider here as intolerance not the average disagreement with laxity but an exceptional prepossession with such problems.)

8. There is no doubt in the writer's mind that the atheistic tendency, surely present behind the facade of the firmest belief in God and revealed religion, can manifest itself in two different ways. It may facilitate tolerance through the medium of a deep realization that there are logical reasons for religious doubts. In another type of person the suppressed revolt against the authority of religion results in a fierce intolerance towards those who are not much concerned with God and his commands as these are assumed by various doctrines.

Clearly, the difference between the two reactive attitudes toward outside objects is based on the quality of intrapsychic tolerance towards the atheistic component in the subject's own psyche. Not all persons' capacity for self-tolerance is equal. We may also safely assume that there are differences in self-tolerance with regard to various elements of the mind. That is to say, a person may have more difficulty with his libidinous tendencies or complexes than he has with his atheistic trend; and the reverse may be the case with another person. It is, moreover, conceivable that a subject may be exceptionally intolerant towards the quite ordinary degree of atheistic component in his mind because of the particular structure of his ideology (*complex* in broader sense, would be the more appropriate term).

9. Quite a number of persons of Jewish origin are exceptionally irritable when members of their race display human weaknesses of a universal character, such as selfishness, impolite behaviour, or mere conspicuity in general behaviour. They feel at such moments as if their Jewish fellowman has committed something for which the whole race might have to bear an irremovable blame. Clearly, such sensitive Jews display a selective intolerance towards fellow Jews because their psyche cannot cope with the realization of their own racial origin and their share in the Jew's social history. However detached they deem themselves to be from the community of Jews, however uninterested they think themselves to be in the fact that races and creeds of various kinds exist, their intolerant sensitiveness suggest clearly a relevant mental conflict and thus indubitably an interest in the whole problem. Their reaction betrays manifestly both that they have not been able to detach themselves mentally from the community of Jews, and also that they are trying strenuously to attain this goal.

10. It is probable that as with psychoneurotic symptoms in general, reactive intolerance, too, serves a psychodynamic purpose. It protests the subject from receiving into his psyche an undesirable, though unavoidable, impression more frequently and more deeply than is absolutely necessary. This intolerant reaction amounts to a rejection of the impression, and it prevents an unopposed assimilation of it into deeper psychic structures. In the case of the atheist who behaves intolerantly towards the belief of the pious it must be obvious that he wishes to fight the element of religious inclination present in himself. There is, as we know, in most atheists, to varying degrees, a thirst for religious experience. If such a person were to allow the impression made by the contented happiness of the believer to sink into his mind, his own repressed religious quest could possibly be stimulated

to a greater extent than would be agreeable to his atheistic outlook. Intolerant objection is a means of preventing such intra-mental clashes. In the case of the atheist it induces the subject to avoid, as much as is feasible, friendly intercourse with the religious. Atheistic intolerance is thus destined to forestall any positive interest of the mind in religious manifestations. The need for this measure exists because a positive interest in anything always implies a degree of liking and even an identification with the cause in question, however temporary and non-committal. For the type of atheist who is not endowed with the mental harmony and calm of a perfect freethinker, such interest in religious manifestations implies an intra-mental threat, that of stimulating a religious conflict. A freethinker, if harmonious in mind, does not consider it below his intellectual dignity to recognize in himself the " weakness " of having religious desires.

11. In view of the fact that a number of tendencies operate simultaneously within the mind, a process of integration has to take place constantly. At any moment there is a resultant dominant trend within the personality, making for the unity of the " self-feeling " as well as a certain consistency in aiming and action. But it is true that the function of integration itself is not always entirely efficient; and there may be various degrees of its successful operation at various times in the subject's life. The factor that accounts for such variations can only be the impact of environmental impressions and the changing character of situations in which the subject finds himself. A person may be known to his friends as calm by nature and incapable of violence or prejudiced reaction. Nevertheless, an incidental difference with a particular person may elicit in him a fury or passion unaccountable to himself. It is conceivable that a certain situation, or a particular person, may activate a complex in the subject that has previously been practically dormant. This small difference in the psychic atmosphere may really interfere with the capacity for integration to a degree making the subject " a different person " for a shorter or longer period.

12. The resultant overt harmony of the personality is not always of sufficient stability. When one of the deeper complexes is stimulated by an impression from outside, the mutual constellation of various elements existing within the mind is altered. The

psyche cannot always stand up to such an event without strain, which is followed by a difficulty in maintaining controlled behaviour. Impressions that stir us, and make us restless or as if paralysed, illustrate this sequence of events. The reactive change in overt behaviour, unintentional and frequently quite inexpedient, is in all probability the result of deeper changes. Let us consider a simple instance. Under ordinary circumstances the individual implicitly assumes the prevalence of peace and safety in his environment. If he suddenly has to witness a quarrel or any improper behaviour of other people, his hypothesis is shaken. This is likely to stimulate in him some fear, as for instance reminding him that his life, too, might be interferred with by unforeseen incidents.[1] This instance is, of course, only one of the infinite variety of cases in which an impression is bound to stimulate certain elements of the deeper mind.

13. In average circumstances there operates instantaneously and effectively a process of intra-mental regulation, which confines the disbalance and prevents such incidents from interfering with the mechanism of overt behaviour. Only on a few occasions, when the incidental trauma is strong, or the psychonervous system is in a lowered state of resistance, does the disturbed balance in the depths extend to the mechanism of overt behaviour.

This is a general law in human physiology. Bacteria or unsuitable foodstuffs do not interfere in all cases with health and subjective well-being. There are defensive processes coping with the emergency, so that practically no disease in the proper sense develops. Only in the case of a lowered resistance, or under the impact of a mass of bacteria or a considerable amount of unsuitable foodstuff, does a definite illness develop. But, obviously, there are individuals in whom such defences do not operate sufficiently. They have to be very careful about their food and physical environment.

14. A comparable weakness exists in certain individuals with respect to coping with impressions that stir their complexes. But here there may develop a specific mode of defence, compensating for the weakness, to some degree at any rate. It consists in a lesser susceptibility to certain impressions as compared with the reaction of average people. Normally, the sight of human

[1] Cf. Appendix II.

suffering leads to a degree of pity, though it is sure that on deeper levels the counterpart of sympathy, that is the aggressive-sadistic complex, too, is stirred. In a number of people, however, this same impression evokes the conscious obsession to add to the suffering of their fellow-beings, for instance, by beating or wounding them. To avoid such reactions of their minds, a number of people develop unconsciously an artificial coolness towards other people's suffering. The impression is not allowed to enter their mind deeply enough as to stir emotional spheres at all, because it would be not only pity but at the same time obsessive sadism that might be stimulated in them. It is probable that persons with an inclination to prejudice and hatred would find it hard to suppress the compulsion to actual aggression at the sight of human suffering, if not for the protective veneer of coolness and apparent lack of human feeling peculiar to them. (Cf. Ch. VII, 7, 9, pages 133–5.)

15. An educated man, father of two children, who suffered from frequent depression, complained that his daughter was cool towards him, whereas his son in most circumstances showed a great deal of sympathy for him. He thought the girl void of fellow-feeling altogether. It was obvious that the two children were different types ; the one easily roused by impressions and the other showing reserve in all situations. But such a difference in disposition does not sufficiently account for such a great difference in sympathy with an ailing father on the part of children, who lived with their widowed father, and who in addition were greatly attached to each other. I repeatedly explained to the father that his daughter has assumed this coolness as a means of self-defence. Should she have allowed her emotional spheres to be untrammelled, too much attachment to the father might have developed, which fact might have interfered with her capacity for work. I was also sure that through her coolness, which prevented a display of sympathy, her mind checked possible outbursts of resentment about the protracted neurotic behaviour of her father. Later developments proved that the girl was of average normality. She married a boy whom she liked and has been a very good companion to him ever since. After her marriage her behaviour to her father also improved.

16. Stekel suggested that in some cases of impotence and frigidity the brake put on the libidinal process exists essentially to prevent

a simultaneous release of aggressive and homicidal tendencies. The fear of *these* patients is, of course, grossly exaggerated; in them no sexual climax would lead on to actual murder.[1] But for the subconsciousness of a psychoneurotic such tendencies are felt *as if* capable of resulting in action. There can be no doubt that the extension of an inhibition from one emotional category into another is one of the existing defence mechanisms in psycho-neurotic conflicts.

17. We should not doubt that, likewise, the full development of prejudice and all types of irrational hatred may be prevented, in many instances, by the deeper emotional function being rendered comparatively unresponsive. From this description the student will recognize the type of personality who is apparently calm and formal, and even to a degree obliging, but who yet appears in a deeper sense rigid and as if void of average sympathy with a good cause or with suffering people. One almost *feels* the operation of prejudice behind the facade of their calm and unimpeachable behaviour, though it is difficult to discover in them unequivocal signs of such a mentality. But on occasions, when for the average person it is impossible to remain unaffected by an event either one way or another, these cool personalities are conspicuous. Incidentally, we are reminded of the "unemotional psychopath" and "schizoid" where, however, in all likelihood there is a genuine inability for adequate response.

The following two quotations will illustrate what is meant by this. Schneider in *Die Psychopathischen Persönlichkeiten*, Ch. 7, states: "There are 'unemotionals' free of any criminal tendency, who are capable of excellent achievements if in leading positions. They are the sort of people who appear inflexible and hard, ready 'to walk over corpses', and whose aims are not necessarily selfish; they may put themselves into the service of

[1] The case of "lust-murder" is entirely different. A person with such impulses does not suffer from impotence, but from a sexual perversion that from the outset aims at murder for the sake of, or in the course of, sexual gratification. In the case of the impotent person with a subconscious murder complex there is *no possibility* of his carrying out the criminal act; for this end the complex is too weak, and the personality of the patient too different from that of the real lust-murderer. The relationship is similar to that between an unalterable, constitutional homosexual, and the vast number of people suffering from a subconscious homosexual complex. The lust-murderer must be classed as a moral defective, that is, as a person who is hardly able to resist the impulse to murder. This is the reason for our statement that "*in them* (the neurotics) no sexual climax would lead on to actual murder". Besides sexual impotence there are other psychoneurotic conditions that are based on the operation of subconscious impulses to murder. Certainly, such patients are not comparable with moral defectives whose speciality is killing.

approvable ideas. Kretschmer refers to them among the schizoids. Their intellect is not only normal but in several cases even above the average."

In *Leaders, Dreamers, and Rebels*, by René Fülöp-Miller, the author writes : " Early in 1793, Robespierre wrote to Danton : ' Nothing but death can weaken my affection for you.' " Yet long ere this, he had been taking careful note of every suspicious action, every incautious word of the " Cyclops " ; and in April, 1794, he ruthlessly sent his friend to the guillotine.

" Robespierre, while still at Arras, resigned the post of criminal judge in the circuit on the ground that this conviction would not allow him to sentence a malefactor to death. As member of the Committee of Public Safety in the early days, he strongly protested against experiments with the recently invented quick-firing gun, declaring that the use of such a weapon conflicted with the principles of humanity."

" The same man had no hesitation in sending his best friends day after day to the guillotine, and he established a Reign of Terror. . . . Yet this did not mean that there was any contradiction, that there had been any change in his character. For, his determination in Arras not to sign a death-sentence, his protest against the use of a quick-firing gun, and his subsequent inauguration of the Reign of Terror, had nothing to do with human feelings. It was ' on principle ' that, earlier, he had protested against capital punishment, and it was on principle later that he made lavish use of it. . . . Virtuality and morality were, by Robespierre the dictator, enforced in the name of reason. . . ."

Both instances, but particularly the second, have an obvious bearing on the problem discussed in Ch. VII (12).

# CHAPTER V

## BIAS AGAINST THE INNER CIRCLE

*A favourable bias towards relatives, friends, and confederates is natural. The opposite attitude is also frequent.—The group represents the inner circle.—Just as one's relationship to the family is not a matter of free choice, neither is one's membership of a religion or national group.—Marriage is no exception.—Negative bias against the group may be based on a process of ridding oneself of family ties, also of infantile fixations.*

1. A BIAS in favour of one's closest circle as well as of one's national, religious, or political organization, is considered to be a natural phenomenon. This can be understood if one bears in mind that the individual extends, as it were, his personality on to his environment; and the same extension occurs with respect to the group of his co-religionists and fellow-nationals. In the case of those of the same faith, the feeling of community and identity may be even greater than that which is felt towards friends or relatives with a different creed. The projection of the individual's self on to large social groups of this kind contains an element absent in his relationship to the intimate circle. It is the feeling that one belongs to a large community representing not only numerical greatness but a revered and superior ideal. From this membership of such communities the individual gains an added feeling of personal significance. This subjective gain is, naturally, apt to increase the favourable bias towards the group in question.

In view of all this it is rather surprising to find so frequently people who are prone to discover or exaggerate deficiencies within the national or religious group into which they were born, and to assume that the ideals as well as the members of other groups are nearer to perfection. This phenomenon invites comparison with the bitterness so frequently felt against members of one's own family. But we realize that the reasons that account for this latter sentiment are obviously not present in the relationship of the individual towards his national or religious community. As described in Chapter I, the members of the inner circle are apt to provoke some resentment for more than one reason. They are, as we have seen, immediate limiting factors ; moreover, the claims on the subject ensuing from family relationships are frequently felt to be burdensome because the relative may be conceived as being only a small creature, and lastly any antagonism or disappointment that comes from those from whom we expect a great deal can hurt far more than the incident in question would in itself justify. All this does not apply to large groups or communities of which the subject is a member.

2. Admittedly, the individual does expect friendliness from the members of his group, and many people are even desirous of an exceptional mark of appreciation from others. Naturally these desires are often met by disappointment, and so there may be resentment enough to create a negative bias towards the group as a whole.

But I feel that this is not the whole truth. Those capable of deeper psychological understanding will recognize in such antagonism against one's group the phenomenon of displacement. Resentment towards close relatives, if to a large extent repressed, disappointment with the amount of love or appreciation received from them, may be shifted on to the larger group to which the individual happens to belong. His membership of these large groups is just as involuntary or accidental as his relationship to his family circle into which he was born, and to his fellowmen who happened to become his neighbours. The process of displacement in the phenomenon under discussion is facilitated by this common characteristic. When there is an occasion for the subject to feel disappointed with a member of his family, or a confederate of his national or religious group, the involuntary character of the subject's relationship to this person enters the foreground of awareness. The impact of the incidental disappointment is reinforced by the realization that the relationship has never been sought by the subject. Personal ties are felt as pleasant if they imply to the subject support and security—after the analogy of reins applied to the infant about to learn to walk. But their inclusive significance as fetters, limiting individual spontaneity, becomes obvious to a person only when a member of his closer or broader community proves disappointing or interfering. There is, it has to be realized, a dormant antagonism to all ties, particularly if they are not chosen from the outset by the subject himself and are difficult to break. Much as the race, nation, religion, and family may mean to the individual, the involuntariness of his ties to these groups implies limitation, and is, therefore, a source of potential resentment.

3. Adherence to a religious denomination or ideology would appear to be the result of deep conviction and thus a matter of free choice. Yet this is more easily said than actually felt. It is no easy task for the mind to dispose of infantile and deep-seated religious elements even though the intellect advises it. They have become, to varying degrees in almost all persons, part of the mental mechanism coping with loneliness, dissatisfaction, and fear. They cannot be removed without leaving behind a wound that is likely to result in some soreness for the rest of one's lifetime.

4. In the case of marriage the element of free decision is more of a hypothesis than a reality. The maintenance of married status once entered into is, certainly to a very large extent, enforced by social rules. But even the very choice of a conjugal partner is much less a matter of free choice than is generally assumed or admitted. In numerous instances of acquaintanceship the man or the woman, or both, feel committed at a certain time to propose, to accept, and to enter into marriage. In many cases of passionate love there *is* a dim or even a clear realization that a deep-seated compulsion is at work, acting in opposition to considerations of logic and common sense. Moreover, the making of a personal relationship into " legal " and " sacred " marriage gives the finishing touch to the involuntary character of this tie.

5. It is easy to realize this element of involuntariness in the relationship to members of the family, as well as to large groups of a national or religious kind. In ultimate analysis, the negative bias towards the group is in most instances based on an intramental conflict relating to close relatives. Hatred towards parents, children, and conjugal partners is generally a hard thing for the superego to tolerate. There is a particular idiosyncrasy towards these elements of the subject's mind. One mode of coping with this conflict is a displacement of the hostile attitude to the group. We may say that in essence the phenomenon of negative bias towards the group is an instance of

intolerance towards the *self* projected on to an external object, since the element that is difficult to cope with is a subjective element, that is, an attitude of the personality.

6. It would be simpler to assume that the group represents the concrete relatives against which hatred is felt ; that is, that in this phenomenon of displacement one external object is exchanged for another one. But this explanation is hardly satisfactory in view of what we know about phobias and obsessive neuroses. In these phenomena, places, objects, and actions appear associated with a considerable amount of anxiety for which they in the literal sense cannot account. The anxiety, as we know, refers to intra-mental tendencies and complexes of the subject, even though these tendencies and complexes *are* related to outside persons. Hence, it is safer to assume that in the case of shifting resentment on to a group, the essential object of intolerance is the subjective conflict, and the group represents both the objective relatives and the subjective element of hatred, which latter is burdensome to the psyche.

7. There is an obvious difference between displacing self-criticism on to the group and the projection in paranoia of prejudice. In the latter phenomenon, as a rule, a human type different from the self is selected for the process of externalization. In the negative bias against one's group the subject's homologous circle becomes the object of attack. In his bias against his own group the subject purports to be better than the other members. Either he feels himself to be the one who represents the ideals of his group more genuinely than the rest ; or, he condemns entirely the characteristics and ideals of his group, in favour of a different type of community. Thus, an Englishman may feel that the French nation is the one most to his taste. A member of the Church of England may be convinced that all beauty and truth lies with the Roman Catholic Church. This type of renegation is particularly frequent amongst Jews, whose social position in the world is rather complicated.

8. Looking at this phenomenon from another angle, one might divine it to be a reflection of the fact that the subject tries to severe infantile libidinal bonds, the group being a substitute for father, mother, and siblings. A growing intolerance of infantile

complexes may thus result in a negative bias towards a larger group to which the subject belongs.

Efforts towards the destruction of subconscious infantile ties is probably the primary force in this process of displacement. Disappointing incidents on the part of relatives hasten this course of events. Just as difficulties in adult relationships may throw the psyche back to infantile aims, disappointing experiences with close relatives are capable of furthering this spontaneous process of breaking away from early infantile bonds. The relatives acting as a precipitating factor for this process are not necessarily those to whom the early libidinal ties refer.

The growing intolerance towards these complexes is probably a process of belated psychic maturation, more or less intrinsic in character. It is as if the mind recognizes that these elements have no proper place in the psychic mechanism of the adult subject, who has to adjust himself to his social environment. It may also be realized by the psyche that these complexes have not fulfilled the pleasurable expectation put into them by the deeper levels. The rather sudden and belated efforts of the personality to rid itself of them cannot remain without psycho-pathological manifestations. Resentment and hostility towards the group may be one of these manifestations.

# CHAPTER VI

## THE ENVIRONMENTAL FACTOR IN CONSCIENCE, PARANOIA AND PREJUDICE

*The individual's fundamental dependence on his animate and inanimate environment.—Existence and function are conditioned.—The subconscious, too, is dependent on environmental events.—The social atmosphere influences the individual's particular attitudes.—The rôle of this factor in complexes.—Prejudice is a " moral paranoia ".—The world at large habitually encourages the hatred of the bad.—Social disapproval of attitudes may amount to a loss in the love that the individual desires to receive.—The organized character of mass prejudice is more than a quantitative factor.—The structure of conscience, its conditioned character as well as apparent autonomy.—Only early influences on the mind are capable of discouraging externalization to a psychotic degree.—The environmental factor in psychoneuroses and psychoses.—Why deeply religious people are less prone to psychoneurosis.—General aggressiveness, as well as resentment of obligations towards family and society, seek abreaction in prejudice.—The competitive complex is another contributor.—Prejudice is not interested in the improvement of the allegedly vicious group.—The intrinsic desire for paranoia and prejudice.—The force of factors leading to psychoneuroses in comparison to those creating prejudice.*

1. Almost everything in the individual's life depends, though to varying degrees, on his closer and broader environment. It is unlikely that the constant repetition of this relationship, which is experienced by the human being from the first day of his life, should have no permanent influence on the psyche. It may be assumed that the knowledge of this relationship—in fact an ancient possession of the human race, and thus a racial inheritance—plays an important part in conscious and subconscious processes alike. The conscious realization of man's dependence on Nature and on his fellow-beings is a distinct concept; it is the fundamental force moulding the growth of the social sense. But the full extent of this dependence cannot be a conscious and thinkable concept. It is in essence a fundamental psychological element permeating the whole personality. Body and mind, both through

racial and individual experience, acquire as it were the awareness that *existence* and *function* are conditioned by the outside world, animate and inanimate. The conscious realization of this dependence on nature and society refers not only to the material, physiological needs of the individual. In a close association with it a mental need for social approval develops, together with its counterpart, a dread of disapproval. Approval is sought not only because it safeguards for the individual the co-operation and agreement of his fellowmen in securing food, protection, and enjoyment for himself; apart from these concrete aims, the approval and friendly interest of the fellowman is a goal of the subject's desire. Disapproval—in essence the denial of friendship and love—is painful just as starvation in a physical sense. This paramount rôle of the society's reaction toward the individual makes the *environmental factor* a force that plays a great part in the formation of the mind and in the influencing of its processes.

2. Not only the processes that are conscious, but to no less a degree the vast and complex spheres of the subconscious are subject to the same influence. We know how incidental impressions in youth may contribute to a person's inclination to psychoneuroses at a later age; it is also a fact that intentional educational measures are never without penetrating effect, however limited in extent. But it is too little realized, alike by authors and by readers of works on psychology, that what we call the general environmental process modifies to a great extent the subconscious processes.

Under the notion " environmental factor " I mean not merely the family or school atmosphere. The concepts about various problems as they exist within society in a broader sense, the general attitude of people towards each other and toward the various types of human groups, are the environmental factors to which I am here referring. How society apparently feels and manifestly acts toward the strong and the weak does not remain without influence on the subconscious processes of the individual. The attitude toward women in general, e.g. the real position of women and children in legal administration, not only implies a fact, " a custom of the world " to the youth in maturation, but may modify various mental processes and " complexes " in the deeper spheres that have no direct bearing on the events of the outside world. To put it briefly, the average health of subconscious spheres depends just as much on the events in the broader society as on impressions by the close and intimate circle of the family.

3. Thus, for instance, a man's attitude toward marriage, its pleasures and its obligations, is to a great extent the result of impressions in his parental home and of his early sexual experiences. But however favourable or discouraging these conditions may have been, it is not they alone that influence the development of the mental complex referring to marriage. If the broader environment in general, and particular experiences in society of a drastic character, illustrate to the subject that the conventional praise of marriage is contradicted by manifested envy of the single man and woman, then in many individuals there ensues a conflict on this point. In some instances the impressions of parental life prove decisive; but in a vast number of people the facts of the broader society prove of superior plastic influence.

4. Another instance is the exchange of the infantile attitude toward parents into one suitable for an adult. Emotional freedom to live one's own love life, and a fair independence of thought as to the fundamental problems of life, are only possible where there is no undue interference by fixations at the levels of the ideals of early childhood. An insufficient breaking away from the influence of the parents is not always based on a primarily strong attachment to them. The dread of mature independence, with all the disappointments it may entail, can delay the process of becoming free from infantile ties. If school and the general atmosphere of society suggest to a sensitive youth that it is hard to achieve personal significance amongst strangers, then an undue persistence of infantile ties to the family may be one of the possible sequelæ. It is really difficult to overlook the rôle of the environmental factor in the development and fixation of the type just mentioned. It is unfortunate that this fact has not been recognized by psychoanalysts of the average type.

No less is the significance of the environmental factors in maintaining an undue persistence of infantile resentment against the adult members of the family. It should not be doubted that jealousy and hatred toward various members of the family occur in the child with such consistency that we are justified in assuming their inevitableness. They seem to be the first attempt of the growing child to "practise" emotional reactions and social attitudes. But we can no longer ignore the fact that much in these reactions is stimulated, almost bred, by the behaviour of the adults. Here, however, I am referring to the *persistence* of infantile attitudes in a later phase of life. And to a great extent events occurring and impressions gathered in the broader environment are responsible for the immature personality seeking as it were "refuge" in infantile sentiments and fixations.

These are but a few instances, and only sketchily described. But the student will be able with their help to grasp the broader problem referring to the substantial rôle of the environmental factor in the strictly subconscious sphere. So many phenomena for which the average psychopathologist has no accurate explanation, though he accepts their existence, may appear in a clearer light if the environmental influences of a more general character are taken into consideration.

5. We have recognized that the formation of prejudice follows a line of development similar to that of a paranoiac delusion. It is one of the possible attempts at coping with difficulties in subconscious spheres. Very probably this difficulty in the case of a prejudiced person is not a particular conflict but rather a strain on the moral process in the broader sense. The intramental awareness of amoral tendencies becomes stronger than average, and it stimulates the process of externalization and personification. It seems in these cases that the wrong, base, and dangerous tendency cannot be repressed to a degree beyond recognition by the conscious mind. It cannot be clouded through a substitute conception as *is* the case in the psychoneurotic symptoms in the usual sense. Here, for instance, the idea of possibly yielding to a sexual temptation may produce agoraphobia.[1] This development takes place because an inability to walk alone on the street is to a certain extent a protection from accepting an invitation by a stranger; furthermore, the street becomes a symbol for freedom and a greater latitude in conduct. Thus, in the phenomenon of agoraphobia the idea of a sexual conflict is repressed, and replaced by the idea of a heart attack that might occur on the street, or simply by the idea that the street and the crowd of people in it are in some way "terrifying".

[1] This is a frequent psychoneurotic construction.

6. In the type of moral conflict that leads to prejudice, the dreaded factor remains to an extent recognizable ; it is still the idea of an *a*-moral tendency, though associated with others who are suspected or condemned by the subject. The essential character of the original conflict remains recognizable, probably because its awareness by the organized ego is strong ; this doesn't mean necessarily that the *a*-moral tendencies responsible for the conflict are themselves strong. In conscious life, too, an event may attract intense attention because the subject is, for some reason or other, keen on observing what is going on around himself, irrespective of the quality and intensity of the impressions received. Likewise, we assume that in some persons the inner *awareness* of their conflicts may be strong, without the conflict itself being really of an extraordinary intensity. Probably, the strong awareness of specific conflicts is due to the very fact that the psyche encounters a difficulty in respect of the postulate for morals in general. The result of this strong endopsychic awareness is that the process cannot be repressed fully and some conscious feeling of a moral struggle remains.

7. This state of affairs cannot be tolerated by the mind, and the presence of the moral difficulties has to be disowned. It is thrown out, as it were, from the subject's personality and attributed to others, just as the case is with persecutory paranoia. Now other people are those who are " base ", " unscrupulous ", " lustful ", and " criminal ". The moral fight to which the subject feels himself prompted by the presence of his amoral tendencies may now go on, but it is displaced to an outside battlefield. The objects of his prejudice are being suspected, abused, and deemed worthy of persecution and even extermination, because of their alleged moral baseness.

8. The world at large habitually encourages the hatred of the bad. It approves the condemnation of sinful and dangerous tendencies. In fact, the amoral tendencies operative within his psyche are disliked by the subject because of his fear of social disapproval. Should the outside world ever know what occurs within the subject's mind, loss of social position and even restriction of personal freedom might ensue. This endopsychic hypothesis is the dynamic element that accounts for the psychoneurotic anxiety that develops when the moral factor condemns a tendency emerging in the deeper layers.

The idea of approval or disapproval on the part of the environment has thus very much to do with the subject's wish to rid himself of the bad and with the tendency to shift the blame on to others. Concrete experience teaches the individual that an accusation of others finds a ready echo in society. People are sensitive to the slightest suggestion of danger and impropriety in their midst; they uncritically agree with the accusing person. It pays, thus, to be an accuser; one receives social significance through warning one's fellowmen that danger is lurking for them near by.

9. Let us also not forget that there is immorality in everybody, and also some difficulty in the moral function in general. With this fact goes the potential inclination to fall in when manifested prejudice singles out an individual or a group for accusation or condemnation. There exists a similar phenomenon with regard to the paranoia proper. Close relatives of such a patient may be convinced that his delusional statements are fully or in part based on facts. This is induced paranoia. In a similar way it is possible for a prejudiced paranoiac to gain a following for his accusations; in fact he attains this very easily and is able to attract in a short time a considerable number of secondary paranoiacs.

Hence, it is on the whole profitable to subscribe to a prejudiced attitude and to the manifest hatred and aggression ensuing from it. The realization of this fact by the subconscious is obviously apt to intensify the tendency towards projection and the creation of certain prejudices. Without the anticipation of some public approval the subconscious mind would *not so easily* decide in favour of forming a certain prejudice in response to intra-mental difficulties. Very likely, the subject would suffer some uneasiness or general irritability towards others, without however developing a clear-cut prejudice.

Nothing is dreaded more by the human individual than disapproval and the denial of friendship and love. If, I suggest, it were to be found that no gain whatsoever results from accusing innocent people, and particularly whole groups of people, organized prejudice in the form known to us would hardly ever develop. What turns the subconscious disturbance ultimately in the direction of manifest prejudice is the prospect of public approval and increased social significance. And conversely, the decided opposition of society to prejudice—that is to say, to group-hatred with no obvious justification—would soon deter the individual's subconscious from creating delusions of this type as an attempt to escape from intra-psychic moral difficulties.

The organized character of mass prejudice is not merely a quantitative factor ; its significance does not lie solely in a multiplication of individual attitudes. It implies, above all, mutual encouragement capable of stilling any doubt as to the logical justification of the prejudiced sentiment. It is impossible that such a critical tendency should be entirely absent, since the average prejudiced person is otherwise of a sane mind. The group of those who are, or are assumed to be, of the same opinion as the prejudiced person, represents to him, as it were, society in its authoritative aspect. Through *introjection* of the approving group, the roots of the delusional element become as if reinforced, and thus more capable of competing with any doubt introduced by logic.

10. It is not superfluous to remind ourselves that the uneasiness and anxiety associated with a deep moral conflict is due to the protest of the unconscious superego. But there can be no doubt that this intrinsic disapproval is closely bound up with the fear of external condemnation.

I am ready to assume that *conscience*, acquired through the complex process of education, in many persons becomes a fairly autonomous factor. We know from analyses that in many individuals their self-imposed moral strictness cannot be traced to a corresponding parental influence. The degree of strictness assumed by an individual's " inner judge " may far exceed the average standard subscribed to by his environment. All this suggests that the ultimate factor at work in the course of moral decision is the individual's moral conscience, and not exactly a fear of environmental disapproval. But, however great an autonomy we are prepared to ascribe to the inner moral judge, it is the imagined approval or disapproval by the subject's superego that decides the extent of mental ease. In other words, it is not so much the *internalized threat*, as the *internalized disapproval* that the subject dreads in the presence of amoral tendencies. For the majority of persons, when making a moral decision, it is impossible to separate from the voice of conscience the idea of the social environment critically observing them. In ultimate analysis, the approval or disapproval by the " inner judge " coalesces with the idea of external approval or disapproval.

If this is so, then a potent threat of external disapproval towards anti-social prejudices should be able to interfere, when the mind feels tempted to solve a difficulty by creating a delusion of prejudice. If the inner disapproval is a potent force capable of causing psychoneurotic anxiety, surely the threat of external disapproval ought at least to be able to prevent the mind from covering up immoral elements by delusional accusation of others. It is easy to see that this act of projection actually increases the amount of impropriety in life, inasmuch as factual injustice becomes superadded to the deep-seated immoral tendency—which by itself is hardly significant for society.

11. Concrete events seem to support our suggestion. The particular social environment, family, and school have at all times been able to modify the frequency and intensity of manifested prejudice. To deny the reality of this extrinsic influence on the subconscious process of creating or rejecting prejudice, indeed, implies blindness ; it almost suggests some sympathy with this evil phenomenon.

It is not suggested that social pressure and threat on the part of the law can entirely prevent the turn of subconscious difficulties towards projection in a very large number of adults. The apt object of this moulding process actually can only be the personality of youth yet in the process of maturation. *If the mind is trained early, in taking resort to externalization, or is unopposedly allowed to do so, then this mode of reaction will become an intrinsic part of the person's psychoaffective structure.* If, on the other hand, the temptation to externalize moral conflicts too readily, and to believe in scapegoats, is known to be unpopular, then only few minds will yield to this infantile-archaic tendency. For the minds of the vast majority of youth the threat of social disapproval would act as a deterrent, a counter-force, and would probably prevent the subconscious from relying on the relieving function of prejudice-delusions.

12. In the field of psychoneurosis proper, too, it appears that general social and cultural conditions have an influence on the frequency of certain syndromes. The relative rarity of " the grand hysteria " as met in past decades, and the increasing frequency of the obsessional forms as well as the character neuroses can only be explained by the influence of changes in the spiritual

atmosphere of society. More scope for individualism, the increased claims for the individual's satisfactions, doubts about religious concepts fostered by a more realistic science, are only a few of the factors that have changed the mental background of society. These changes substantially clash with the subconscious processes of the individuals, because these spheres have retained some measure of primitiveness, and, as it were, have had no time yet to adjust themselves to the radical alterations in the outward structure of life.

" Seligman noted that delusions of a religious nature with a sense of guilt were practically absent in Japan where religion is cheerful and assumes primitive virtue rather than original sin.

" Malinovski believes that psychoneuroses are rare among the Trobrianders in comparison with the inhabitants of neighbouring islands, on account of the family organization of the former, which is characterized by the virtual absence of any one in the rôle of father " (cf. Henderson and Gillespie, *Textbook of Psychiatry*, 1940).

Whatever the real reasons may be, the influence of different cultures on the psychopathological processes appears supported by these and similar observations. It is, of course, possible to assume that the cultural pattern accounts for the form and content of the illness rather than for its existence. But there are observations that speak in favour of a more essential rôle of the cultural pattern in neuroses and psychoses.

It appears to be a fact that the incidence of neuroses amongst people who are wholeheartedly religious is comparatively smaller than amongst those who doubt. This cannot be taken as an unequivocal proof of the theory that religion might protect persons of all types from neurosis. It is more probable that a structure of the mind that is capable of religiosity without much interference by the element of doubt is less prone to psychoneurosis. The doubt is there ; it cannot be absent, owing to the obvious contradictions to religion originating in empiric realities and logic. Yet, the inner awareness of this element,[1] as well as its dynamic opposition to the fundamentally religious trend of the personality, is not strong enough to lead to a substantial conflict. This suggestion is no contradiction to what has been stated above with regard to the changes in the general social atmosphere and their rôle in the increased incidence of deep-seated neuroses.

[1] Cf. on this point, Ch. IIIA (12).

13. It is well to remember that intrinsic general aggressiveness welcomes every opportunity and pretext for its manifestation. If a subconscious moral difficulty tends to seek relief through projecting intrinsic " baseness " on to others, then this mode of abreaction finds a ready support by the general urge for aggression.

In addition, the obligations and limitations associated with family relationships are no small factors for the individual to manage. They imply a mental burden, not always easy to cope with. Even though there may be a *general* tendency in the psyche to assume a dutiful life and to enjoy the moral satisfaction associated with it, *particular* claims on this point prove burdensome. In conscious aiming, too, there may be an unequivocal desire to reach a certain goal ; but, if the way leading towards it presents too many obstacles, uneasiness is likely to result which may lead even to the abandonment of the goal. A comparable course is imaginable with respect to the moral process. The attainment of self-restriction may, at a certain phase of life, be the genuine goal of the youth's personality. But since this aim implies struggle with the self, some difficulty is bound to be felt. Nevertheless, this difficulty is not yet coloured by the element of personal resentment ; just as a person does not actually resent the toil needed for the gardening he carries out as a hobby. Occasions arise, however, when the rôle of particular persons in causing intra-mental moral difficulties becomes an object of distinct knowledge. The feeling of *general difficulty* changes into *personal resentment* when the psyche begins to doubt whether the persons in question fully deserve that for their sake the subject accepts limitation. Obviously, relatives are human creatures with faults of their own. Resentment and hatred felt by the subject are referred by his mind to the fact that relatives do not always behave properly and pleasantly, and, in more general terms, though less clearly, to the fact that the subject has not freely chosen them to be his relatives. In view of all this, self-limitation becomes an object of personal resentment, the psyche assuming that these relatives are solely responsible for its necessity. The mind conceives of the general mental difficulty implied by self-limitation in terms of a burden caused by a number of persons.

14. The resentment spreads on many occasions to the wider environment or, as in the case of prejudice, to a certain group of people. These victims are made to represent society as a

whole, in serving as targets for the subject's hatred. The subject actually hates his relatives, and also society from which the compulsion comes to love and help members of his family even though the subject might not find them loveable. The subject also resents his duties toward his employer, towards his friends, and towards the various institutions of organized society. But not having the courage to admit all this to himself, his resentment might be directed towards scapegoats. The hatred towards them is a displaced sentiment ; the original objects are those towards whom obligations of any kind exist as well as the obligations in themselves. The condemnation of the scapegoats as base and dangerous corresponds to the realization by the subject of his own social and resentful tendencies. Should the world know about the subject's reluctance to co-operate, and about his resentment against ties and duties, he himself would be considered mean and culpable. This realization is expressed by the belief that scapegoats are " low and dangerous ".

15. It is obvious that the competitive complex, with all its implications, has its dynamic share in the formation of prejudice. The large variety of limitations to which the individual is subjected is indubitably associated with the existence of his fellow-beings. Resentment of a compulsive social order implies the idea that it would be good to remove a number of people from the horizon of the subject. The phenomenon of externalization, in itself a product of moral conflict, may become a fitting servant of the competitive resentment. Obviously, groups of people who are deemed to be base and culpable do not deserve the food they eat, the air they breathe, and the status of ordinary human beings they usurp.

If a number of people are singled out as unworthy of being included in society, this implies a prospect of getting rid of a number of competitors in life. Any limitations imposed on such groups is likely to increase the share and freedom of the prejudiced subject. Moreover, if the members of a group to be excluded suffer a loss of personal esteem this fact theoretically increases the chances of the prejudiced subject of becoming more prominent at some future time and in some way not yet specified.

There is, thus, an additional reason for the mind to yield to the temptation of projection. Not only can subjective immorality be shifted on to others, and repressed hatred against close relatives be given vent through displacement ; but what is perhaps even more significant and closer to the world of concrete events is the fact that the competitive aggressiveness of the subject likewise gains a certain measure of imaginary satisfaction. Should the world at large follow suit and array themselves behind the prejudiced leader then a large-scale elimination of human beings from the enjoyment of the rights and pleasures of life might really occur.

Every resentment implies hatred, and hatred is an imagined destruction of the subject. This implicit promise of the ultimate destruction of fellow-beings is, perhaps, the most decisive factor in the formation of prejudice when intra-mental difficulties require some relief. Here lies the deeper reason why discouragement by public opinion and law is the only measure that is likely to interfere with the subconscious processes in prejudice. Explicit disapproval and the definite absence of any prospect that competitors in life might be got rid of by violence, are two factors capable of countering the temptation of employing prejudiced hatred as a means of mental relief.

16. Anyone who wishes to see clearly must recognize that prejudiced hatred differs manifestly from other resentments. It is blind, and generalizing, and prefers as its object people whom the subject does *not* know personally, or of whom he has little intimate knowledge ; prejudice desires, in fact, anything but the moral improvement of those accused and condemned. In the case of a real enemy, or of a person who has insulted or harmed the subject, there is, in most cases, a readiness to accept apology, compensation, and even friendship. It is true that hatred following concrete personal grievances is often enough as passionate and implacable as that observed in prejudice. But in such cases the justifiable resentment is greatly mixed with irrational passion remindful of prejudice ; it is sure that this admixture of the irrational with the intelligible resentment is supplied by subconscious sources comparable to those at work in prejudice.

In the case of prejudice there is a marked desire for maintaining blind accusations ; there is an obvious wish to see the condemned objects as mean and dangerous, beyond any chance of moral improvement. Prejudice proper is not open to enlightenment, explanation, or discussion. It is against its very nature to admit that a correction of its outlook is possible. In this aspect the analogy with paranoia becomes more obvious. Kraepelin and Bleuler assumed that in paranoia there exist an intrinsic desire for the delusional belief.

Why, indeed, should a projection that offers relief, and implies promises, be given up for the sake of objective truth ; particularly, if these explanations, as usually, come from those—or on behalf of those—who are the targets selected by that particular prejudice. In the resistance of prejudice there is an element of the possessive instinct, so strong in children and " archaic " types of adults. Their formula runs : " Whatever I have in my possession, whether rightly or wrongly, whether I need all of it or not, is unalienably mine. Even though some of it has been taken from fellow-beings by violence, their attempt at recovering the means for their elementary subsistence represents, in my opinion, nothing less than robbery." For the prejudiced paranoiac his very wish amounts to fulfilment, just as a psychotic delusion has the strength of reality for subjective experience. The prejudiced person has, as it were, attained the destruction of his fellowmen and the gains ensuing from their departure. Enlightenment would deprive him of his imaginary booty. Writers advocating an objective outlook are thus his enemies ; and people who try to side with the prospective or actual victims interfere with his rights and possessions.

17. It is suggested by the writer that appropriate environmental measures are capable of decreasing the proneness to externalization of this type of prejudice. This assumption might allow the inference that the intrinsic pressure to create a symptom in response to intra-mental difficulties is lesser in the case of prejudice than in that of a psychoneurosis proper. This difference, however, does not entirely exclude the extrinsic factor from psychoneuroses. It has been at all times thought by psychologists of a broad outlook that the general external circumstances of the individual have a definite part in determining the overt manifestation of a deep psychoneurotic condition. Both the timing and the particular syndrome of the manifestation, and also the intensity of its interference with life, are influenced by social-economical and personal circumstances. *The individual's psychoneurosis has not only emotional roots and causes, but concrete goals and targets.* It is, therefore, equally true that environmental factors may contribute to the success or failure of therapeutic measures.

On the other hand, we must not fail to recognize an important difference between the condition of prejudice and that of psychoneurosis proper. The latter incapacitates, in various degrees, the subject. Agoraphobia, impotence, obsessional neurosis, sleeplessness owing to anxiety dreams, imply restrictions of life and work in well defined fields of human existence. Prejudice, on the other hand, merely restricts the general scope of social intercourse. Within the restricted field the manifoldness of life is allowed to go on ; the proportions of the component spheres of individual life remain the same as in the normal. This fact may confirm the suggestion that prejudice is indeed a lesser degree of psychoaffective illness, and that its prevention at least might be an easier task than that of the psychoneuroses proper.

# CHAPTER VII

## THE MANIFEST ASPECT OF SOCIAL PHENOMENA

*Social manifestations, however undesirable, appear to be a variety of normal life-phenomena.—The relationship to psychoneuroses is in general unrecognized.—The voluntary contribution of the average masses to the normalization of society cannot be considerable.—Only an indirect approach to subconscious mechanisms is feasible, and a dependable factor.—A prejudiced teacher.—An advocate of justice who is not free from all prejudice.—Dormant sadism often invokes the principles of justice.—People too easily put up with concentration camps for others.—Too little genuine indignation about the mass torture of human beings.—The psychology of this phenomenon.—The psychologist who is unfit to be a healer of abnormal people.—Lack of sympathy with suffering fellow-men may be a defence of the mind against aggressive tendencies.—The idealist-criminal.—Why people sympathize with this type of aggressor.—Mass phenomena are prompted by deep emotional processes.—The individual's metamorphosis in becoming a member of a group.*

1. THE social psychologist, as distinct from the expert in psychopathology, must not overlook any manifest aspect of human and social life. To him the concrete and tangible manifestations of life are just as important, or even more so, as are the deeper psychological processes. For the analytical psychotherapist the symptom in itself is a minor matter [1]; the patient, too, finds it alien and is keen on its removal. The average psychoanalyst has assumed a somewhat biased view of life through shifting the emphasis of his interest on the deeper roots of conspicuous manifestations. But one must not do so where social phenomena constitute the problem. These manifestations are much more

[1] It is, however, true that in the psychotherapeutic technique of Stekel or Adler the manifest form of the symptom, with its dynamic significance for the patient's practical life, receives a great deal of attention. The question which a follower of Stekel or Adler has, sooner or later, to answer is against what or whom is the particular symptom aimed by the subconscious. In comparison with this recent goal of the symptom, the deeper roots of the psychoneurotic disturbance, including traumatic impressions in early childhood, may, in some cases, have only a secondary importance. Nevertheless, the literal significance of social phenomena, however psychoneurotic in their foundation, is even greater.

F

"substantial" than are the psychoneurotic symptoms, which we have learnt to look upon merely as peculiar consequences of primary events.

Social phenomena, too, have their background of which the individuals are unconscious; but however unsatisfactory some of these overt manifestations are, the masses do not realize the anomalous character of these events, whereas psychoneurotic patients usually do show some degree of insight into the abnormality of their symptoms. A symptom strikes one as an unreasonable deviation from the normal routine of life; social phenomena, on the other hand, appear as a variety of mass life, and not as a foreign element in the fabric of social structure. People are accustomed to the fact that in political conceptions and modes of social administration, groups fight each other, at times even violently; but they are sure that the difference is only that of views, right and wrong ones. They do not think about these phenomena in terms of degrees in mental integrity. The opponents of a particular system consider it rather a variety of social manifestation than a psychoneurotic one. Even if the attributes of "madness", "stupidity", or "brutality" are applied to the others in the course of argumentation and propaganda, this is not taken too literally.

2. Obviously, the *mass character* of social phenomena must impress both participants and outsiders. The picture strikes one as different from the psychoneurosis of an individual. This difference in phenomenological quality itself makes it difficult to recognize the psychoneurotic or quasi-psychotic element in a social phenomenon. Moreover, as suggested above, in the social phenomenon normal life and abnormal features are much more interwoven into a unitary phenomenon than appears to be the case in the psychoneurotic symptom of the individual. And in the instance of the psychotic proper, however deep his own conviction in the reality of his delusional belief may be, the environment definitely recognizes the extraordinary change in him. Here two facts help in the recognition of the abnormal. The one is the conspicuously peculiar character of speech and behaviour in the psychotic; the other is the isolated instance of such patients amidst the crowd of those who are different and apparently "normal". A similar realization by people at large of the psychopathological facts cannot sufficiently operate where mass phenomena are concerned.

3. Consequently, it is too optimistic to place confident reliance on the active contribution of the masses in general in combating prejudice, whether racial, religious, or political. It is even less justified to expect that people should realize the irrational element in all types of economic struggle. It is easy for a person who is outside the competitive struggle to state: "Whether we have a little money more or less, and even the existing gross inequality in possession, should not prevent us from knowing that there are sources of satisfaction available also to the poor man." It is, likewise, easy for the detached social psychologist to explain the genesis, and psychoneurotic character, of secondary personality traits. There is, clearly, no possibility for the average masses to realize fully these scientific facts; and it is even less possible for them to let their feelings and conduct be influenced by such theses.

The only practicable way of influencing society is the adoption of an indirect approach to people's mind. Large scale alterations alone in the concrete spheres of communal life are capable of imparting to people the message of humane progress. Only if it were possible to persuade the *subconscious* of the masses that the social leaders, and above all the wielders of worldly power, really aim at freeing people from unnecessary pain, and are really determined to protect people from unnecessary attacks by prejudice and exploitation, only then would their minds really attempt to change in outlook and programme. We shall cite a few instances showing the problem and the difficulties involved.

4. It happened in 1939 at a school for little girls aged about 5–10: the teacher spoke about the bad climate in Kenya, and the risks to the health of prospective immigrants. Then she said: "This is the right place for Jews." An inquisitive pupil asked: "Why only for Jews?" The answer was: "I mean the bad ones." "And where is she going to send the bad people who are not Jews?" asked the little girl who told me the story.

This instance—one of many—illustrates that a person of fair education and unimpeachable conduct may have a particular paranoia. It would have been difficult to suggest that this teacher was in general unfit for this vocation.

The next instance shows how the element of prejudice (an unfair judgment) may creep in into the thinking of a person during the very process of deploring irrational persecution committed by others.

5. The writer of an article, known to his friends as a just and kind person, said with reference to the horrors in the German concentration camps : " . . . crimes committed in cold blood against people *who in most cases* had done no wrong at all. . . ." Note the qualifying phrase " in most cases ". What is the limiting clause to suggest ? and how great a proportion of the ten million civilians murdered by the regime is it intended to exclude from the majority who were *entirely innocent* ? It appears as if thousands or even tens of thousands are implicitly excluded by the above writer from the total of victims, because they did deserve, to some extent, their horrible destiny. Yet, in all probability, they, too, were only human beings of average type ; not less virtuous or more vicious than were and are the many millions of average people in Great Britain and America, who were fortunate in being separated by the seas from the centre of organized mass murder. If the exclusion refers to those victims who were originally incarcerated because of petty thefts, black-market, homosexuality, and other comparable vices, these can hardly be a justification for their humiliation, starvation, torture, and ignominious death.

Quiet sadism and latent paranoia are always ready to invoke *Justicia*. When a person is exposed to maltreatment, because he is one of those who are singled out by prejudice, or because he belongs to a group too weak for self-defence, many a man is only too ready to gloat over his sufferings if it can be pointed out that the victim is, in any case, of insincere character or even on occasions deceitful. It has at all times, however, been sufficient for finding " political maltreatment " justified, if the victims were merely successful in the competitive race for social position. People easily put up with a system of questionable justice when they think that it will not apply to themselves.

It is, at the same time, generally overlooked that throughout the world millions of individuals hurt and exploit other millions with impunity, because they do so within the limits of formal legislation, or because there is no law forbidding every type of conduct that causes unnecessary pain to defenceless fellowmen. Not only do these tolerated trespasses against human peace remain without retribution, but the perpetrators continue to be looked upon as respectable citizens, enjoying the full protection and privileges that an organized society affords. In view of these largely inevitable inequities, certainly there can be no justification for persecution committed by political or " ethical " paranoiacs, under the disguise of ridding society of " undesirable elements ". It is only the sadistic or paranoiac element in people at large that can make them complacently acquiesce in such events.

6. The sudden indignation of the western world after the discovery of the German murder camps betrays a very deficient social sense. It appears that unimaginable brutality has to take place before men concern themselves about the lot of millions of their unfortunate fellow-creatures. Let us assume that no more happened than that people were herded into concentration camps; that homes and families were broken up, human beings deprived of their freedom and the opportunities generally afforded to average people; but, at the same time, these prisons were hygienic and tidy and characterized by discipline of a machine-like precision. Was then the brutality and crime not condemnable enough? . . .

We have read during the war accounts of certain detention camps, in some countries, where in the eyes of the visitor the " cleanliness and the discipline were exemplary " and where " no torture was applied in so far as information on this point was available ".[1] I cannot help recognizing in such observers their sadism and dormant psychopathy. What is, however, most pitiable in all these instances is the fact that the general public, simple and educated alike, accept such reports as satisfactory and forget the elementary standards of life which they apply to themselves.

7. Prejudice and all its masked forms are paranoias. Those affected by it can have no sufficient insight into the irrational character of such a sentiment. The responsibility for its possible consequences rests on the remaining part of society, on those who, in certain cases or periods, are not really affected by the popular psychosis and can remain detached onlookers of improprieties ensuing from the paranoiac attitudes of others.

Yet, the number of those who are unable to feel genuine indignation on occasions where unimpaired social sense expects such a reaction, is admittedly great. Contemporary events have shown this phenomenon so frequently that a social psychologist cannot afford to ignore it. People of culture and of undoubtedly correct behaviour in ordinary walks of life, and persons who are

[1] This did not refer to a German camp.

upset by the slightest suggestion of interference with individual freedom by *state control*, have remained apparently unmoved at the news that masses of innocent people were suffering imprisonment and death. Men and women, to whom the classics of literature and music, to whom the beauties and harmonies of art and nature were sacred, showed no manifest response to the fact that families were disrupted and tender children led into slavery and gas-chambers. One would have expected them to revolt against the unparalleled extent of destruction of social and individual harmony, just as they are wont to become excited if a masterpiece of music or drama is robbed of its majesty by a deficient performance. Not only the present writer but a number of observant persons have met people of otherwise excellent character and education who simply stopped conversation if somebody happened to lament the fate of his friends or relations deported to Auschwitz, Lublin, or Belsen, or if another member of the party expressed concern about his relative in Japanese hands. What these things meant in the years 1939–1945 was sufficiently known to all who did not make a point of not knowing.

8. Indignation on the part of the fair-minded when faced with such strange phenomena is not enough. Certainly it is not enough, and in many cases even unjustifiable, to say that " these people, though educated, have no heart ". The phenomenon referred to rather invites a searching inquiry from the social psychologist.

The fact is that people in general are unable to eradicate all potential cruelty and prejudice from their own psychic structure. Consequently they have to build a mental *cordon sanitaire* around themselves, which prevents their taking too deep an interest in contemporary events of a distressing nature. If they allowed themselves to be influenced by the full realization of appalling news their dormant sadism and prejudice might be stimulated to a degree which would be " too much " for them to bear consciously.

9. There exists a similar phenomenon in an altogether different field of life. Not everyone is fit to be a psychoanalyst, though he may be a person interested in the subject, and even possess talent for psychology. If the repeated meeting with more or less

pathological personalities stirs the psychologist's complexes unduly, he is likely sooner or later to feel uneasy, become irritable, and unfit for his professional activities. It is thus better for him to leave psychoanalysis alone, both its literature and the patients who need this particular treatment.

An analyst of substantial gifts has recognized his repressed dissatisfaction with his own marriage through the fact that one of his patients " got on his nerves " though he was a pleasant and sincere man. A great part of the session was occupied by minute descriptions of scenes between his patient and his wife, and the analyst had soon to admit to himself that his own marriage-complex was stimulated to an extent interfering with his work.

In other instances analysts, themselves not sufficiently analysed and not yet experienced enough, found it impossible to understand the case and the dreams of some patients, though the problem in question was not difficult to recognize. This happened when the analyst himself had not recognized in himself the presence of a complex from which his patient was suffering. As long as the blindness of repression with regard to a complex continues to operate in the analyst, he is greatly incapacitated for discovering a similar complex in his patient.[1] His blindness towards the patient's complex exists in order to maintain his own repression. There is an obvious analogy between this reactive ignorance of the analyst and the artificial coolness of many people towards large-scale human tragedies. Their attitude, however, does not exclude an average degree of sympathy with suffering people in general.

10. It is not the problem of sympathy in the narrower sense with which we are concerned here. It is possible to be rather reserved in emotional reaction, and still to know clearly how much response and action a situation may require from the individual in case of social emergency. Moreover, there is a difference between merely recognizing the pains other people suffer, and assessing clearly the social crime committed against them. This latter faculty is mainly the point with which a social science of an intelligent standard concerns itself.

If we have once recognized the deeper cause of the insufficient fellow-feeling displayed in times of large-scale human tragedy, we might be nearer to mending the deficiency than if we deal merely with the aspect of sentimental sympathy. We must,

[1] Stekel called this the *psychoanalytical scotoma.*

thus, keep in our minds that the very fact of a human tragedy on a large scale has for many people a specifically unpleasant significance because those impressions might stimulate their worst instincts. They like, therefore, to forget about it as much as humanly possible. Their coolness is, to some extent, a protective wall in the service of their conscious ethics.[1] Should, however, society as a whole, with all its administrative, scientific, and religious representatives stand up in an organized manner, actively protesting and fighting on behalf of the victims, all cool hearts would be carried by the general attitude, and such social enthusiasm would prevent a substantial stimulation of aggressive-sadistic elements. But if sympathy remains a matter of individual reaction, a great many people cannot help responding with the emotional defences described.

For the social psychologist, as we said, the phenomenon under discussion can be only a subject of calm and careful reflection. The most important conclusion to draw from such observations is that relying solely on the ethics of individuals is a rather primitive social attitude, in fact an unresponsible principle of government. There are too many harmless people whose decency and social value is barren, incapable of producing warmth and dynamic humanity. Were the affairs of the world left to them chaos and ruin would most likely follow.

11. A scientific discussion of social phenomena must not confine itself to subtle and intricate psychological problems whilst ignoring phenomena that appear obvious. For this reason a short discourse will be devoted here to the " decent " aggressor. I refer to the large number of persons, in power at various times and places, who as a matter of course used their legal and social authority to the detriment of innocent human beings. Kings and governors who purported to be, and even were in many ways, guardians of justice and general ethics, kept in prison under most inhuman conditions human beings, young and old, husbands and fathers, for no real crime but from prejudice, suspicion, and revenge. Clergymen of various denominations, some of them even of scientific accomplishment and most of them undoubtedly genuine about their concern for religion, persecuted masses of families unto death, or in more recent centuries into social and economic ruin. In quite recent times supervisers and henchmen of notorious extermination

[1] Cf. Ch. IV (14), (17).

camps could, in their self-defence before the courts, refer to acts of mercy and kindness which they very probably did carry out on occasions. Not a few of them were reputed to be devoted husbands and fathers. Such and similar phenomena puzzle the average masses. People like to think on rather simple lines and to believe that a person is either good or bad.

The first thing for a proper appreciation of social phenomena as well as all manifestations in life ought to be a comparatively unbiased approach. A *double aspect* presented by a phenomenon may be confusing at first, but nevertheless an undoubtable reality. A person's criminal significance for society remains a sad factor, however numerous might be the proofs that he is at the same time not entirely void of a sense of decency and ethics. One could even conclude that the responsibility of such a " pious monster " is the greater, the more certain it is that he is not one of those suffering from what is called moral deficiency, that is, an organic lack of ethical capacity. But this need not necessarily be the viewpoint of a critical scientist. It may be safer to take the two contradicting attitudes of such a " decent " criminal separately, without judging the one in the light of the other.

12. It is of paramount importance to realize that partial decency does not preclude a person from being a dangerous adversary of society.[1] Obviously, the popular attraction of a demagogue advocating hatred and prejudice of whatever kind is likely to be greater if he is reputed to be a man of principle or a devoted son of his faith, or otherwise decent in various walks of life. We can guess the psychological background of this popularity. It is the general tendency to fall in with " sanctified " violence. The decent attributes of the demagogue-aggressor supply the element that satisfies the claims of conscience in the misled masses. All-round criminals have indeed little chance of becoming a danger on a large scale.

It is an indubitable fact that people have considerable sympathy with the great criminals of society and are reluctant to ignore the few good deeds of such individuals. And the attitude of the masses is at least as influential as the temperate wisdom of a few scientists and officials.

This sympathy with the demagogue-aggressor is largely due to destructive tendencies as well as to the revolutionary element

[1] Cf. Ch. IV (17).

always present in the mind. But it is probable that the concern for justice and fairness also has its share in these attitudes, which from a higher point of view are obviously harmful for general social well-being. Sympathy implies a measure of identification with its object. And every person would like to be treated by others in accordance with his own good aspects rather than with his moral and intellectual deficiencies. People, therefore, like to forgive the aggressor's attacks aimed at others, and to focus their attention on the few favourable aspects of such a person.

For the social psychologist the problem of aggression is not so much that of guilt or innocence but rather a task of protecting society. Aggression and all its sources, such as prejudice or lust for exploitation or revenge, occupy the sociologist because these manifestations interfere with the lives of harmless people. Consequently no amount of intellectual gift combined with pleasantness and kindness in a person who is in certain ways dangerous to others makes him less fit to be an object of preventive restraint.

13. Politics, and to some extent also business, are based on the clear realization that social phenomena have an irrational background. It is not rare for a proposition to be made by a group solely with a view to arousing indignation to it, and employing this public passion for another goal. In this type of manœuvring all calculation relies on the fact that people are unable to see beyond the surface of manifestations. Even if hidden motives *are* suspected and discovered, they do not belong, as a rule, to the category of deep psychological processes we have in mind with regard to public passion. In view of these circumstances it is well-nigh impossible for the most straightforward programme to dispense with an admixture of what is called diplomacy; and it is inevitable to plan practical measures mainly with an eye on the manifest aspect of events.

All this may be found unsatisfactory by the few who prefer to look at things objectively and would like logic to be the supreme force in public decision. But there is no prospect whatsoever that this might ever be the case to any substantial degree. Even where the voice of sanity seems to be listened to, the favour of the masses of people is, in fact, directed by emotional forces. *Vox populi* can never be more than the expression of mass sentiment springing from the subconscious. Should, however, an environmental process succeed to any substantial extent in introducing rational elements into the subconscious spheres of people, the spontaneity of their thought is bound to be influenced in desirable directions.

It is not the individual but the member of the group who is so greatly subject to this subconscious irrational factor. The working of the mind in prompting attitudes is modified, once the subject becomes involved in manifestations of a mass character. There is no getting away from this fact, even though the establishment of it may appear uncomplimentary to the individual of the race *homo sapiens*. The subject cannot become a member of a "crowd" without some change-over within his psyche; but this psychic metamorphosis, though partial, is not limited to the fact of mere adjustment.

## CHAPTER VIII

## MASS PREJUDICE IN CRITICAL TIMES

*The scapegoat theory is unsatisfactory.—The burden implied by personal ties and duties, and the amount of general satisfaction.—In critical times there is less satisfaction and more reason for difficulties in the moral process.—Soldiers have more liberties and less personal obligations than civilians.—This fact influences the mind of the civilian.—The rôle of the sexual urge as well as that of death wishes in critical times.—The revolt against necessary sacrifices.*

1. Mass prejudice against Jews and their bloody persecution have often followed wars, financial crises, and, in the Middle Ages, also the outbreak of epidemics. This has been a stereotyped recurrence in various periods of European history. The habitual prejudice against them was cherished by religious fanaticism, and made possible through the prevailing primitiveness of people's minds and a cultural atmosphere of superstition; but on the whole, this attitude was qualified by toleration in periods of comparative peace and economic prosperity. But no sooner did a critical situation begin to develop than the manifest tendency to mass persecution emerged. Besides Jews, any group of foreign nationals might have become the object of violent public disfavour in critical times; there are numerous instances of this phenomenon.

The customary scapegoat-theory does no more than describe the phenomenon without really going more deeply into the matter. It is not so simple to grasp why the masses—not all the members of which are devoid of intellect or of the sense of elementary justice—should so readily "fall for" a scapegoat offered to them. *They* cannot, indeed, be so much interested in substitute victims as are those who, perhaps, have led a country into a ruinous war, or are held responsible for a bad turn in economic or political affairs. Where is the force that makes the masses blind and leads them into wanton persecution?

The statement that aggressive tendencies wish for blood is not a sufficient explanation; certainly not enough to explain why the particular occasions mentioned are apt to bring out such outbursts of prejudice and persecution.

2. Let us not simply compare these things with the unparalleled crimes of the German regime and its satellites in the recent past. In these events the crude economic element and lust for power played the dominant part in so far as the masses were concerned. Since ruthlessness had been made a principle, and crime the law, there was no reason why as many as possible of the joint claimants for the good things of life should not be eliminated. People were promised an increased share, and many of them did receive it. That traditional superstition and "induced madness"[1] played their part, too, and mass prejudice was deliberately exploited for rational aims, does not alter the central rôle of the principle at work of brutal selfishness. But in almost all the other instances in history, and in the so frequent cases of mere local outbursts, the gain promised to people, or actually attained after riotous looting, was not proportionate to the passion and crime involved in these outbursts.

All that has here been said so far may or may not be right; it does not logically affect what follows. The chief problem for our discussion will be constituted by the undeniable fact that critical times are apt to increase a passion arising from prejudice against groups, whether political, religious, or racial.

3. The prototype of the scapegoat phenomenon is the case of a husband or father who comes home displeased from his office, and is irritable and even unfair to his family; or, that of an employer or manager who comes from his home annoyed, and cannot stop nagging and finding fault with his innocent employees. I think the psychological background of such a phenomenon is not very obscure, as the following analysis will show.

The reader is referred to the statement that the maintenance of the moral aspect of the personality requires the constant operation of a particular endopsychic process. Any duty or other customary limitation of personal autonomy implies the simultaneous presence of a resistance against this. The necessity for a constant moral process, in fact, implies that the unpleasantness associated with dutiful feeling and conduct is realized as such by the mind and, therefore, a moral process is called for to

[1] *Inducierte Paranoia*, or *folie à deux*.

maintain the moral standard. The moral process has constantly to neutralize the realization of the burden implied in self-limitation, and to make this moral aspect an approved element satisfying the integrated *self*.

Any event in life that makes the person suffer may render the moral function more difficult. Thus, an insult or a mere unkindness suffered in the factory, office, or club, or, likewise, a disappointment in business or other sphere of planning, decreases the general satisfaction of the subject with his life. This temporary loss in the amount of *fundamental satisfaction* makes the burdens implied in morals, duties, and social customs more difficult. It is as if the expenses of a business, hitherto accepted in a matter-of-fact way, were suddenly to loom large in the mind of the owner because he has recently lost a substantial part of his savings. The deficit in the experience of satisfaction with life through upsetting the psychoaffective balance makes the toleration of natural sacrifices a conspicuous task. Since family life always implies the fact of being tied down and of having to seek pleasure and satisfaction in accordance with these ties, and largely even within these very bounds, it is intelligible that a loss of satisfaction from other sources may make the compliance with family duties difficult, although in average circumstances they may be easy to bear and even a cause of happiness. I remind the student of my thesis that the self-perception of actual human insufficiency, or of habitual analytical complexes, may become too marked and thus cause trouble.[1] Hence the same may apply, as we see, to the perception of the burdensome aspect of obligations ; they may come to the fore of awareness and push back the pleasantness associated with duties, if, as described, there occurs a loss in satisfaction from other sources.

4. It is obviously possible to extend this conception to the larger problem of society. When general conditions are more or less stable, when there is a certain order and regularity in communal life, the majority of people can, with comparative ease, put up with the burden implied by various duties, private and communal. But in times of war, for instance, external conditions interfere with this stabilized routine of men's minds. Restrictions of various kinds come into operation and repeated sacrifices are required. Fear for relatives or friends in the forces is a constant undercurrent in the mind ; and in up-to-date warfare the life

[1] Cf. Ch. IIc (1), (8).

of practically everyone is exposed to aerial attack. Through unavoidable circumstances the sexual tension of those under military discipline is increased, and the same is the case with the wives and fiancées left at home. Moreover, through the absence from a regulated civilian life, the sexual manifestations of the men in the forces become poorer in self-restrictive and refined character. It is also inevitable that the member of the army is, to a large degree, freed from many of the responsibilities of the ordinary civilian ; indeed, he could not devote himself to his military life if this were not so.

Those still in civilian life do not escape the influence of such changes in the members of the armed forces. Half conscious or fully conscious envy of all the liberties afforded to the soldier stirs the minds of many people at home ; and what takes place in the strictly subconscious spheres is clear to the psychoanalyst, though almost incredible to the rest of mankind. But it is inconceivable that such vast changes brought about by wars should leave these deeper spheres of the mind in stability and quiet. The relative indifference to the integrity of life, a central feature of war, must stimulate the aggressive complexes in all strata of the population. And though the average person is, perhaps, in practice just as far from wanton murder or robbery as he has been in ordinary circumstances, his *moral process* is exposed to a greater strain in retaining the habitual standard.

5. However firm in his or her sexual morals a person may be the clear knowledge and day-by-day observation of the liberties brought to the fore by wartime creates acute conflicts deep down or even consciously. Irritability, proneness to fatigue, or frequent colds may be the result. Obviously the very opposite also takes place. The actual sight, and additional imagination, of licentious behaviour on a scale generally impossible in ordinary circumstances opens new avenues for phantasy, and imagined freedom may give the individual a measure of satisfaction. This lifting of repressions can and does give to many people the additional energy necessary for coping with other wartime changes of a burdensome character.

On the other hand, in exceptional times there is less order, less constancy, less security, less peace and comfort. All this means a *deficit in satisfaction with life* ; and this, as suggested, may render the deep moral process difficult. Thus, two phases make for this increased difficulty of the moral process. The observation of aggression, of sexual liberties, and of the ignoring of the obligations of ordinary times, creates envy of all this and emphatically stimulates *in all minds* the impact of the anti-moral factors. On the other hand, the universal loss of comfort and ease afforded by average peacetime conditions is a factor in itself lessening the amount of general satisfaction that usually compensates for the burdens of a dutiful life.

The very insecurity due to the circumstances of war, both for individuals and for families, and the unpleasant excitements caused by instability in the supply of food, fuel, transport, etc., upsets the balance of the psyche and renders the moral process difficult.[1] In consequence, anti-moral tendencies—aggressive, anti-social, and sexual—threaten to emerge, breaking through the barriers of normal repression ; and this frequently results in an increased proneness to externalization and to manifestations of prejudice. The accusation levelled against the chosen objects and the call for their persecution provides an outlet at the same time for subconscious hatred against authorities and relatives who in essence are those responsible for the burden of the duties and the necessity of moral behaviour on the part of the individual.

6. The soldiers, exposed to continuous mortal danger, and subject to military discipline, cannot but develop resentment against civil and military authorities. Patriotism and intellectual realization of the vital necessity for sacrifices do render easier the subordination enforced by martial law ; but nothing is able to prevent entirely the welling-up of resentment, frequently

[1] *Social Order and the Individual's Psychoaffective Economy.* The deeper layers of the mind apparently take a serious view of disturbances affecting the fundamentals of the existing social order ; the writer thinks, indeed, that the character of this intra-mental concern may, in some people, be more " panicky " than the feeling in response to personal mishap and individual frustration. An upheaval in society suggests to the mind a danger to social morals, to communal peace, in brief to all that in which the individual finds reassurance in face of human inadequacy. Hence, a general disturbance of social life has a potent influence on the deeper moral process.

In addition, a problem of psychoaffective economy in general is involved. An upheaval in social order robs the personality of the feeling that a dependable stability of conditions prevails in the human world. The prospect of having to cope with a quick succession of changes strikes the psyche unfavourably ; it appears as a task beyond accomplishment. Thus, the capacity of large-scale disturbances for interfering with psychic efficiency is intelligible ; and in particular the presence of an added burden on the moral process in such circumstances must be obvious. This explanation may throw some light on the phenomenon that the average masses prefer stability in clearly unsatisfactory conditions to a gradual progress requiring from them a substantial period of effort towards a desirable goal and the successive short-term adaptations involved. The average masses are ready to revolt in an irregular way but they find it difficult to take part in a gradual progress, because such a rôle heavily taxes their desire for stability.

bitter resentment, against the state administration. And even after the hardships of actual combatant service have ceased, and the individual has returned to civilian life, the memories of the recent past remain for a long time a source of passionate resentment. (Add Ch. IIIc, 8.)

Those who have lost a dear relative, or supporter of their existence, envy and even hate those who have been in their eyes more fortunate ; they can hardly repress their rebellious antagonism against Government and administration. All these emotional forces seek for an outlet ; and the channels of prejudice are very fit for this end.

People who consciously subscribe to duty toward their country or universal humanity obviously *cannot* openly revolt against the leaders whom they have followed. The pain associated with the fulfilment of their duties, and their resentment of it, must find another, a pseudo-moral, outlet. Those who participate in a war solely through force, without any ideals, merely *do not dare* to revolt against the authorities ; and their revengeful aggression manifests itself toward substitute objects even more readily than in the case of the former group.

7. In the recent war when the life of each civilian was in danger from aerial attacks, the idea of relatives and competitors being killed appeared in the dreams and day-phantasies of almost all people. I feel sure that a disappointment of such " hopes " will constitute an additional source of proneness to prejudice. This assumption may also briefly explain the passionate outbursts in time of epidemics in the Middle Ages. The constant threat of death had probably increased the working of death-wishes, and had thus created difficulties in the moral process.[1]

In addition to this, a threat to the life of the masses seems to increase unbridled sexual lust ; this has been described by historians of certain periods. It is obvious that not all individuals yielded fully, or at all, to this sudden urge. For them the amount of ensuing repression constituted a burden beyond average endurance. Thus, in times of epidemics and plagues there were

[1] It is clear to the psychoanalyst that also necrophil tendencies, stimulated by the sight of corpses, might have played their rôle. The dynamic influence of such tendencies on intra-mental stability could not but be a disturbing factor. This is, however, not the place for elaborating this aspect of the social phenomenon under discussion. It is only necessary to add that in a well-organized army the individual is properly cared for both physically and mentally ; in such circumstances archaic tendencies of the type of cannibalism and necrophilia are likely to emerge only in minds psychoneurotically undermined.

in the main two sources of threat to the moral process ; the one associated with the welling-up of libidinal tendencies, and the other based on the increase of death wishes. In addition, the universal deficiency in ease and peace of mind was bound to decrease the stability of general mental balance, which fact led to a difficulty in maintaining self-restraint both in feeling and behaviour.

The increase of libidinal pressure at times when the life of the masses was threatened has been explained as a simple psycho-biological phenomenon. The danger of imminent death, so it was thought, created a reactive urge for life in the elementary sense. There is no reason for denying this causal connection. But it must be obvious that to the social psychologist's mind a somewhat modified explanation for such phenomena offers itself. The general upheaval and disappearance of the average feeling of security upsets the functioning of the minds, and there is very little to support the continuation of the moral process. Consequently the elementary libidinal urge becomes isolated (in the sense described in Ch. III, 67) and can manifest itself nakedly.

8. The greater or lesser measure of stability in external conditions has its repercussions within the individual's psyche ; it may contribute to his inner harmony, or stir up the subconscious struggle of tendencies, as the case may be. A frequent change in day-to-day circumstances is a burden to the average mind, just as frequent changes in outside temperature are not easy to withstand without some indisposition. Cf. footnote in (6).

We know that a fair mental balance is the result of complex interlinked psychological processes ; very little is thus required to upset this balance. The more complex a mechanism is the greater is the possibility of a disturbance within it. The human mind is, more than anything else, far from possessing perfect homogeneity ; its working would not be intellectual in the fullest sense in the absence of its complexity. Undesirable results in the course of its functions are just as natural to occur as those mental manifestations that *are* desirable.

The very complexity of mental processes allows for various corrective modifications in circumstances that in themselves are precarious. Thus, for instance, if a heroic struggle, such as that of underground partisans, occupies men's minds, there is something in the situation of hardship that is apt even to support the moral process. The devotion to such a struggle implies a subordination of the personality to a moral principle. Consequently, here the instability of external conditions does not interfere so crudely with the moral process as in the case of ordinary masses who are mainly passive participants in a large-scale upheaval. In the latter case the difficulties in the moral spheres become dominant within the mind, because of the absence of a corrective factor.

# CHAPTER IX

## HAS MASS PREJUDICE A USEFUL FUNCTION?

*Is a homogeneous composition of society absolutely desirable?—The necessity of a constant defence-mechanism is an unhealthy sign.—Democratic and scientific leaders denounced as "paid agents of the Jews".—This is always a sign of the renunciation of uncompromising humanity and logic.—Intolerance of heterogeneous elements is a symptom of deeper fundamental weaknesses in a group.—The writer does not think that mass prejudice has actually any relieving function.—Social paranoia does not confine itself to the original field of its manifestation.—The imperceptible social atmosphere.—Preference in social intercourse for the fellow-believer is not yet a prejudice; it is the consequence of a limited capacity of the social sense.*

1. We have recognized the symbolic value of anything *new* for the deep intra-mental spheres.[1] It has been easy to understand that an impression, too strange to the feelings of the subject, should stimulate the impact of subconscious complexes tabooed by the superego. The *ugly* and *unharmonious* become disturbing reminders of what is disharmonious within the mind. For practical life, the avoidance of such impressions seems to be the logical line of prevention; and the prejudiced individual, indeed, knows no solution other than the removal from his horizon of people whom he cannot tolerate. Of course, about such measures he thinks in terms of purely objective justification.

2. For the broader problem of large social groups the question presents itself whether their more homogeneous composition would make for greater peace within such communities. Undoubtedly too frequent stimulation of a "complex" cannot be as healthy a condition as a comparative absence of such reminders. A sheltered condition of the subject has, likewise, proved beneficial in the case of potential threats to the individual's physique or mind in the medical sense. The biologist and psychiatrist will, however, be able to point out that through

[1] Cf. Appendix II.

avoiding specific stimuli the bodily or mental constitution has not yet ceased to be of an inferior quality. The essence of the deficiency in resistance obviously remains.

Doubtless if a person has always to bear in mind the avoidance of a certain food, or if he must not expose himself to the day-by-day changes of weather without having to adjust his clothing, he is limited in his life potential. The actual escape from indisposition is paid for by an extra amount of self-limitation. Yet I suggest that such a person may still be capable of a comparatively satisfactory life, as long as his mental potentialities are not limited. Enjoyment in the emotional and intellectual spheres is able to make up for the restrictions, and thus a fair balance of life in a broader sense may be secured.

This satisfactory result cannot be expected if it is the psychoaffective spheres that require constantly preventive measures. An artistic personality whose senses cannot tolerate without a feeling of irritability, a picture or a musical composition that is not of a " high-brow " quality, as a rule suffers from a psychoneurotic condition. It is not the limitation of his likes alone that renders him a neurotic, the truth is rather that his intolerance is as a rule a symptom of a more fundamental instability. The same is the case—and even to a more marked degree—with a person intolerant of groups singled out by his prejudice-paranoia. He remains deep down a paranoiac even though not meeting any member of his disliked group. He is, so I have observed, hardly ever in a state of fair mental harmony. Any limitation of an intrinsic nature in the psychoaffective functioning amounts to the narrowing down of the personality as a whole. This fact implies suffering, and a substantial restriction in what I have referred to above (p. 143) as the general satisfaction with life. The paranoiac of the prejudiced type may be spared many outbursts of intolerance if he has the chance of avoiding the objects of his specific intolerance. But the sum total of his " satisfaction with life " remains in all events below the fair average, and in the long run he is bound to realize that he is intrinsically unhappy.

3. In certain European countries where the passion of prejudice (national, racial, and religious) was habitually high, there prevailed on the whole a social atmosphere of deficient stability. Their internal affairs in general were conducted in a manner lacking the calm human dignity of the type considered desirable,

at least in principle, for instance, within the British parliamentary system. Periods of economic or political crises—of which there have been many in Europe since 1914—elicited manifestations of particularly uncouth character. What is even more significant is the fact that in such times the political influence of broad-minded and level-headed personalities had become negligible. It was not very rare to hear that this or the other politician or writer—previous to the crisis acknowledged as a "cultural or political hero"—was actually a "Jew" or a paid agent of Jews; and this in face of the fact that the person referred to had no more or no less in common with Jews than all average non-Jewish citizens. The people and newspapers spreading such statements did not even mean literally what they said. The aim was to discredit intelligent, humane, and tolerant attitudes, through employing a clichée, a symbolic expression, capable of conveying much more to agitated minds than any objective description might do. The words "Jew", "Free Mason", "Socialist", or "Bolshevist", etc., were used in a symbolic sense, just as are the phrases and figures of speech of a paranoiac proper, not clearly intelligible to the layman but suggesting a wealth of content to the psychoanalyst.

The habit of attaching the above names preferably to persons of political or scientific significance had a symbolic meaning of its own. In the opinion of the writer it signified the denunciation of principles that imply the rule of logic, civilization, and peace. The observant social psychologist recognized that there was no longer a question of one or more particular prejudices; for him it was obvious that on the whole a semi-psychotic atmosphere prevailed.

A society is mentally ill if it cannot tolerate a certain measure of variety amongst its members, whether the heterogeneous elements imply enrichment of culture and enterprise or merely represent naïve, peculiar but innocuous types.[1] There are no potentials of sufficient vitality for humane progress within such an ethnographic group, even though concrete reforms in administrative and economic fields are adopted. The social paranoia is bound to destroy in the bud the desirable psychological effects that might be stimulated in people's minds by the concrete environmental changes.

4. What has been said so far is not necessarily the end of our

[1] Cf., however, pp. 153, 154, and 239 footnote.

inquiry. It is possible to go further in the discussion of the problem. In view of the psychological character of prejudice as expounded above, it may be asked whether this phenomenon has not a useful function; whether it should not be considered rather as a means of relieving mental tension in a large number of people. Even if this were so, there would still remain the question of how to protect the potential victims of such psycho-neurotic reactions. Persons of an excessively realistic outlook, up to the point of believing in a life-philosophy of cynical rationalism, might easily point out that the prospective victims are a minority and should be sacrificed for the sake of the masses who need this particular mode of abreaction. In addition, the objects of prejudiced attacks are as a rule groups belonging to a party, religion, or race different from that to which the ruling majority belongs. They are thus, at any rate, not "equals". Hence, in the opinion of cynical politicians, our modern knowledge about prejudice ought not to be allowed to interfere with the status quo.

The present author was for a great number of years aware of this question, and was not able to come to a definite answer as to the actual psychological value of prejudice on a large scale. He admits that he was determined to keep the dangerous truth to himself in case he had to come to the conclusion that mass prejudice, if tolerated, has indeed a useful function, beneficial in the long run, which may justify the exposure to it of a certain number of his fellowmen.

After having struggled with himself regarding this problem for years, and observed closely a number of prejudiced people, and also having studied the social history of various periods, he is now certain that mass prejudice possesses no psychological function that could convince the expert, and the authorities, that it is better to abstain from interfering with such social phenomena. Prejudice is a reactive mental element that enables the subject to "rationalize" his aggression; but this state of affairs cannot give the subject any substantial relief. In this connection it is apt to refer to the compulsory system of obsessional patients who gain relief through compulsive actions or omissions only for a brief moment, but who remain at the same time very much under the influence of forces depriving them of mental ease.

5. I am now certain that in the ultimate outcome it would be better for all concerned to suppress the full development of this

type of reactive formation by the masses. Once created within men's minds, and assured of public approval, the element of prejudice becomes a stimulus to further intra-mental disharmony. A hypothesis that creates, as it were, enemies must, if nothing else, increase the dynamic power of the *competitive complex* with its aspects of resentment, fear, and suspicion. Apart from this, a hypothesis so flagrantly untrue cannot satisfy the mind, since the inner enemy cannot be ignored or eliminated through adding to it a great number of alleged external adversaries. Anything in the nature of mere analogy can only further elaborate this theme, but can add nothing to what is known about the essence of the problem. Therefore, I do not wish to enlarge further on the explanation of my thesis. All practical experience from various periods and places, where prejudice has been discouraged, shows uniformly that the general social standard of the people suffered no harm, but rather gained through this artificial suppression of a psycho-pathological mass process.

It must not be forgotten that, as historical experience shows, social paranoia does not confine itself to a fight against obviously heterogeneous elements, but extends its intolerance to other layers. This force creates a political division of the population far in excess of what is the healthy democracy of a few parties.

The writer is aware that many a reader might find it difficult to agree with the fundamental thesis arrived at in this chapter, considering it to be a biased opinion. These readers, whether expert psychologists or persons of good education in general, are referred to Chapter XVII in *Man and His Fellowmen*. The careful perusal of it may prove helpful in understanding the discussion here. From what has been described there, it appears almost certain that the basic material of a specific prejudice is an accumulation of universal human complexes in repression. It is therefore hard to believe that a reactive delusional formation should be capable of mending the wrong. Once the mind has assumed the mechanism of externalization for screening a deep-seated disturbance, the latter is likely to retain its dynamic force and continue in generating further similar products.

6. In the foregoing discussion a deeper view has been taken of the problem. It would, however, be futile to deny that a relative separation of heterogeneous groups is a measure that limits the frequency of aggressive incidents. And it is certainly not a wise

thing to make prejudiced people mix with the objects of their particular intolerance, in the absence of other comprehensive socio-psychological measures capable of modifying the deeper layers of people's minds.

It is, in general, a mistaken conception to rely solely on the introduction of concrete reforms without having a congenial spiritual atmosphere. We may replant in a garden a flower or tree grown elsewhere and expect it to thrive there, provided that the new soil is not foreign in composition to the nature of the transplanted organism. It is true that improvements in all spheres, if they be attained in a comparatively short period, are carried out by what may be compared to grafting. But, obviously, there must prevail conditions that will result in the acceptance of the graft.

The fundamental atmosphere in which planned reform is likely to work must be such that it would be capable of producing spontaneously, in a slow development, the new institution. If this is not the case, then the general atmosphere itself needs altering to become capable of keeping alive the concrete reform. It is true that the introduction of new manifest elements in social life may in turn stimulate the general atmosphere towards progress; yet if the fundamental composition of the social atmosphere is allowed to contain dynamic elements hostile to the goal in view, this reflective stimulation cannot take place.

7. It is no good asking the individual to appreciate the significance of his fellow-beings, whilst the fundamental structures of economics and politics consider the human being rather as a passive object of administration. It is hopeless to demand from the citizen a firm belief in the validity of social ethics, whilst in politics and diplomacy the goal justifies the employment of otherwise condemnable means. There is an imperceptible social atmosphere, the components of which cannot be explicitly defined in terms of concepts though they are nevertheless dynamic. What emanates from this ethereal atmosphere into the regions of perceptible social processes is stronger than all attempts to introduce particular reforms, however just and sensible.

For these reasons it may remain necessary to supplement genuinely progressive steps by old-fashioned remedies of anomalous phenomena. It is not easy sufficiently to modernize and humanize the socio-psychological atmosphere referred to here; to ameliorate it to a degree resulting in its full harmony with the individual reforms introduced. But it remains indispensable continually to purge at least the perceptible social atmosphere from archaic elements that are expressive of the significance of crude power, possession, and the cheapness of human life. For, as pointed out, a graft cannot thrive in a soil where elements hostile to it occupy a substantial place.

It is not prejudice in the exact sense if people prefer to meet their likes, or if they feel more or less uneasy in the presence of heterogeneous fellow-beings. The capacity for friendliness, and even more for familiar relationship is not unlimited and not independent of certain conditions. If we bear in mind the various aspects in the significance of the fellow-being for the subject, as discussed in Chapter II, it must be clear why the functioning of the social sense is not unconditional. Anything strange in the impression created by a newcomer is apt to intensify the impact of archaic misanthropic tendencies at the cost of the elementary interest in friendliness discussed in Chapter I.

The structure of personality in most individuals contains a certain pattern for the desirable or tolerable type of friend. The prospect of having to put up, for an appreciable period, with people different from this pattern may create distinct uneasiness, which is indicative of a disturbance in the function of tolerance. This individual limitation is a sign of an under-developed psychoaffective function in the broader sense, or even of a faulty trend imposed by the environment upon the maturing mind. Our psychoaffective processes—actually all human faculties—are concerned to a large extent with the task of social adjustment and the enjoyment of a community with others. The more rigid the intrapsychic pattern relating to the subject's tolerance or to his capacity for life in the community, the less is the freedom of the psyche to employ the social sense for its satisfaction.

It is an indubitable fact that many persons are capable of a fair degree of ease in social relationship only if they mix with their homologous fellowmen, whilst avoiding those whom they feel to be different in fundamentals dear to themselves. Such a limitation in social life has a semblance of aggressive prejudice in the sense referred to in this work, but there is no real identity. It is, however, sure that a social community, the various layers of which are distinctly separated, may become a fertile soil for a dynamic prejudice. Nevertheless, it is advisable to know that the two phenomena referred to are different, in spite of the points of contact between them. In both cases the motive of attitude is the defence of the personality from uneasiness, but there need not be a manifest element of aggressive projection. The fact of separation—in itself a sign of people's emotional immaturity—develops into mass-intolerance only when prejudice and social aggression are approved tendencies.

# CHAPTER X

## FROM IRRATIONAL PREJUDICE TO PASSIONATE ETHICS

*As the paranoiac* suffers *from his delusion, so the prejudiced person can never be fully at ease.—What is to happen if the tendency to prejudice is suppressed?—Early psychological advice might prevent further pathological developments.—Differences in degree of indignation and concern at undesirable social phenomena.—A proneness to prejudice might be changed into a somewhat passionate concern for problems meriting it.—The turn of attention from the criminal to the crime; from the particular to the general.—The progress implied by this metamorphosis.—Freedom of thought is an unreliable factor; reasons for this.*

1. We know that the patient with persecutory paranoia *suffers* because of his delusional experiences. It is, therefore, very probable that the prejudiced person likewise feels uneasy because of his belief that certain people are a danger to himself and to those near and dear to him. On the other hand, we have to assume that for him, as for many people, the belief in other people's baseness is easier to bear than would be the realization that the evil, and the difficulty in coping with it, lie within the self. Besides, so I suggest, both the paranoiac and the prejudiced subject deep down know that the imagined danger is a symbol. Thus from this reason alone, in both cases the delusional formation is preferred by the mind to the undisguised clear realization of what is actually going on in the psychic depths.

2. We cannot avoid the question: What is to take place with the moral difficulty if public discouragement of the kind suggested were to prevent the formation of a well-defined prejudice. The subconscious difficulty and the associated tension within the psychic system remains in full. Very likely, some irritability and emotional instability would in many cases constitute the alternative symptoms.

If ever there is a human community in which a young person may have an expert at his disposal to discuss all his conflicts at a time when the psychoneurosis is yet in the making, a short analytical exploration and appropriate advice might result in the most desirable outcome : in the realization of the existing moral conflict. So prepared, and living in a society that ridicules prejudice, the subject might prefer his somewhat unpleasant knowledge about himself to any delusion his phantasy may offer him later as a model of relief.

As things are, this type of preventive psychiatry is not available, and to an adequate extent, probably, it will never be a reality. Only people of psychological inclination think that the science of psychology ought to be the foremost factor in regulating life. The substantial majority of people would certainly not seek psychological advice very frequently, even if such advice were as available as bread in ordinary circumstances. It requires a particular kind of intelligence and self-criticism to feel the need of some psychology in periods or situations where average people blame outside obstacles and think only in terms of removing these external factors.

3. We have, therefore, to view the question posed above in the light of existing conditions. There are many things that in all objectivity deserve our suspicion and condemnation. There are the indubitable manifestations of crime in the usual sense ; and it has to be admitted that a variety of attacks on human lives and minds are committed in a form more or less legally tolerated. There are a number of idealists who display a passionate hatred of these deplorable events. This passion contrasts with the apparent calm attitude of other people who equally deplore these phenomena. In all probability the conspicuous concern of some persons about these deplorable events is fed by deep-seated affective processes in their psyche, independent of the social evils in question. There is, however, no real harm in this fact. Such a " psychoneurotic fear " of moral and social evil can lead only to an improved care for the welfare of humanity. The calm attitude of average people without the enthusiasm of a few is as a rule insufficient to give weight to progressive ideas advocated by men of vision.

I believe that in the wake of suppressing customary prejudices through such public measures as suggested there would occur nothing worse than an increased sensitiveness towards existing evils. The number of those who fight against injustice and crime, and do so on battlefields where such enemies do exist, would be greater ; the number of deluded persons in proportion smaller.

4. The emotional reaction at the news of murder, rape, etc., is in fact small or short lived in the average individual. The response to the knowledge about social injustice and mental suffering of other people is hardly emotional in colour, it is rather an intellectual realization of the existing wrong. On the other hand, the sight of a multiple murderer or political gangster as a rule evokes a genuine interest with a definite tinge of admiration, and people utter their indignation more from conventionalism and a sense of duty than from an appropriately deep sentiment. The intensity of prejudiced hatred towards its object and the insistence of the hostile attitude in these matters is conspicuously different.

A great deal of the passionate antagonism manifested in militant prejudice would, in all probability, be directed towards concrete dangers of social harmony, should the social process interfere with, and restrict the development of, mass prejudice. The tendency to project inner conflicts on to external objects would still operate ; but the ultimate objects of the projection would preferably be those who are by all logical standards condemnable in the interest of general welfare. More probable than not, the concern of such psychoneurotics would be ultimately directed to the problem of crime and immorality in general, rather than to the concrete human beings associated with such a disapproved conduct. This displacement of interest is likely to take place through the fact that it would be society as a whole that suppresses the formation of prejudice and is the medium that directs the intrinsic desire for passionate condemnation into channels of concrete reality. And since the concept of " society ", with all its implications for the individual mind, is to some extent *abstract*, besides its reference to the concrete community of people, the redirection of the projective tendency is likely to assume some feature of abstractness. This, as we suggest, would consist in the emphasis on the problem of crime and immorality, instead of on the criminal and immoral person. This displacement makes prejudiced accusations against concrete people impossible.

5. Such a metamorphosis in the elementary tendency of projecting self-condemnation would represent a progress that goes beyond the immediate elimination of violent prejudice. The basis of prejudiced attacks on fellowmen is a substitution of external victims for the subject. An excess of emphasis on the individual

*self* is never a healthy phenomenon. It is the prerequisite for psychoneuroses as well as for character-neuroses and prejudice-paranoias. Obviously the metamorphosis of a concern for the self and the specified persons respectively into a concern for the community and its problems is a victory of higher intellect over elementary emotional forces. There is no need to discuss the potential value of such an event in further developments of a beneficial character.

6. But we might be permitted to indulge in another more optimistic assumption without being suspected of lacking in critical faculty. Should there ever exist a society decidedly opposed to the emergence of organized prejudice, this change would imply an era of a higher spiritual level in general. Other simultaneous reforms of penetrating character in education, production, and work, as well as administration, might indicate a general change in human life.[1] In these circumstances, perhaps, the very weakness of the mind favouring projection would be a less frequent and a less potent propensity of human beings. It cannot be overlooked that the amount of real extrinsic threat to his personality and life process that the individual has to suffer, both in childhood and maturity, is a factor greatly deciding the strength of his *ego* and its capacity for coping with moral conflicts. Surely environmental factors, responsible for this source of pressure, are still capable of improvement, and in the case of its materialization the *ego* is bound to become stronger.

7. Knowledge and a relative freedom of thought have at all times been, and will remain, factors capable of countering, to a degree, the tendency to projection. There have been a number of writers and lecturers who have recognized the necessity for more freedom of thought, and encouraged people to change in this respect, without, however, realizing that such progress is not possible by mere encouragement and by the wish to follow the advice. Admittedly there are a number of individuals who through deep study of their experiences have been able to throw off some of the fetters that their thinking has acquired during the formative period of their life. Yet this corrective process takes years; and besides, it certainly cannot occur in the masses of individuals. The ideal in view would be a freedom of thought

[1] Cf. Ch. IX, 6, 7.

that is the natural share of all average people and is the immediate result of early education and the general social atmosphere.

The fear of economic insecurity in a system of large-scale competition renders the development towards intellectual independence well-nigh impossible for the masses of individuals. The fundamental dependence and insecurity in spheres vital to life restricts the function of the mind. The great deal of secrecy that has to surround libidinal wishes in youth, and in people in general, is another factor fettering the freedom of the psycho-affective processes ; but ideation is a function that takes place in close association with the non-conceptual affective currents.

On the other hand, a system of economic equality (perfect communism), as long as it is only enforced by political measures and associated with an isolation of minds from outside influence, is likewise a condition in which ideal freedom of thought, in the sense envisaged here, can hardly develop. And how to find a less repressive and, at the same time, relatively safe system for coping with the forces of libido will remain a thorny question for a long time to come.

For all these reasons it is difficult to imagine that a large-scale revolution of human thought in the direction of more freedom—a dependable freedom—might become practicable within a human society and with a human type we know or are able to think of.

# CHAPTER XI

## THE PROBLEM OF AGGRESSIVENESS

*References to the problem in the psychoanalytical literature.—Aggressiveness is in part a derivative of the instinct of self-preservation.—The struggle of ideas and psychoaffective currents is the basic process of primary aggressiveness.—Factors responsible for a superfluity in this tension.—Spiritual values.—Formality of Civil Administration and unsatisfactory international relationships are arresting genuine progress.—A new element has to be introduced into the deeper affective processes. Education in childhood illustrates the fact that foreign elements may become assimilated even though at first there is a resistance to them.—The appeal to the libido of a new element is indispensable for success.—The hypothesis that a-social attitudes are abnormal, and a pretence manifested by society in its confirmation, should be able to influence the deeper processes of the mind.—The personal significance of all human beings is a concept with a certain appeal to the mind, even though archaic, misanthropical elements are in opposition to it.—The psychological effect of a concrete reform is not always as dynamic as expected.—What is given to people might also be taken away from them.—The value of inanimate objects compared with the significance of human lives.*

1. There are numerous references in the psychoanalytical literature to the problem of aggressiveness. It cannot be doubted that the rôle of various factors and aspects suggested by authors of this literature are vindicated by therapeutic analyses. Thus we are justified in assuming that frustration in general and that of libidinal forces in particular may activate aggressive tendencies ; and it is equally true that aggressiveness is a primary tendency of the human personality. It is true that after a successful analysis some of its manifestations may disappear, and it is also true that to a certain extent this force is capable of sublimation.

For a decrease on a large scale of social aggressiveness very little can be achieved solely through utilizing the results of psychoanalysis proper. It is hard to visualize a future society in which libidinal repression, personal frustration, motives for jealousy in family life, etc., will be reduced to an extent sufficient to dry up the wells of irrational resentment in the individual psyche. The spread of psychological knowledge through literature and individual education is a measure that is unable to fulfil even a small fraction of the expectations put into it by enthusiasts.

Whatever results enlightenment in the course of individual psychotherapy may achieve, this is possible solely because the patient *suffers* from his symptoms ; for him a change in his mental functioning is urgently desirable. Moreover, the intellectual enlightenment does not do the work independently, but only within what is called the psychoanalytical situation. In the absence of troubling symptoms, and outside the psychoanalytical situation, there is in the deeper spheres hardly any effort to change, even though a person may feel consciously that he is *too prone* to resent and hate. Intellectual enlightenment on analytical psychology has, in fact, very rarely helped an individual towards a change of his psychic functioning that included a decrease of his aggressiveness. Much more often has this miracle been performed by a satisfactory love relationship, without any explicit knowledge of " how to do it ". In the comparatively few instances where an intelligent grasp of, let us say, Adler's Individual-psychology has helped a person to become more balanced, there was a sufficient anticipatory readiness towards a mental rearrangement. There appears no hope whatsoever that libraries and lectures might achieve a similar effect in the masses of people who have no such deep desire to be converted. Popular approval of psychological theses as to aggressiveness refers as a rule to the desire that others should take the lesson to heart. The fact that knowledge, however extensive and deep, does not decrease aggressiveness has been sufficiently proved by the militant attitudes taken by psychological schools not so long ago.

2. Elementary aggressiveness cannot be compared to symptoms or reactive character traits. The psychoanalytical notions of displacement and substitute formation are not applicable to a factor assumed to be of a primary character. Admittedly, aggressive behaviour manifested in response to frustration of a natural tendency *is* reactive ; but the propensity on which this reaction is based is as elementary as any of the fundamental forces within the human personality.

The secondary character traits are in a different category. If, for instance, a person is habitually suspicious or quarrelsome this being his way of coping with his feeling of "inferiority", we may assume that such traits are dispensable. We can imagine him capable of dropping such attitudes should he learn to reassure himself in a different manner. But it would be against elementary nature to abandon aggressiveness that is called for by the frustration of fundamental needs. This aggressiveness exists in the interest of life. It pertains to the mechanism of self-preservation. Thus resentment felt at being interfered with, together with the ensuing aggressiveness, decidedly springs from an elementary propensity.

Apart from these reactive manifestations, there must be a primary urge and capacity for pursuing personal goals. This in itself implies aggressiveness, which is comparable to that employed by a predatory animal in the process of attaining its food. The extension of this "instinctual aggressiveness" to an infinite field of personal aims is able to explain much manifested aggressiveness that might appear objectively dispensable.

The extension of "instinctive aggressiveness" is intelligible if we keep in mind the psychosomatic duality of the human personality. Its needs extend far beyond elementary desires and the aversion of pain. The mental aspect of life permeates the sum-total of physiological processes, since the psychoaffective currents appear to be closely associated with practically all somatic functions.[1] This results in the psychosomatic unity, as well as in the fact that the elementary pugnacious instinct is put into the service of the mental personality, too.

The complexity of mental spheres implies a large variety of psychoaffective currents which are interwoven with an infinite wealth of conceptual elements. Ideas are even more definite and specific than tendencies and affective currents. In the latter processes the phenomena of bipolarity and amalgamation allow on their peripheries for an almost smooth link between two of them. Ideas are, on the other hand, of a more defined character and, therefore, distinct and independent. This distinctness throws up the intrinsic differences existing between various ideas. The emphasis attached to each of them implies as it were a negation of a number of others; this, in terms of dynamics, amounts to an attempt on the part of one idea to eliminate the others. Thus, a constant polar tension prevails within the psychic system; more exactly, a vast number of small areas are charged with a polar tension between an idea and its antitheses. The tendency

[1] Cf. the discussion of this thesis in the author's *Psychological and Biological Foundations of Dream-interpretation*, and in Chs. VIII, X, of *Man and his Fellowmen*.

of each idea to maintain itself must thus imply an *aggression* against a number of other conceptual elements.

Impressions from the outside always have their impact on the process of ideation. The behaviour of an environmental person is bound to influence some or other of the intra-mental processes concerned with the competition of ideas, either through adding to the emphasis of the one pole or through contradicting it and thus indirectly siding with the other pole. Thus there is a constant interactivity between extrinsic and intrinsic mental elements. This blending of the external and internal may be followed by a turn of the intra-mental aggression against an environmental person. The polar tension, which on the intra-mental level represents the fight for the maintenance of one idea against another, becomes more or less extraverted ; as if the idea has to defend itself against an external concrete factor.

Prejudice, and intolerance in general, are magnified distortions of the normal process just described ; they develop from there as a tumour does from the matrix of normal tissue.

I submit that outward aggressiveness may be the result of a " superfluity " of aggression within ; just as hatred with an outside object, if suppressed, turns more or less towards the self. It is this phenomenon of recoil that is uppermost in the minds of psychoanalysts when they speak of *aggression against the self*. (Cf., however, in (5).) But if it were not for a pre-existent mechanism, as for instance the one suggested above, a turn of outward tendencies towards the self could not occur to the extent and frequency it actually does.

3. It must be obvious to the reader that our conception of aggressiveness is capable of throwing a new light on the phenomenon of " self-aggression " so often referred to in psychoanalysis. It is, likewise, *primary* in a sense, and not merely a recoil of outward tendencies. In addition to what has been said so far, the following consideration will explain this.

The human personality is faced with a large number of tendencies which require continuous regulation. Moreover, every moment of life is unique ; the sum-total of endopsychic processes at any moment is hardly equal to that of another one. Increase and decrease of processes, deflection to various " degrees " of tendencies, a changing variety of mutual proportions and constellations, are going on continually. All this amounts to a struggle against the general *status quo* of a particular moment and thus against the resistance of the tendencies to be altered. These events obviously imply *intra-mental aggression aiming at elements of the subject's psychoaffective structure.*

An explorer who travels from place to place will not infrequently find the parting with a particular town or region painful, though there is no question that in pursuing his aim he *has* to proceed. We may compare this case to the intra-mental processes that are concerned with the continual metamorphosis. There is a decided urge to carry them out, but implicitly also a resistance offered against these processes. Each recent intra-mental process thus represents " aggression " against the *status quo* of the mind, though clearly this takes place in the interest of personal existence. Here we have the fundamental mechanism of *aggression against the self.*

Processes of alteration go on in biochemical spheres, too ; but these are rather concerned with restoration of a pre-existent condition, that is, of a physiological standard, and they are on the whole stereotyped. Only the process of adapting the organism to new physical conditions implies a breaking with the accustomed *status quo.* A new climate or new diet requires an appropriate adjustment in the physiological functions ; and the success of maintaining average health in the new circumstances depends on the capacity to change the accustomed routine of physiology. Likewise, the regulation of the blood circulation and nervous currents, in accordance with the changing requirements of life, represents a breaking away from the previous status. We know how important this particular capacity of the organism is for efficiency and a proper economy of life energy.

4. It is necessary to inquire into the factors that might be responsible for a superfluity of inside aggressiveness and for its direction outwards. It is justifiable to assume that there may prevail a real over-production of polar tension between ideas and affective currents respectively ; and if the position is beyond the capacity of the psyche to be dealt with intra-mentally, then something has to take place to enable an abreaction.

Constitutional psychopathy does indeed cause in a number of people an abundant flow of conscious ideas which they find obsessive. One has to assume that in such cases the underlying trouble is an over-production of affective elements. Just as in the somatic spheres there is the phenomenon of hypersecretion, something comparable is likely to exist in the psychoaffective regions. It is easy to apply this knowledge to the particular element of aggressiveness.

It is, however, justifiable to assume the existence of a further possibility. Superfluity may be relative, in that the psychic mechanism, owing to some dynamic weakness, is unable to bring about a balancing of polar tensions. It appears to be a basic propensity of the psyche to redirect accumulated elements and suppressed tendencies, particularly if there is a preformed path for this secondary process. Extravert aggression in the service of self-preservation is such a pre-existent elementary tendency, employable also for the externalization of intrinsic tension.

Moreover, an inability to bring currents of tendencies to an even balance is in itself bound to increase aggressive propensities within the psychic system. For the sake of analogy we may be reminded of the irritability and anger felt by people who are unable to cope with a task, particularly if they encounter difficulties in combating an adversary. Thus the *feeling* of the difficulty in coping with polar tensions is an additional cause for the increase of aggressiveness, up to the point where a redirection towards specific objects enforces itself.

A further link appears to be interpolated into the process that turns unspecified " inside aggressiveness " into an objective extraverted tendency. As suggested, the relative " superfluity " may be caused by a difficulty to attain balance in a vast number of polar systems. But it is obvious that the stimuli, giving rise to a vast number of endopsychic processes, actually come from outside. The continuous impact of impressions, together with the general necessity for the personality to take into consideration the " outside ", greatly accounts for deep psychoaffective currents and particular constellations of ideas. Consequently the concrete outside in general *is* in fact responsible for intrapsychic difficulties. Hence the turn outwards of an intra-mental tension not only represents an " outlet ", a process of necessity, but there is some logical meaning in the course taken. Projection and persecutory delusions are thus psychologically logical phenomena.

5. The primary character of aggressiveness is suggested by the fact that psychoneurotic characters (psychopaths) are greatly prone to resentment, hatred, and prejudice ; as if they grasped every opportunity to associate environmental events with the accumulation of intrinsic aggressiveness. In a descriptive sense we say that they react too readily with resentment and aggression.

The counterpart of this type is the person with an "over-strict superego". It has been recognized by Freud that many of these people have never been subjected to a strict educational regime; the exaggerated degree of their "self-aggression" is therefore endogenous. A turn of internal aggression towards the outside is illustrated by the militant prejudice. We have recognized this phenomenon as developing from an intra-mental condemnation of the subject's part-ego.

It must not be forgotten, however, that Freud's system of psychology provided for the existence of a "death instinct". All living matter tends to return to a non-living state, because the living matter developed from the inanimate world. Life is at the same time a process leading to ultimate death. The force of self-destruction is thus implied in the very process of living. In the opinion of the present writer it would be possible to imagine that a subconscious awareness of the fact that death is daily approaching, may in some cases be undesirably strong and cause a vague fear as well as reactive outwards aggressiveness.

It appears, however, that the conception suggested here on fundamental aggressiveness within the psychoaffective spheres represents a more comprehensive view; to those with a critical inclination it must have long appeared advisable to attempt a new or additional approach to the problem under discussion.[1] The application of the writer's concept of intra-psychic aggressiveness to the problem of practical reform is dealt with later. (Cf. Chapter XII 13, 14.)

6. The old formula that men need outlets for aggressiveness receives a new viewpoint for its examination. We can understand why it is that a lessening of outside pressure and a widening of individual liberty does not substantially decrease irrational aggressiveness. There is no need to adduce instances of individuals and groups revelling in crude persecution when in power.

A larger degree of intra-mental peace and harmony (homeostasis) appears to be the essential condition of a decrease in aggressive tendencies. *And only those environmental influences that are capable of easing the intra-mental struggle in general are likely to result in a more peaceful attitude of the personality.* Not all concrete reforms in society are of a substantial benefit for this socio-psychological end. More accurately, the intra-psychic value of reforms may not be as great as suggested by their significance in the world of concrete realities in the narrower sense.

7. Here we cannot avoid turning our attention to "spiritual values". The belief in God's wisdom, in the absolute justice of all events however painful and confusing to ordinary thinking, has assuaged at least as much aggressiveness as have the reforms of our era granting more equality of opportunities through diminishing class distinctions.

There must never, of course, be a return to the times of sanctified slavery of the minds and legalized exploitation of bodies. But the task still awaits the thinker and sociologist how to help modern man, freed of many fetters—concrete and intellectual—in his intra-mental battle.

The question is to find ways that might decrease intra-mental unrest and charm the forces of aggression, without slipping back into a devoted acceptance of a rule by intimidation and oppression.

We cannot fail to recognize the paramount value of a religious ideology that promises infinite forgiveness by heaven in exchange for faith and devotion. Were this ideology not so closely connected in human minds with the potential horrors of the after-life, it would deserve explicit support by the social scientist, however great may be the intellectual sacrifice for him involved by such an attitude.

We cannot close our minds to the actual experiences mankind has had throughout history with organized religion.[1] There has prevailed a contemptuous attitude towards the believer of other creeds, an inclusion in religious life of passionate hatred and prejudice, and even official sponsoring of bloody persecution. Admittedly, these characteristics of mass religion have with the passing of time lost a great deal of their crudeness. But it is hard to deny that the progress attained in this field is due to intellectual enlightenment in secular spheres. Without the growth of the secular sciences and the modernization of political concepts the practical programme of powerful religious organizations would have hardly developed on such refined lines as the case has actually been.

[1] The reader whose scope on this point is limited to his closer, perhaps even idyllic, environment, as well as to the experiences of his generation, will find this statement unfair and entirely unintelligible. The writer, however, as well as many other readers, has in mind a substantial number of historical data referring to various ethnical regions. They know that organized power, coupled with what is indubitably a purely subjective strong sentiment—without any corrective foundation in the empirical world—has proved to be too often an irresistible temptation to aggressive manifestations. In the writer's opinion, the case of pure religion might fare much better without powerful organizations. Admittedly, this could only be the case within a secular system that is more fair than the present one, since prevailing forces in social life are definitely hostile to all programmes that are idealistic and unsupported by some kind of bargaining power.

8. There must be a search for ways of imparting more peace to people's minds, without relying greatly on the social work of religious authorities. And there can hardly be any doubt that the feeling of security and personal significance is a factor that should be able to work the miracle. Economic security is not the magic formula, however important it is in the link of events. What is meant is a feeling by the masses of individuals that they are important and appreciated. Clearly it is no easy matter to impart a genuine belief of this kind to the masses, particularly to those people who are not credulous. Facts contradict assertions in this sense ; proclamations by statesmen and scientists have no more effect than sermons on the scepticals. They may be interested in the blessings and promises of religion, but they are unable to believe in the reality of these things.

As long as civil administration has to be carried out with much formality, and the citizen feels himself to be a passive object of a powerful agent—in fact of several powerful agents—he cannot very well believe in his personal significance. Unfortunately it is difficult to imagine that this state of affairs could easily be altered. To blame the Civil Servant for his habitual attitude of being " an authority " should, in the eyes of a thinking person, be outright ridiculous. The Civil Servant is the embodiment of the prevailing administrative spirit, which exists without his individual contribution. To expect the Civil Servant to remodel his whole thought and to assume hyper-progressive concepts of social psychology is pious optimism and unfair, too. He in general cannot do so, however much he may try to be sympathetic and considerate on individual occasions.

9. To a great extent international relations are responsible for arresting genuine humane progress. It is so far impossible for governments to adopt a foreign policy based on mutual trust, with the elimination of suspicion, secretiveness, and all that goes with it. International relationships are, at the best, governed by a spirit peculiar to men who are actual or potential competitors in the economic spheres and from opportunism carry out their business under certain recognized formalities.

Since governments are obliged to adhere to such a policy of craftiness, whilst carrying out the defence of their countries' elementary interests, the same spirit of " diplomacy " and " suspicion " is bound to dominate in all respects the minds of the leaders. The aim of out-smarting other countries and, where feasible, of dominating them, are the guiding motives of foreign politics. This cannot fail to obstruct attempts at improvement *within* the country. Economic necessities for such a struggle undoubtedly do exist. There appears at present little prospect that this basic cause may undergo any genuine alteration. Whether a more even distribution of natural products would really change international affairs, it is not possible to foresee. Age old tradition has so greatly poisoned the life of nations and individuals that power-politics would not easily be eliminated even though gross inequalities in economic supplies might have ceased to exist.

The tragic fact remains that to this day responsible statesmen and their advisory scientists are not sufficiently aware of their belief in archaic conceptions on politics. If they were, probably they would have to withdraw into the background of popular disfavour or would lose much dynamic influence ; many others would be ready to take up the trend and to serve their country on the old lines of ridiculous competition including occasional crudeness of mentality.

10. The widespread significance of power and prestige, coupled with economic difficulties in several countries, is thus, so I suggest, obstructing the reduction of aggressiveness in the average individual citizen. Admittedly, there are many who do find the principles of existing politics ridiculous and archaic, and who have a contempt for " diplomacy " in the deplorable sense, as well as for sheer bureaucracy. But they are largely persons without any strong appeal to the masses. Those groups in society who are influential consider philosophers of this kind to be weaklings. Thus, their humane wisdom is of no social consequence.

The real test of an ethical attitude is a potential power for domination and exploitation, which is, however, not taken advantage of. Therefore, people who apparently could gain a large following for savage aims, but show a disregard of such a rôle and its methods, should be most apt to further the cause of progress. In the case of the passive and weak personalities who stand up for the " good " the fact is that they may have the benevolent consent of their fellowmen, but hardly their admiration and active co-operation. Their example is not convincing enough and therefore not really stimulating. It is in the nature of things that soft idealists and personality types incapable of domination swell the crowd of those who object to aggressive methods. On the other hand, comparatively few in number are those who are of a forceful personality and with a considerable following, yet who are independent enough to revolt against the general trend that complains against oppression and at the same time adores it.

This is a problem that is easier to describe than to solve in practice. No amount of logical reasoning against the popularity of power-politics in the widest sense can be of any help. Human behaviour is essentially based on events in the affective spheres; and their character is not sufficiently in agreement with common sense and intellectual principles. People in general, though to varying degrees, appear to have *libidinal ties* to phenomena of power and domination. It is not possible to interfere successfully with this direction of the libido without enabling the psyche to have other preferable objects.

In our search for new ways it is of no avail to adhere rigidly to the sum-total of results yielded by a careful analysis. After having established the outline of a problem as a whole with its implied details, the steps to follow are a selection of component problems fit for practical measures and the search for compromise where total solution is impossible.

In the case under review it is obvious that international relations, both political and economical, will continue to necessitate competition and the craft of diplomacy in its aggressive and defensive aspects. It also remains unavoidable that the internal affairs of a country will reflect this fact; the elements of domination and crafty competition will continue to infiltrate social life. Therefore, there can be no remedy other than a corrective one; no other way of progress than by sustained efforts at balancing the deficiencies and smoothing out the incongruities created constantly by the interactivity of processes.

11. Any attempt at altering the course of an existing process has to introduce a new element; it is expected to modify either the rhythm or composition of the whole phenomenon. In matters of social life the same rule holds good. Propaganda and practical measures are the means employed here. Experience shows that both means are complementary. Through apparent gifts and privileges, or alternatively, through threats of deprivation, it is possible to influence the mentality of the masses in favour of a political programme; and through an appropriate appeal to their emotional preferences it is equally possible to alter the

course of production and economic situations within a national group.

Common sense and principles of justice are motives generally acknowledged as human values; but their dynamic power is comparatively small if in clash with the irrational elements of the mind. The peculiar mode of classical psychoanalysis in presenting its theory is responsible for the difficulty of the general reader in realizing the significance of *libidinal economy* in life.[1] Yet it remains a fact that a number of attitudes and concepts that logical thinking recognizes as "foolish" or "ignorant" have a strong appeal to the masses. The intelligent person, too, if involved in mass life, readily submits to these infantile and archaic influences. A large variety of "stupid" or "absurd" or inhumane scenes in a picture or play hold the public spellbound. This observation must not fail earnestly to occupy the social research worker. The impressions referred to undoubtedly satisfy the *libido*. From the ubiquity and extent of the favourable reception of such products of art we can infer the paramount rôle of a corresponding desire for them. More important than merely to know that "foolish" and "crude" impressions have a great appeal, is the realization that a libidinal desire for such experiences is independently pre-existent in the mind. No wonder then that the victory of the rational and intellectual factor is not always secured for individual as well as group life.

12. Nevertheless, education of behaviour is a feasible measure. Its essence is the introduction of dynamic elements into the automatism of psychic events. The growth of the individual "super-ego", that is, the sense for order, refinement, and ethics illustrates the scope of educational influence. In the process of individual development a number of elements, introduced from outside, become part and parcel of the personality. Beliefs at the outset only taught, as well as modes of behaviour at first merely enforced, are transformed into principles and tendencies. In the course of development the psyche will even assume a strong liking for not a few things—ideas and performances—that were in childhood adhered to merely from fear of painful consequences.

This transmutation of the extrinsic and burdensome into the intrinsic and desirable implies more than the overt phenomenon itself. A thing cannot change into something different unless

[1] Cf. Appendix II.

a new potent element has been introduced into it, or, alternatively, unless it was from the outset potentially capable of developing into its ultimate form. This latter is the case, for instance, with regard to the relationship between the flower of the apple tree and its later fruit.

It is justifiable to assume that the human individual is endowed by nature with a faculty for the development of his super-ego. This holds true of the human race as we know it since historical times ; it is, however, probable that this faculty owes its existence to phylogenesis. The fact that concepts of the super-ego satisfy human nature corroborates, perhaps, the assumption that a corresponding fundamental disposition exists, independent of later individual education. Also the fact that some kind of super-ego has been an aspect of the human personality of all races, confirms that the capacity for ethics is an elementary propensity. Obviously, the training of the infant to regularity and cleanliness helps to develop a capacity for the super-ego (Ferenczi).

The particulars of the super-ego are nevertheless extrinsic elements. The fact that they are advocated and enforced by the individual's fellowmen—who in essence only wish to transmit human traditions—does not make the acceptance of restrictive rules any easier. Intrinsic resistance has constantly to be overcome. It remains nevertheless true that a transformation of foreign principles into genuine tendencies of the personality takes place. This, as we may realize, cannot occur without far-reaching changes in the deeper elementary processes of the mind. In all probability spheres other than those of the ultimate super-ego are involved. One thing appears sure. The elements introduced by education have to receive narcissistic libido in order to be fit for their satisfactory assimilation. A libidinal cathexis of the super-ego as a whole has been postulated by Freud.[1]

Obviously a new element to be introduced in human life

[1] Cf. *Zur Einführung des Narzissmus*, Ch. III.

Freud suggests : " The development of the *ego* consists in the subject's parting with primary narcissism, at the same time creating a strong tendency to recover it. The former process occurs through displacing the libido to an ego-ideal that has been imposed upon the subject from the outside ; the satisfaction of the latter tendency is achieved through fulfilment of this ideal."

It appears, however, possible to discover a close relationship between the narcissistic cathexis of the ego-ideal and object libido. Since educational precepts originate from environmental persons—parents, teachers, and society as a whole—elements of the super-ego are in a way representative of members of the subject's environment. Thus, the libidinal cathexis afforded to the elements of the ego-ideal is to a certain extent a derivative of object libido. In liking the precepts of his super-ego and fulfilling them, the subject pays tribute to his human environment. He cannot accept education without some love of educators and fellowmen in general. In turn, the acceptance of social morals by the psyche leads to the further development of the capacity for love and friendliness.

with a view to ameliorating social behaviour has to be of a kind capable of attracting libido. Moreover, it has to be capable of altering the total distribution of libido within the psychic system so as to diminish the proneness to *a*-social reactive traits. If these fundamental pre-conditions are fulfilled, even an idea or practical measure that is at first foreign to people, is likely to find its place within the mechanisms of behaviour. In this way the reactive conduct of the individual amidst various situations of life may be altered in the direction of altruism, this fact constituting a genuine satisfaction to the subject.

13. What kind of factor might serve as a new element capable of altering the traditional modes of inter-human behaviour? It is difficult to imagine that the existing body of ethical principles could be made to work better by the discovery of a brand-new striking conception. It is also unjustifiable to hope that a growing knowledge of social and psychological sciences might ever penetrate people's minds to such a degree as substantially to alter the quality of processes responsible for behaviour. It is, lastly, rather uncritical to assume that there is a potential capacity for individuals and organizations alike to increase, by sheer will, their efforts in adherence to ethics and combating anti-social tendencies. It needs hardly to be mentioned that mere economic measures of whatever type known to us have shown so far little result in improving deep-seated mental mechanisms.

14. One feasible way might suggest itself if we have in mind what takes place in the course of children's education. Principles of a regulated life, in which children are trained, are purported by the adults to be all-important and indispensable. At first alien and indifferent to the child, these principles later appear essential to him; above all because the world of grown-ups puts a great stress on their significance. Adults are so successful in presenting these principles as of absolute validity that children suppress their own observations suggesting that these rules of behaviour are not actually inviolable laws to the educators themselves.

There is a phase in the life of the maturing individual in which various principles are already recognized, even though frequently ignored in practice. Many a child will shirk from having a good wash, though at the same time he considers cleanliness a proper thing for human beings. We know of a large number of children who occasionally steal, even though at the same time they feel that in a world of decent adults such acts ought to have no place. The yielding to temptations does not exclude the recognition of principles trespassed against. Also in the world of adults many vices are committed in secrecy to the accompaniment of a moral protest from inside. And a large number of tendencies are entirely suppressed mainly because society pretends that they are " abnormal ". Most individuals who, for instance, feel distinct hatred and death wishes towards close relatives, or, for that matter, incestuous interests, suppress such wishes with the aid of the idea that " average people do not have them ".

An attitude of society pretending that certain tendencies are " abnormal " and " impossible " has a strong influence on the psyche of the individual. It is not only the fear of consequences that diverts thought and action away from disapproved aims and towards permissible directions. The hypothesis that certain attitudes and tendencies have no place in society, the imagining that they do not exist, is a complementary force modelling the deeper levels of the mind. The automatism of the psyche accepts as a dynamic element, and as a quasi-reality, a hypothesis implied by universal pretence.

It is, however, sure that not all " social hypotheses " would be capable of becoming dynamic forces of general behaviour. Only those are likely to find a place in the mental automatism that appeal to deep-seated tendencies, as is for instance the aspect of the mind called the super-ego. Cleanliness does appeal to the child ; he prefers the look of people who are clean and smartly dressed, and likewise he loves himself to appear clean and neat. The act of stealing may appear even to a child of school-age genuinely improper, on the ground that such an act by others may deprive himself, or his parents, of valuable things. In the eyes of a child parting with property is a very serious thing, his belief in possession is deep-rooted ; thus, anyone who interferes with it commits a crime. Though this conception refers mainly to the child's or his family's property, the act of stealing may become a condemnable notion also with regard to himself, in spite of the fact that the temptation might on occasions prove stronger than the principle.

15. The personal significance of all human beings is likewise a conception that has a definite appeal to the deeper spheres of

the mind. Admittedly, against this there is a distinct realization that people are not equally clever, good, pleasant, and above all not equally useful and impressive. There is also the archaic desire for superiority, exclusiveness, and domination. These factors stand in the way of acknowledging the personal significance of all well-intentioned fellow-beings. The existence and powers of one's fellowmen represent to the archaic depths of the mind hostile forces, a threat to the personal significance of the subject. But this interpretation, archaic it may be, is not a natural one ; that is to say, it is not one indispensable for human life. In savage cultures the individual had no personal significance in a true sense ; moreover, the great hardships of existence would not even have allowed such a feeling to develop. Fear and ignorance as to the forces of nature made the human being an ever trembling creature. The idea of mutual human relationship did not include the members of another tribe ; they were but potential enemies.

To-day we know well that actually there is room on earth for every human being ; that existing limitations are not entirely unavoidable but are largely a matter of imperfect organization and circumstances and not of lack in natural potentialities. We also know that science and social organization have been capable of relieving to a considerable extent the burdens of life as compared with human existence in primitive historical periods. Hopes of further improvements are thus reasonable. Hence, part of the competitive aggressiveness in present day man is but an archaic element, with no roots in actualities. Successive reforms in the social organization may be capable of decreasing the other source of fear and aggressiveness which is the actual deficiencies of economic and administrative life throughout the world. However halting this progress may be in fact it appears to the average mind as humanly feasible. Proof for this belief is the fervent desire of people for the establishment of certain systems, social or religious, in which they put their hopes.

Consequently the idea of each other's personal significance should have an appeal to psychic depths, sufficient to render a corresponding " social pretence " a workable factor. But the unequivocal manifestation of this principle in practical spheres of life would be indispensable for the end in view. Granted this, the desired influence on the deeper psychic levels is very likely to take place. To the writer it appears sure that this suggestion is in the domain of the humanly possible. A number of modern schools,[1] in which children enjoy certain autonomy under the guidance of enlightened pedagogues, have succeeded in creating an atmosphere of fairness and sincerity, which resulted in the improvement of difficult children. It is an unfortunate fact that the members of such artificial communities are bound to be disappointed—or puzzled—when later entering the society of adults. But, perhaps, they are better equipped for their life than they would be without their experience in these schools. Whatever the further course of development in these pupils might be, these schools definitely illustrate the possibility of creating a better social atmosphere through a " behavioural hypothesis " and its embodiment in manifest life.

16. The practicable application of this knowledge to adult society is admittedly not easy. However great the progress in social legislation may be, as shown by customary concrete measures, the psychological effect on the average individual must lag considerably, because these measures alone do not strike at the root of human fear. Democratic ways of settling internal affairs by parliamentary majority certainly give satisfaction to those who are the victors of the day's politics. But, behind the façade of their satisfaction, there is bound to exist the knowledge that what has first to be given to men, might just as well be taken away.

The concepts of right and justice are interpreted so differently that people cannot feel that the principles in question are natural laws of human evolution. The infant does feel, very probably, this his parents' help is always at his disposal. Likewise, aging parents may, in most cases, rely with certainty on the support of their children, if this should be necessary and the required means available. There is no feeling comparable in naturalness to these instances in the average citizen with regard to his position in society. A social order by a majority vote is unquestionably more adequate than a system of dictatorial administration. It at least acknowledges the justification for change if expressed in freedom by the masses. But where is the guarantee that the

[1] Cf. *Children's Communities*, edited by The New Educational Fellowship ; *Making Citizens*, a review of aims and methods of the Approved Schools, H.M. Stationery Office ; and the works by A. S. Neill.

The reader may also be interested to read a brief but graphic account of the success attained, more than a century ago, by Robert Owen in " creating a model settlement, in accordance with the principles of harmony, which should serve as an example to the whole of mankind ". Cf. Ch. V in *Leaders, Dreamers, and Rebels*, by Rene-Fülöp-Miller.

resolutions of the majority are the best possible ones? A vote by majority expresses the genuine *emotional preferences* of people, provided the voters are comparatively free from influence; thus, the practical measures following from such decisions are not always to the advantage of order and justice. Besides, the majority vote is, even within a brief human period, far from being a constant factor. For these reasons all that is being given to members of a society can also be taken away from them.

The individual's physical characteristics, such as strength or good looks, are his inalienable property, unless an unfortunate accident interferes. A capacity for the appreciation of beauty and science, once acquired by a person, cannot be taken from him as long as his mind remains in health. But the economic and social position of the masses of individuals depends on a system of laws, on politics and ideologies of those who, at a given period, are in power to direct both public opinion and actual administration.

A feeling of security in the deeper psychological sense cannot yet prevail. In general the individual cannot face the administrators of public affairs, and even less his private employer, with the same ease as, for instance, a person booking a ticket for the train. He may be pretty sure of receiving it and assume with certainty that the booking clerk has neither power nor interest to deny it to him. Should, nevertheless, such an unexpected event occur, it might suggest to the would-be passenger that a mental disturbance has suddenly come upon the clerk.

In fact, the individual cannot face his fellowmen in general with natural spontaneity and trust. People know about each other's very limited significance in society. They clearly realize how much in life depends on chance or craftiness, and how little on the personal significance in society of each individual. So much success or failure clearly follows the presence, or absence, of certain conditions required by custom or law; but many of these rules appear arbitrary and not at all postulates of justice or necessity. For these reasons the fellowman in general is envied, feared, and at the same time looked down upon for being a weak dependent creature, at the mercy of superior forces, because he is supported so little in his manifold needs. All these facts are largely inevitable. They are not pointed out for the sake of deploring them, but with a view to showing their rôle in generating fear and aggressiveness. The establishing of casual connections, or at least the search for more knowledge in this respect, might prove equal, if not superior, in practical value to the traditional way of appealing to the individual to be decent.

18. The appreciation of the human personality is much smaller than we like to admit. During the last war there arose the question whether works of art and buildings of great historical value should be spared destruction, at the cost of human life. There were one or two sincere persons who, in their letters to the press, favoured the sacrifice of life for saving historical places of religious character or artistic value. I call them sincere, not because I agree with their opinion, but because they have expressed an undisguised human attitude. People are so much attached to *inanimate objects* capable of satisfying their religious sentiments or sense of beauty, that the life of a few or a few hundred soldiers means to them a negligible price for the continued existence of the objects they adore or admire. Should we ask the soldiers to be sacrificed or their families about their opinion in this matter the decision might be different.

Nevertheless it is sure that a picture, a piece of music or sculpture, or for that matter a building, awakes much more genuine interest in people than does the idea of the lives of human beings who are not objects of their personal attention. The same preference exists, in fact, with respect to all the good things in life. The thought of one's fellowmen in general inspires no comparable interest, since there is so little attached to this concept that strikes one as admirable and pleasant. Miserably dependent on major forces for all the essentials of life, burdened with family ties, threated by illness, and with no exceptional personality, the masses of individuals appear rather inexpensive and dull articles on the motley market of social happenings. Apart from the few people of emotional-libidinal significance for the subject, only a person backed by power, money, or a marked public interest, is able to attract attention, and his existence may be felt as valuable to a degree that competes with the attraction of material goods in life.

## CHAPTER XII

## THE NEW ELEMENT IN THE SOCIAL PROCESS

*The enactment of the hypothesis that all individuals are equally significant for society.—The psychological and economic aspects of the scene.—The owner of a business is merely a privileged user of opportunities given to him by society.—Authority and control are necessary, but ought to be coupled with an appreciable degree of personal significance for the employee.—Most individuals as we know them to-day are not eager to be really free.—The attraction which the performance of domination has for many people makes them even like a passive rôle in the act.—Early education has to insist on submission and obedience.—There is an inertia for assuming attitudes different from those practised at an earlier age.—Difficulty in realizing the existence of the tendency to submission.—The higher interpretation of emotional complexes, processes, and impressions decides the ultimate rôle of the element in question.—Intra-mental struggle is, likewise, capable of a more and a less favourable interpretation by the personality.*

1. The new element to be introduced into the social process would thus be the manifested assumption that the individual has a personal significance, and this in both instances, as the subject and his fellowman. It is obvious that both aspects of this personal significance require an equal emphasis in order to secure the double aim in view, the prevention of unreasonable fear as well as of aggressiveness. The personal significance of the subject makes reactive fear and aggressiveness unnecessary. The simultaneous realization of the fellowman's significance removes much of the temptation to externalize intrinsic tension ; but it also helps the subject to believe in his own significance, through the medium of identification. The implicit idea in question would be : " If society really protects my fellowman from my aggression and I have no chance of public approval for such an attitude, then society will surely do the same service for me."

The enactment of the hypothesis would have to start with all representatives of offices and organizations. By purporting that the individual is as equal a factor as any concrete authority, and that no capital, group, or person in office has more weight than the life of the individual and his family, the impression may be conveyed that the genuine acknowledgment of personal significance is something general and natural. This in turn would result in the fact that all tendencies the individual might feel to the contrary would be considered by him as something to be ignored, hidden, and suppressed. The manifestation of the social hypothesis in question ought to be so unequivocal that a doubt as to its genuineness and spontaneity would be difficult, in spite of our knowledge that in reality there *is* an artificial plan and law behind it.

2. We may recall the phenomenon of fashion and public propaganda, which are greatly capable of directing mass sentiments. Things considered desirable, as well as behaviour deemed " normal " by the public and particularly by those who are in leading positions, may appear essential to the individual though previously he did not feel so. Should the enactment of the hypothesis that the individual is important, ever become reality, we were bound to know much more about human nature and the possibilities of social improvement than we do now. The writer feels that such a large scale measure, carried out sufficiently long—for two or three generations—could not remain without beneficial effect. He dares to say that the results of such a large-scale experiment would be on the whole better than those of the Russian experiment in the economic sphere.

It is not easy to envisage the measure suggested here without an economic counterpart of a substantial extent. It would not be easy for people to believe in the average person's significance if the elementary prerequisites of a fairly pleasant life—luxuries included—were not safeguarded for all who are ready to work for them. It would prove impossible to secure for the masses of average individuals the genuine recognition of their personal significance, if big business or any profession should continue to be a source of personal privileges to those associated with it. It is, therefore, obvious that the economic spheres cannot be ignored if the social hypothesis referred to were to vindicate the hopes put into it. Yet the writer thinks that a substantial beginning could be made by carrying out equalization in all fields where personal significance is in question. This would result in a considerable amelioration of the social atmosphere, even though the economic organization of society were not communistic.[1] One

[1] It is futile to deny that an ideal communistic society, existing all over the world, would represent a high degree of progress in human affairs. It might be enough for

of the essentials would be a large-scale educational programme, enabling much more people than so far to cultivate their intellectual aspect. By this fact it ought to be easier to attain the recognition of personal significance for millions who, at present, do not impress favourably those accustomed to an exclusive circle of friends. In the economic field, the provision with well-tailored dresses of all working people must support the suggested reform, from the same reason. But the main thing would be the insistent display by the administration of its appreciation of the individual, as well as an enforcement of this attitude in all spheres of occupational life. It is not only the wealthy, educated, and influential who, as a rule, look down on an average fellow-being. The members of the average masses themselves do not really believe in an ordinary person's significance, since they take over the standard of valuation from the others. But there is an added reason for asking the influentials and well-to-do to co-operate in the creation of the new outlook ; they owe a particular debt of gratitude to organized society. This will be shown in the following paragraphs.

3. The right of free competition automatically prevents the acquisition of excessive economic power by a few ; and in this way, too, the social system aids the individual enterpriser. He owes all his opportunities to the very fact that a few would-be lords of industry and business are to some degree limited in expansion. There is, in brief, hardly any aspect of occupational life that is secured by the self-sufficient power (autarky) of the individual. The idea of private ownership is, therefore, a rather arbitrary principle, provided we do not believe that crude power is the real source of rights. We must, however, realize, that in many aspects the existing legal concepts are undoubtedly based on the archaic significance of crude power. That is to say, the modern social system approves of some types and degrees of possession through power (this word referring also to abilities). But at the same time it is clear that it is the consent of society, and its help, that maintain these rights. Consequently the individual is indebted to society for all he is allowed to have and to do in his capacity as producer and employer.

It ought to be sufficient for an employer to be allowed to

its creation if the best and most educated members of the human race felt a genuine desire for it, and a vast majority of people had at least a proper understanding of its value. Undoubtedly, these prerequisites are not in existence.

enjoy his relative independence and the profits of his enterprise, without being in the total sense an owner and the personal "boss" of his employees. He ought to be responsible to society for all that is going on in his factory, on his farm, in his office, etc. Once a person who is in need of employment for his subsistence has entered a business the employer has become his guardian, responsible for his economic life and also for his mental life in so far as this is connected with his occupation. The capital invested and the implements used are personal property. But the employment of these means in production and business makes them an object of public concern, almost public property. Moreover, it is the right of an organized society to know that materials, money, and labour are used for desirable ends.

4. Were a large-scale improvement in social sense ever to take place it is indispensable that there should first of all be a new conception as to the position of the employer, and owner of properties in excess of his needs. It is obvious that all opportunities of producing and making profit are given to the individual by the existing body of laws and customs. There is no individual powerful enough to secure his business, trade, or profession without being aided and protected by the social and economic system. If a person is allowed to make a certain amount of profit this is simply a gift from society; and it is merely the power of the police that protects the individual's property from being taken away by some one who is stronger, and wishes, from some reason or other, to acquire more than he has.

There were times when tyrannic squires were able to keep their own army and a host of serfs, and thus secured their income and luxuries and protected their property. But their army and serfs alike were primitive human beings who, from fear, from traditional reverence towards crude power, and from lack of another type of subsistence agreed to serve the squire. To-day we can no longer believe in the "sacredness" of possessions in any absolute sense, even though considerations of peace and order require a practical adherence to this principle. It is a *modus vivendi*. Before unprejudiced common sense a person has *absolute right* to no more than what he and his family need for a fairly satisfactory life. All other type of possession is an arbitrary gift by society. For the time being the state is content with the taxes and customs, and temporary measures regulating economic life in times of emergency.

5. The employer, as we have said, remains the receiver of the material benefits derived from his factory or business. For his gift of organization and management he receives the privilege of his independent economic position and of earning more, and frequently with less hard work, than he would if he were an employee. But in respect of the fellow-citizens who are employed by him, and of the public interest in his production, he ought to be no more than the humble administrator of affairs acting on behalf of society.

A social system that tolerates the subdued position of the employee puts up, in fact, with remnants of ancient slavery. Trade unionism is admittedly a large step towards the protection of its members. But the position in general is nothing else than a dormant or open tension between the class of capitalists and employees. The superior social power of the employer, and for that matter of the head of an office, still remains, in spite of the possibility of strikes, arbitrations, and appeals. These institutions imply no more than some degree of economic and physical protection. All this hardly alters the fundamental fact under discussion, which is the individual's too deficient feeling of self-significance, and the capacity of this complex for generating aggressive potentials.

6. Admittedly there must be authority and some educational pressure for securing organization and team work. Individuals in general are far from being dependable if released from control and the pressure implied by authority.[1] But it would be futile to deny that in our society the pressure emanating from superiors and employers far exceeds the requirements for efficiency. A larger equality of social significance would in its turn make for more decency and spontaneity in carrying out the task allotted to the individual. This assumption is not merely the pious wish and optimistic promise of idealistic writers. It is a well-nigh established fact, unless all that we experience during psychoanalysis is deceptive. In fact, there is nothing more sure, more generally valid, than the fact that the deep feeling of being appreciated can decrease aggression and evoke a desire for collaboration. But it must be a feeling coming from the depths, a conviction penetrating the core of the personality. In the course of analytical psychotherapy this feeling is allowed to develop, because every detail of the analysand's personality appears of

[1] Cf. p. 188.

interest to the analyst ; and also because the subject's elementary desire for symbiosis is allowed to come to the fore by the very technique of psychoanalysis. In social life such a feeling might exist only if the actualities of life would impart it as convincingly as is the certainty that day is followed by another day. This feeling does not mean actual paradise for all ; jnst as for a number of mortals, in spite of their expectation, to-day is not succeeded by a to-morrow.

No doubt these suggestions will strike many a reader as strange, and not a few will even feel strong opposition to them. The writer does not expect a world to come easily into being in which these conceptions on property are elements of social morality.

Nevertheless they ought to penetrate the minds if a decrease in aggressiveness is ever to take place. There is, indeed, no other measure from which a favourable change might be expected, if not from a more equable distribution of power and personal significance.

7. The State organization ought to become, much more than now, the devoted servant of the individual and his family ; the country must become the home of the citizen. The atmosphere in public offices ought to change its traditional character so much so that the citizen should love to call there. The individual should be able to look upon an official with a sentiment not dissimilar to that which people feel towards a skilful medical man who in the past relieved the sufferings of many and is ready to do so at any time. *The change in the administrative atmosphere cannot come from the civil servant; his goodwill and civility is insufficient to recreate the social atmosphere.*

8. There is a source of difficulty with regard to genuine progress that people particularly like to overlook. The vast majority of human beings, as we know them, are *not eager* to be free in the deeper sense ; they admire power and superiority and even domination. One may account for this fact by more than one cause. In the superior position and domineering behaviour of the other person there is a fulfilment in imagination for people of what they themselves would like to do. Little boys are from the same motives enthralled by watching a football match, a fight on the screen, or by the mere presence of a fully-armoured stern figure. It may be that another reason, which is a readiness to

be dominated, ensues from this imaginery identification with the powerful. To the unbiased observer, the fact is obvious that there operates in human beings, to a substantial degree, a tendency to look with awe at the display of power, even if the subject himself is the one who is being dominated. It thus appears that the performance of domination is attractive to people whether they play the active or the passive rôle. Their submission to being directed and ruled enables the process of domination; and, owing to this contribution on their part, they are able to enjoy it.

Moreover, for many individuals a passive rôle in the social organization appeals from inertia; they are reluctant to assume the initiative and make the effort required by the assumption of some leadership. And this relative passivity prevails also in their relationship towards many of their fellowmen who though not actual leaders, yet like to act as superiors and guides.

9. There are also a number of people whose manifest desire for active domination contrasts with their practical inability to achieve the submission of others to their will. In this case the presence of a psychoneurotic stimulus for wishing to dominate is obvious. A vast number of individuals, however, feel at their easiest when directed and ruled by a few who give them the impression of being born for leadership or for the privileged positions they hold at the cost of their fellowmen. Certainly for this type of submissive personality a dependent position itself *does not* amount to a frustration generating in them reactive aggressiveness.

It appears almost as if pre-existing aggressiveness, coupled with the practical inability to dominate, would create the readiness to submission in order to enjoy the enactment of domination. Nevertheless, it is probable that periodic bouts of inner revolt against the fact of being ruled and restrained occur in the psyche of such individuals. The very pain implied by the subject's inferior position may be indispensable for having the full experience of domination. These currents of resentment in their turn intensify the pre-existent aggressiveness, and this, in fact, contributes to the attraction of submission. The desire to throw off the yoke and to triumph over the domineering partner finds, as suggested, its satisfaction in the very continuance of the tension implied by the inequality of positions; the ruling partner does the job on behalf of the other one.

10. The pre-existent aggressiveness which is thus assumed to initiate the process of yielding, is first of all an endogenous one. It has been assumed (page 164) that the sum-total of psycho-affective metabolism implies struggle, and might suggest aggressiveness. Elementary processes of the physiological category are not only *perceived* by the self but are followed by an *interpretation* on a higher psychological level. The same applies to the psychoaffective processes on a deeper level, where the elements and their action are yet amorphous as compared with definable ideas and complexes in the psychoanalytical sense. These processes, too, are associated with the interpretative products on a higher conceptional plane. (Libidinal currents, e.g. produce sexual or anxiety dreams, as the case may be.) *It is through interpretation of the psychoaffective metabolism as a struggle, that primary aggressiveness is created.*

It is a fact that in the majority of people the psychological processes are not so precise and smooth as to result in what we consider perfect health. Inborn weaknesses of the psychic function, and difficulties ensuing from environmental influences on mind and body, give sufficient cause for disturbances in the course of intra-mental metabolism. One general idea associated with these processes must, therefore, be the realization of *human inadequacy*. We may compare this realization of psychic insufficiency with the feeling of helplessness in face of a difficult concrete situation; then we shall be able to imagine that it is natural that a feeling of frustration, a sort of resentment, should follow this deeper realization of general psychoaffective imperfection. It will be easy to assume that a similar course takes place when intra-mental difficulty on the amorphous level is interpreted on a higher plane. It is here that the feeling of intra-mental, i.e. subjective inadequacy, creates aggressiveness of the objective external category.

11. It is obvious that education in early childhood and youth insists on obedience to the adults; the compliance with their wishes is, as a rule, associated with receiving their care, praise, and love. Education of children in freedom is a comparatively new principle. Its results will only be seen when a large number of those having it have become adults. The infantile type of subordination for the sake of expediency remains a fundamental pattern of social relationship in the adult. It is, however, unavoidable that in many individuals it continues to occupy

a place that cannot be considered ideal. Very likely it is easier for the mind to employ a well-ingrained pattern of behaviour than to acquire a new one that is, in essence, the opposite of the earlier attitude. It is more than mere natural inertia which accounts for this. We can imagine that a development towards freedom cannot be a very easy matter if past experience has proved that to comply and yield is safer than to insist on an independent choice of action. A course of freedom resulting in success and pleasure is dangerously near to reckless independence which is likely to invite restraint and trouble. The inevitable realities of life, as we know them, continually bring home the risk of defying tradition and the will of those in position. Only few persons are so gifted by nature to find, without special training, the way of wisdom that leads to a practical combination of independence and yielding.

Systematic education in freedom given to youth simultaneously with training in necessary yielding, might bring about results in the vast majority of individuals that would be different from those attained by traditional education. But as things actually are there is a substantial readiness to retain the infantile pattern of symbiosis. The child, as a rule, proudly thinks of the power wielded over others by the adults to whom he belongs ; though, undoubtedly, he greatly resents the exercise of their power over himself. When the infantile attitude of submission is carried over into adult life this bipolarity takes a modified shape. The servile individual admires the power exercised over and against himself, and at the same time resents it. In essence, thus, he enjoys the act of domination whilst he himself is the suffering partner in the drama.

Many a reader of this discussion may doubt that this readiness to submission is so widespread as is here suggested. But those who have exercised and exploited power have always realized this fact, and abundantly employed their untutored psychological knowledge.[1]

[1] A large proportion of employees do not respond favourably if the personal distance between them and their employer approaches the relationship of two independent individuals. They work with less conscientiousness than average, and might even take advantage of the trust put in them. This occurs so frequently that it must not be ignored by social scientists. It appears that the relaxation in personal relationship makes this type of people more aware of the inequality in economic and social position ; and this feeling tempts them to make up for their deficiency. Employers, naturally, draw the conclusion that the best policy is to be firm and keep the customary distance. I have heard this opinion expressed during psychoanalysis by several employers who basically were friends of the labourer and fully aware of the hardships for the wage-earner implied by existing economic conditions. As long as there is no change in the *fundamental social atmosphere*, the anomaly under discussion is bound to

12. With regard to this phenomenon, a substantial self-deception operates, particularly in the minds of educated people who might nevertheless have in their make-up a substantial share of the tendency to enjoy submission. Their pride may consequently induce them to overlook the phenomenon in general and to fail to allow for it both in practical planning and scientific interpretation.

In giving, for instance, too much independence to a person in charge of an office, there is always some risk that he may lose interest in his work and become indeed less conscientious. Should he also wield too much power over his subordinates their servile tendencies might help to screen the undesirable state of affairs.

The tendency to submission—just as that for domination—is one of the factors making the belief in all people's equal personal significance difficult. Through projecting one's own submissive tendencies on to others, the subject may feel inclined to deny to his fellowmen the significance of individual personality.

13. The source of primary aggressiveness lies, so it has been suggested, in the psychoaffective processes, which imply struggle against elements of the *self*. An absolute or relative superfluity in polar tension is bound to lead to a deflection of internal aggressiveness towards environmental objects. It has been assumed [1] that an increased personal significance for the individuals in society is likely to improve mutual social adjustment. We now have to show how this reform may dispose of primary aggressiveness in ways other than through irrational aggression towards fellowmen.

There are many phenomena in nature and society that are capable of being influenced. This means that to some extent they are not yet fully defined in composition and contour. Like plastic material they are capable of being moulded, and even their dynamic is capable of modification. If you convince a child that all his dashing and daring makes him just a nuisance and a miniature criminal, he may combat these inclinations in himself, or, alternatively, he may become an enemy of all that is stable and

exist. An employer's exceptional kindness or informality does *not* improve in essence on the current position of the individual. The amount of threat and fear to which he is exposed remains, and occasions in response indecency of social behaviour. Comparatively few are the people in whom the friendly relationship with the employer is capable of reducing intra-mental tension, and induces them to reciprocate for the gift received, by added conscientiousness.

[1] Cf. (1) of this chapter.

quiet in society. If, however, you train a child to use these propensities for sport, the result will be quite different. The attitude of adults may, in many cases, be the decisive factor in making of a disposition one thing or another.

Something similar may occur where two different interpretations of a phenomenon are possible. In the course of my research on dreams I have come to believe that, on rare occasions, the interpretation we give to a dream material may determine the ultimate shaping of a *complex* to which the dream refers. The dream may correspond to a comparatively amorphous element in the mind, which has not yet been detailed to operate on either side of a conflict. Such phases exist in the course of mental life in general, but they are clearly observable during protracted treatments. The analyst's interpretation may, in such cases, decide the definite rôle which this emotional element is to play, for a limited period at least.

Likewise, there are phases in a mass movement where it is not yet determined whether the popular forces are to array themselves in the service of progress and construction or in that of reaction and destruction. The explicit interpretation given by suitable leaders to the masses is capable of giving a final direction to the developments.

14. These few instances will also enable us to see the point under discussion here. Primary aggressiveness is, as explained in Chapter XI, in essence but the operation of forces within the complex personality. Much depends on the secondary interpretation as to their natural rôle, whether they are to contribute to an increase or decrease of social aggression. If the position of the individual in his environment suggests to his mind that what is going on in social life in general represents, for the most part, aggressive struggle with too little admixture of justice and fairness—then the mind may conceive of its deeper processes in a corresponding way. It may ignore the fact that by the law of nature all that is going on inside, actually aims at balance and positive life, even though there may be an absolute or relative " superfluity " of tension in the psyche. It may overlook the fact that these intra-mental difficulties are nothing more than obstacles in the way of the principal aims of psychic-function, and that they do not necessarily prove that the essence of psycho-physiological processes is a destructive struggle.

Because of the indubitable fact that environmental events to a large extent stimulate the psychic processes, it is inevitable that the mind should tend to assume a correspondence between what is external and what is internal ; logically this is not entirely unjustified. Hence, as it were, the reference is drawn that the intra-mental processes imply aggressive tendencies.

In a person of average psychoaffective health—that is to say, with the exclusion of psychopaths—we may assume that his interpretations are not entirely void of truth. If there is in him a tendency to *a*-social reactive traits, to suspicion, fear, and pessimism, then it is unlikely that he feels to be of sufficient personal· significance. And this indicates that environmental circumstances are unable to give him a more satisfactory feeling in this respect. Constitutional differences in interpreting what is going on in this human environment undoubtedly exist.[1] There are persons whose interpretation is much more pessimistic than is objectively justified. Summarizing, we may say : Whenever the intra-mental interpretation of external events suggests social danger and unsurmountable difficulties—whether rightly or in part wrongly—the mind conceives of its deep psychoaffective struggle and associated difficulties in terms of hostile aggression ; and in the wake of this the employment of these aggressive intramental potentials in overt social hostility is inevitable. This is, so the writer feels, a fundamental thesis deserving further study by other authors.

[1] Cf. Ch. Ia, 1–4 and Ch. Ic, 1.

# CHAPTER XIII

## EDUCATION OF SOCIETY

*Inborn mental dispositions also become the soil of secondary reactive traits.—Envy is probably associated with the faculty of self-preservation.—Pride and sensitiveness.—In spite of resistance to educational regulation, the ultimate acceptance of rules for behaviour proves the presence of a disposition for it.—Extrinsic elements introduced by education may lead to a decrease of intra-mental tension; their acceptance is thus intelligible.—The application of these observations to the broader social sphere still encounters great resistance by the public.—The analogy with popular resistance to hypnotics.—The working hypothesis of the supremacy of social decency.—A bipolarity with regard to the problem would exist, but not necessarily cause disturbance in the spheres of behaviour.*

1. The assumption is not unjustifiable that all the personality features of the adult, acquired through education in the broader sense, have been present from birth as potential nuclei in the mental disposition of the individual. Likewise what throughout this work we term *secondary traits* are clearly either desirable elaborations or distorted exaggerations of fundamental and vital tendencies. Thus envy, for instance, is closely related to the defence of one's own fair share. A comparison with what others are and possess, is *one* mode of ascertaining the subject's situation and justifiable claims. But in envy proper the whole process shoots far beyond the mark. What is only of secondary importance —the other person's share—becomes the point of central concern. In this case the element of self-insufficiency is unduly stimulated by the realization of an asset possessed by one's fellowmen. A similar relationship between fundamental dispositions and their distorted offsprings might easily be described with respect to all other secondary traits, however anti-social, unjustifiable, and even detrimental to life.

The same relationship exists with regard to approvable reactive traits on the one hand and fundamental tendencies that are presumably the matrix of these secondary elements on the other. Self-esteem and moderate pride are obviously related to the instinct of self-preservation. These two feelings, and the ensuing sensitiveness to insults, are the mental corollaries to the concern for physical integrity. Proud sensitiveness to slighting attitudes on the part of others, or to lack of response to the subject's friendly approach, is a secondary trait; it develops during maturation and is obviously stimulated from the feeling of insufficiency; but in essence it is a manifestation of the instinct of self-preservation.[1] There is frequently a surplus of these manifestations, both in children and adults, going beyond what average human *dignity* should require. But in a moderate degree they are desirable "normal" manifestations; they are meant to condemn the unjust attitude of the other person, and to result in a possible change of heart in him. These particular instances should illustrate the more general thesis that all that can be instilled *through education* must utilize a fundamental disposition of the human psyche. Consequently all that may be acquired in the course of individual life is in a certain sense "natural".

2. Nevertheless when the education of the infant begins, and throughout the years of development, the principles of a regulated life are in flagrant contrast to the automatism of the original personality. All conditioning goes against the grain, even though the final results appear to be accompanied by the feeling of satisfaction. Cleanliness, regularity, adaptation, and civil conduct in general are enforced upon the child; but once attained, and maintained for a limited spell, this state of affairs appears to be enjoyed by the child. This is true in spite of the fact that the repeated return of unbridled automatisms betrays resistance to "order". The temporary satisfaction, it may be assumed, points to the existence of the dispositional nucleus of the later acquisition; the much more manifest and repeated preference for the opposite state of affairs suggests that this innate disposition still possesses too little dynamic independence both in the child and the infantile adult.

3. In effect all education consists in the process of introducing into the subject's personality a working hypothesis; that is, of the assumption that the educational principles in question are "good" and necessary. Through *accepting* the working hypothesis

[1] W. McDougall refers pride to an instinct of *self-assertion*.

the subject pretends to possess as a quasi-autochthonous trait of character what is actually an importation, a foreign element. Experience shows that ultimately such an element is, to various degrees, assimilated into the self. However great may be, even later, the resistance offered by tendencies that obstruct the new principle, the adult subject may feel that both conflicting trends are genuine, and both are components of his *self*. In brief, a working hypothesis can become in the fullest sense of the phrase a *working principle*. This takes place because, in reality, many of the elements introduced, even at first enforced, contribute to a decrease of the intra-mental tension that ensues from the dynamic competition of a variety of tendencies. The fact that planned secondary processes of the mind do smooth out intra-mental storms is one of the motives for their acceptance by the self. In terms of classical psychoanalysis, even restriction and strictness can be enjoyed by part of the self, since these experiences satisfy the claims of the *super-ego*. Any reader of my works must, however, understand that this reference to a well-defined concept is only a limited view. The satisfaction is not solely due to the appeasement of the super-ego ; it is more accurate to say that the psychoaffective process in a broader sense, requires regulative elements for reduction of its tension ; and there is much in this auto-regulation going far beyond the principle of morals (super-ego). Moreover, the reader should be reminded of a concept advanced in Ch. I, 2 (4) [1] according to which it is better to consider the moral idea operative in the mind, as a notion much more comprehensive than that in the narrower sense of the expression. All that is felt to be appropriate, pleasant, impressive, and harmonious in the manifestations of the human personality is implied by this notion.

4. If the urge for automatism requires, for instance, that the individual should not wash, but his being dirty makes an unpleasant impression on others, then the realization of this social fact combats the former tendency. As things actually are in the sane adult, the acceptance and approval of the subject by his environment is too precious a gain to be sacrificed through stubborn adherence to tendencies of autistic nature. And thus not only the positive performance of washing and the cleanliness attained, but the implied overcoming of the resistance to the efforts involved may become for the subject, a member of society,

[1] Cf. pp. 31–2.

a source of pleasure. This admittedly simple instance may well illustrate the thesis advanced above.

Through the introduction of a working hypothesis genuine mental satisfaction can be gained, if the hypothesis in question represents a cultural or humanitarian principle of a highly developed society.[1] To mention only one other instance—if it were a genuine wish of society that people should not oppress each other merely for the sake of primitive satisfaction, then the subjects should be genuinely able to enjoy their self-limitation in the aggressive tendencies.

5. It may be assumed that the statements made so far will meet with no objection from the average reader. The instances referred to are of too common occurrence, and the theoretical implications involved in them are unquestioned principles both in children's education and in political propaganda. Yet there seems to be a marked resistance in the minds of many educated and influential persons, if it is suggested that a broader application to social reform of these very principles is desirable and may be profitable. Even critical readers and authors of sociology and psychology shake their heads with a condescending but disapproving smile at such suggestions. People find it possible and right to educate children ; it is also deemed natural to carry out propaganda in favour of certain interests, or in favour of ideologies adhered to by influential people. But when the problem of social attitudes is the object of discussion, suddenly some mysterious fear of " interference " comes over people's minds. It appears to me to be akin to the fear of many persons of taking a sleeping drug ; it is not natural sleep, they say, and prefer to suffer the unpleasantness of insomnia, which is indeed an even less natural condition.

6. The writer has been an advocate of the reasonable application of hypnotics from an early stage of his career ; this at a time when the great majority of his colleagues more conservative in outlook have been holding the view that such things are " not natural ". I feel to-day surer than ever about the deep motive of such reluctance. In the, perhaps, too concrete phraseology of

[1] The writer feels that the more advanced and refined a society is, the more capable are its dynamic principles and forms of satisfying elementary tendencies. Cf. *Man and his Fellowmen*, Ch. XI (4).

sexual-analysis, the motive is a subconscious fear of an assault. In a more comprehensive, and, I think, more accurate definition, we should speak about the reluctance to have one's intra-mental constellations changed; this implies also an alteration of subconscious libidinal preferences in favour of other complexes which are brought to the fore by the activity of the drug. But such a change of intra-mental constellations is obviously called for where insomnia exists. Even at the risk of temporarily accentuating an element in repression, and also temporarily reducing a desirable one, such rearrangements prove in their entirety to be curative. After an improvement has been attained through interruption of the conditions existing during insomnia, the desirable composition of intra-mental processes restores itself.

7. It is not only for the sake of a superficial analogy that this detour has been made in the course of this discussion of the social problem. The full aim of referring to the problem of sleep and hypnotics was to point out that interference with the spontaneity of the mind can indeed, if properly carried out, result in the improvement of the psychic functions. In other words, a planned interference may lead to a condition in which the amount of satisfying processes actually increases, and that of those causing solely intra-mental tension decreases. This ought, in reality, to have very little to do with dictatorial regimes, with suppression of human liberty and with obstructing the development of individual variations, as feared by some readers of my previous book. The suggestion is, in fact, concerned with the improvement of the human race, of the social and individual aspect of its members; just as the gardener tries to improve the character of flowers and plants, to suit a refinement in taste and new modes in using them. Through measures suggested below, the social aspect of the individual should be modified to the satisfaction of *all* concerned. The outlines of the programme referring to this are as follows:—

8. Let us create for the affairs of society a working hypothesis that unreasonable selfishness of the individual and also unnecessary and officious interference with human happiness is something that is " not done ", something of a low category, comparable to burglary or wanton adultery. A similar hypothesis has been

maintained in children's education—partly usefully, though very much in excess—through pretending to deny the universality and naturalness of libidinal tendencies. Well, all who know the realities of life and its psychoaffective laws, know how untrue this hypothesis is and always was. But on the other hand, its actual influences—beneficial and otherwise—cannot be overrated. Thus a hypothesis, if insistently applied in the conditioning of human character, can have far-reaching effects, and this even in the case when the agent to be modified is such a potent force as the libido with all its ramifications. (Cf. Appendix II : The Libido ; also The Libido and the Social Faculty.)

9. It is only too true that selfishness and the psychoneurotic desire for domination, as well as officious narrowness of outlook, have the appearance of quasi-natural tendencies, being strong and widespread. For all practical purposes they strive for manifestation too intensely to be really negligible. But this is the very reason for the necessity of the programme here suggested. In this way a hypothesis is to be created, implying not only that such tendencies are despicable in principle, or in moments of leisurely devotion to ideals, but that their manifestation is indeed harmful to the social reputation and even to the material interests of the subject. Of course such a working hypothesis can be of no value if it is not perceptibly manifested in spheres of concrete life. That is the reason why I speak of a *working hypothesis* and not merely of a religious principle or ethical ideal.

The individual, each individual, will of course realize that there is a gap between the naturalness of such a hypothesis and what he occasionally does feel to be striving within himself for manifestation. But, as elsewhere in education and social conditioning, the working hypothesis referred to should be capable of becoming potential agent, a factor of considerable reality.

10. The reader ought to be aware that so great a thing as the social approval of the subject is involved in this conflict-laden process. Love overcomes so many things ; and so does the desire for love, and the prospect of attaining it through adherence to certain modes of thought and conduct. It is simply impossible that a working hypothesis such as that under consideration here should fail in its effect on the human mind, both in its conscious and deeper spheres. It is probable that the attitude of the mind towards the new element would be bipolar, as is the case with all human tendencies. There is no practical harm in this ; there is

the possibility of fair and even pleasant mental harmony, in spite of the presence of bipolarities.

The soundness of an enterprise is not actually affected, though its management may be complicated, by very heavy expenses, if the ultimate profit is satisfactory. Bipolarity does not, of course, make the working of a desirable intra-mental factor simpler.[1] But this cannot be helped. A number of psychic processes are concerned with tasks ensuing from this fundamental bipolarity, and even multipolarity, existing with respect to practically everything psychological. In the same way men's minds will certainly be able to cope with the contradiction existing between individualistic tendencies and the social hypothesis under discussion. If in the wake of such a reform society should become more balanced, more calm, more capable of offering peace and stability to the individual, the aforementioned intra-mental conflict or contradiction should easily decide itself in favour of emphasizing the one and, as far as possible, neglecting the other.

To conclude in words manifesting a keener sense of realities and possibilities than perhaps shown by the discussions on this point so far, I should like to state :—

Improvements in human life depend on the degree to which the above suggestion is being or will be carried out. To the extent to which the above conditioning proves to be incapable of materialization, things will in essence remain the same as they have been. And this, so I feel, will be the case in spite of any progress in the formalities of the social administration and distribution of the existing material resources.

[1] In some instances, however, bipolarity is put in the service of intra-mental counterregulation.

# CHAPTER XIV

## THE PROBLEMS OF RELIGION AND INSTINCTUAL REPRESSION

*Compliance with religious morality and the desire for liberty of behaviour.—It appears that traditional morality is indispensable, though the number of its casualties might be diminished.—A feasible way of relieving mankind lies in a general increase of personal significance.—This has to be a political principle, not a religious or charitable one.—Over-sensitiveness towards instinctual elements of the* self *may not occur if the feeling of personal significance be satisfactory.—Human genesis of morals, and the additional element of their absoluteness.—Metaphysical craving is universal.—The purely objective mode of thought and judgment might have disastrous consequences for society.—For this reason an intentional cultivation of the spiritual element appears to be indispensable.—The struggle between " good " and " bad " creates a dynamic* conscience.—*Cultivation of the religious element goes hand in hand with the potentials of prejudice.—The function of the mind is impossible without undesirable by-products.—Intolerance of the intrinsic " bad " makes aggressive projection possible.—Repression of religious tendencies may, likewise, produce prejudice.—The " ethnic soul ".—The prejudiced free-thinker.—The mental scotoma of the psychologist.*

1. Psychoanalysis of people suffering from psychoneuroses could not fail to stimulate the question whether our moral conceptions and the ways of enforcing them might not require an overhaul. There has been much justifiable discussion on the rôle that might be ascribed to sexual forces by unbiased research, as well as on the customary measures of interfering with this sphere of life in the name of social discipline and morality. A comparable interest has been devoted to the universal phenomenon of religious thirst and to the feeling of moral guilt preceding or following the acceptance of a theocratic ideology. The cry for ridding mankind from the burdens of both categories has not ceased to be heard both in scientific and popular quarters. A large number of psychoneurotic sufferers, as well as social misfits, are held up as illustrations of unhealthy " repression " and " sense of guilt ".

The realization is, however, growing that there is no easy way for a substantial increase in sexual and religious freedom. Mankind is not mature enough for dispensing with our traditional morals ; and, perhaps, by dint of human nature not even capable of such a radical change.

2. In human life with its needs for social organization there is no scope for the exclusive rule of one alternative principle. There will always be a necessity for compromise between the forces of freedom and those of suppression in the psychoaffective spheres of individuals. A number of psychoneurotics and misfits have to be considered as inevitable casualties in any system, should its advantages greatly outweigh its injurious effects.

Attempts at diminishing the number of such casualties remain a legitimate aim, and its materialization may be possible without really harming the moral potentials in society. There seems to be no sense in continuing, for instance, to foster the idea that masturbation before the age of sexual maturity is abnormal and harmful. Neither can we, with responsibility, deny the exclusive right of each individual to such a degree of sexual or religious freedom as he feels appropriate for himself, provided no encroachment on other people's life be involved.[1] Even less must we pretend to believe genuinely that homosexuality, for instance, is a particularly damnable vice, since we know with certainty that it is either inborne or a psychoneurotic symptom over which free will has no omnipotent control.[2] Fundamental morality in society will not decrease if people no longer believe that sexual activity in whatever form may be the cause of all imaginable

[1] Admittedly, the personality of an individual subdued by the personal obligations of marriage, as well as the needs of his family, is welcome in society ; the repressive influence of his status makes him more law-abiding, and concern for his family more cautious. A fair measure of order in society safeguards the welfare of those near and dear to him ; and from this altruistic motive, which is reinforced by fear of complications, the individual accepts social restrictions, even if as an unmarried person he might feel more as an individualist and behave in a more adventurous way. Thus, the principle of sexual freedom on the one hand and that of communal interest on the other, are more in clash than it would at first appear. It may be argued that in the interest of social order it is preferable that the individual members of society should have rather less than more emotional, and particularly sexual, freedom. No doubt this holds true for a large number of people of our era who have not been reared in the art of appreciating freedom as a means of a better development of the *self*.

The claims of religious ideology are, obviously, ignored in this discussion. However, it is only fair to realize that one of the strongest motives in the creation of religious ethics has been the aim of subduing the individual and securing the p ace of society. But through the metaphysical-mystical concepts of religious systems this utilitarian motive and its significance are greatly overlooked.

[2] Cf. Appendix III, pp. 290–2.

illnesses, or that unspeakable punishment awaits an individual in the after-life for having satisfied an urge, for the existence of which he is hardly responsible. We need not lament the passing of times when theological mistakes and the threat of imagined or invented consequences were the main buttresses of sexual ethics.

3. Notwithstanding all this intellectual progress sexual limitation and repression as well as a certain compliance with religious ideals will remain essentially part of human civilization ; at the same time people will continue to find religion, its dogmas, rituals, and restrictions, an interference with the spontaneity of life and ordinary common sense. And because this is so there will always be a number of people who have psychoaffective difficulties and who even develop psychoneurotic symptoms, either passing or of a permanent nature and disabling if not treated. No writer does a service to mankind who ignores the deep-rooted desire of an organized society for ideals and practical ethics. It is even necessary that certain principles become deep-rooted in the individual in order to secure their dynamic power through the phenomenon of conscience. This, nevertheless, need not exclude the clear knowledge by a person of average education that ethical principles are not of a dogmatic, revealed absoluteness. No dread of the after-life, nor threat of physical ailments, need be associated with the compulsory strength of moral tendencies. It is possible to be influenced by a *categorical imperative* without projecting it on to a heavenly judge.

We realize, however, that the belief in God will remain indispensable for millions both as a source of consolation as well as a source of conscience. And a substantial exercise in self-restraint, backed by the firm voice of conscience, will have to continue to be part of human civilization.

4. The feasible way of relieving mankind of unnecessary burdens lies elsewhere ; it has been suggested in various contexts throughout this work. An increase in personal significance of the average individual is called for. The feeling of significance ought to be the unalienable property of the individual. This change would be capable of eliminating many undesirable manifestations which current psychoanalytical conceptions have attributed to instinctual *repression* and the influence of *religion*. In order to be effective this personal significance of the individual ought to manifest

itself unequivocally in practical life. It ought to be a natural element in the dealings of all persons with their fellowmen. It has to be a political and economic principle and not a charitable religious one, if it is to be believed firmly enough by the masses of individuals and relied upon by them at any moment when their mind suggest their weakness in a given situation.

Psychoanalysis assumes that a person may feel uneasiness or even strong anxiety because, unconsciously for him, in the psychic depths there is an emergence of non-moral tendencies and these are perceived by the psychic apparatus as dangerous. It has been recognized by Freud and others that a particular strictness of the *super-ego* is not necessarily the outcome of a strict education in childhood. We have, therefore, to assume that there may exist a weakness of the psyche that results in unjustified anxiety when certain repressed elements exert their pressure. The anxiety is unfounded in so far that there is, in such cases, no risk at all of the tendency being translated into an apprehendable action. I suggest that the intolerance towards such unconscious processes would be much less were the individual's psyche stronger through having a firmer feeling of personal significance amidst his fellowmen.

A vast number of persons react with the feeling of jealousy, or hurt vanity, in response to events that do not objectively deserve their concern. We are wont to say that their " sense of inferiority " makes them so touchy. Were they in a position to enjoy a firmer feeling of personal significance than they do their exaggerated sensitiveness would probably not exist. A large number of *a*-social reactive traits would have no suitable soil for their development in people who feel socially secure in the sense indicated.

This assumption can be supported by individual cases where, owing to changed circumstances, or a new outlook imparted through psychological treatment, the social personality of people has improved. This is suggested with equal clarity by experiences of educationists gained in modern children's communities. The increased feeling of personal significance might work a miracle where previously neither strictness nor lenience was able to improve the social character of a difficult youth.

The phenomenon of an unreasonable sense of guilt, or of an overstrict super-ego that has developed without appropriate external pressure, becomes intelligible if we keep in mind the factor under discussion. Oversensitiveness towards instinctual elements, and an overstrict super-ego are secondary mental phenomena. An unsatisfactory feeling referring to the subject's personal significance probably creates a compulsion towards ejecting all traces of tendencies reminiscent of immoral conduct. The general sense of social smallness seeks for compensation in various ways ; and one of these may be a psychoneurotic intensity of self-purification.

5. The human genesis of our morals can be realized by anyone who dares to face such a conception. If nothing else then the obvious variations in legal, religious, and otherwise ethical notions throughout history and in different geographical regions would suggest this fact. Absoluteness of a moral principle can thus imply no more than its actual ability to further a fair distribution of opportunities, to protect men from unnecessary suffering and to give them some uplift of spirit. A metaphysical absoluteness of any ethical principle is merely a working hypothesis, no matter what system of philosophy has endorsed it. Even those who wish to have nothing to do with the commands of a divinity consider as *fundamental principles* of society the " sacredness of life " of every harmless individual, or the right of every human being to share in the opportunities of life. But they will have to admit that the validity of these fundamentals is based on no more than an arbitrary acceptance by common sense. If there is a feeling of " absoluteness " about these useful principles, it is as " religious " in its essence as any religious dogma in the customary sense. In other words, a common-sense judgment and an arbitrary acknowledgment of a principle may be surrounded by the additional sphere of " absoluteness ".

6. The introduction of such metaphysical elements into utilitarian morals in all likelihood answers a corresponding need in human life. What is felt to be in a sense absolute is adhered to more deeply than any principle where the subject's agreement with its usefulness is too obvious to the conscious mind. The halo of absoluteness safeguards the practical rôle of a principle. Apologists of religious customs and dogmas were at all times at pains to explain the sense and wisdom immanent in them. By this the unavoidable critical attitude of the believer's mind towards the extra-logical and extra-utilitarian elements in a religious system were to be countered. But the essential force that has secured belief in these things has been the element of extraneous revelation

ascribed to them. Men are likely to doubt the perfection of what is a product of their own mind, assuming that their self-made principles cannot be of a higher category than they themselves, being weak human creatures. From this feeling of human inadequacy, they are too prone to abandon their principles which, however greatly acknowledged by them, are representative of their own intellect. Great as the need may be for universal increase in objective, purely scientific thinking, the exclusion from life of quasi-religious elements may have dangerous implications.

7. There is on the purely objective level of thought no place at all for genuine ethical attitudes towards one's fellowmen. There can only prevail a strictly utilitarian view on action and omission. It is, for instance, quite legitimate for a person, who does not wish to be a saint, to strive for his aims in a competitive manner. A scientist is applauded if he succeeds, in a heated discussion, not merely in proving his point but also in disclosing the weaknesses in the statements of others. He is considered as being right in doing so, though no harm at all might befall the world if he refrained from emerging victorious in what is only a theoretical question. It is also approved if a writer or actor draws to himself the attention of the public through his superb performances, though inevitably several other writers or actors to some extent have to suffer a defeat through this.

These instances have been cited to introduce the problem under discussion, because the legitimacy and even loftiness of the aggressive conduct in these spheres might be the least controversial. The exercise of skill and ingeniousness in all walks of life is encouraged, if for no other reason than for the sake of the highest achievements in production, science, art, and sport. The inevitable defeat of the less successful is tolerated and legalized even though limited by a few regulations. What is thus legally limited is, however, not the spirit of aggression but the number of acts and to an extent the crudeness of their form. On the strictly objective level of thought there are only restrictions as well as deterrent measures agreed upon, but no principles absolute in the metaphysical sense.

There appears indeed no logical reason why the person who in a certain situation is the stronger partner should refrain from proceeding recklessly to his heart's content. To comply with the law implies for him an escape from the punitive restrictions of his life, and secures for him the advantages that an organized society offers to its free citizens. But there is in all this no element of *absoluteness* as felt by " moral conviction ". Where the individual is not likely to incur disadvantage, and when no bias of love interferes with his decision, purely objective logic should militate in favour of ruthlessness.[1]

Unquestionably there is also in those who do decidedly believe in absolute morals a perceptible tendency to ignore the claims of the ethical principle. Yet, even with a stronger emphasis, a self-directed moral indignation compels the subject to abandon the " temptation " in favour of the ethical alternative. It must not be doubted that the subject's preference for the ethical alternative *is* genuine. But his love of the ethical cannot spring from the spheres of objectivity. There is, apparently, no objective and logical motive for feeling happy about our virtue of self-restraint.[1]

Admittedly there is one trend of thought that may link the genuine love of the ethical with the utilitarian viewpoint. The law-abiding and ethical attitude of others, it is true, is a practical safeguard of the subject's own life and ease. Hence, so it may be argued, the subject likes to shroud the utilitarian principle of social adaptation with a loftiness of absolute ethics in a metaphysical sense, in order to contribute to the validity of laws regulating life.

It may also be assumed that the tendency to please one's own conscience is an heir to the infantile tendency of pleasing the adults for the sake of receiving their care and love and avoiding their displeasure. Thus the ultimate preference of morals for their own sake develops from an originally utilitarian situation.

However convincing this genetic analysis of morals may be on the objective level of thought it does not vindicate this transformation from the utilitarian into the irrationally absolute. This transformation is, obviously, a function of quasi-religious forces in the human being. From a purely utilitarian viewpoint there is no necessity for the individual habitually to adhere to ethical principles for their own sake, considering them as " absolute ".

8. Obviously the domination of minds by pure science and objective truth in general might have serious implications, anti-

[1] See, however, pp. 273–7, the discussion of the social sense.

social and anti-cultural. Such a frame of mind would advise against the ethical alternative in the vast majority of people on most occasions ; and often enough even in the few exceptionally just persons. The objective truth is that advantage and pleasure are overriding forces in feeling and action, provided that untoward consequences are unlikely to ensue. In borrowing Freudian terminology we might speak of a combination of the pleasure and reality factors.

Admittedly, spiritual experiences may likewise give satisfaction to the subject, a satisfaction that is comparable with pleasures of a concrete nature. Impressions of artistic character are enjoyable to such a degree that, for their sake, gains of a less refined type might be readily ignored. Nevertheless, on the purely objective level of experience and thought, self-discipline for its own sake is not by necessity enjoyable. This occurs only in compliance with mental forces of a quasi-religious nature.

We should be reluctant to trust the future management of human society to an outlook governed solely by " rational facts ". Conscience, to a degree that is necessary for the maintenance of average peace within society, cannot develop on a rational soil sterilized entirely of illusions of the ethical-religious category. The logical contradiction between the outlooks of objectivism and spiritual illusionism will always exist. But this contradiction will never enforce an exclusive decision in favour of the pure objectivism in human life.

9. The recognition of these facts should lead inevitably to an attitude towards the " illusionistic " aspect of mental life that goes beyond sheer tolerance. What is important for human life has to be an object of intentional cultivation. Ethical ideologies of various types, as well as the " religious " element of the mind in general, will have to be developed by individual education and general literature. The growth of moral conscience must remain part of the programme in the education of children and youth. It is no use ignoring this fact, and certainly, the objective social scientist in particular does well to assess this aspect of social life appropriately. Any attempt at leaving it out of his equations must render his formulæ of dubious value, as they will not be in line with present facts and coming events. He may annul for himself the significance of religious currents in society ; but life will continue to produce and to rely on this form of human " energy ". It is better from the

outset to include the intentional cultivation of metaphysics in social programmes and social administration.

10. But this implies, inevitably, so it appears, that at the same time mechanisms of potential prejudice are actively stimulated and helped along in their development. The careful reader of previous chapters will have guessed this, and the discussion to follow here links up directly with what has been suggested in Chapters III A and C.

The function of conscience is essentially dependent on a struggle between "good" and "bad". This process of competition goes on subconsciously at least as much as in the conscious spheres. There is sufficient reason to assume that the extent of this process in subconscious regions is, in fact, far superior to that consciously realized. This accounts for the unexpected emergence of moral scruples insistently vetoing a thought or a step that has already taken place irrevocably.

The dynamic rôle within the psyche of what is felt as "bad" is not inversely proportionate to the extent of the forces of "good". The dynamic pressure within the mind of "tabooed" tendencies does not always decrease in direct proportion with the growth of the "good". It was pointed out by Freud that the adoption of a strict moral measure (stern super-ego), leading to an extensive repression of instinctual currents, may actually increase the sense of guilt; instead of bringing moral peace to the subject extensive repression may render the claims of the super-ego increasing. That is to say, the pressure on moral harmony of a condemned element may be strong, despite its quantitative attributes having been cut to a minimum so as to render it non-existent in practice. This implies that the pathogenic strength of any element classed as "bad" and "dangerous" depends on the degree of tolerance displayed towards it—or its very shadow—by the integrated personality. Endopsychic intolerance in this respect may be very substantial; and the ensuing reactive process may lead, amongst other phenomena, to the growth of social intolerance manifested through prejudice. (See Chapter III.)

On a purely objective level of thinking there should be no opportunity of reacting with prejudice formation. Not only because the imaginary character of such a formation would be recognized and the prejudiced attitude rejected. But chiefly because from the outset there could not be that irrational fear of the "bad" dwelling within the mind; consequently there would not emerge from this source an incentive to projection and symbolism of the " bad ".

11. As long as " conscience " in the individual is socially desirable its growth cannot really occur without the intrapsychic moral bipolarity as described above. It appears that the tension implied by this bipolarity is the very source of the pressure exercised on the subject by his " conscience ". The positive desire for the " good " is not enough to secure its victory against the claims of the opposite tendency. There might be a passivity, as if giving up at times the enjoyment of the " good " and allowing the alternative feeling or action to assert itself. In other spheres of life, too, there are moments of quite sensible passivity that result in the person's remaining content with a lesser achievement, if the much better thing, originally desired and preferred, could not be attained without strain. In the bipolarity of " good " and " bad " the latter partner plays an important rôle in the service of the former. It is necessary to feel not only the difference between the two alternatives, but at the same time the impact of the " bad ", by which experience the possession of the " good " is made more precious. Anything valuable becomes more appreciated if a threat of having to part with it appears on the horizon. This is, in approximate terms, the reason why pressure of the " bad " is necessary for the maintenance of " conscience " in a sufficiently dynamic rôle.

On a purely objective level of thought the " bad " is not necessarily dangerous for the integrity of the personality. What is considered inferior, and in addition unavoidable, as for instance a particle of dust or a measure of noise, is likely to be ignored or merely tolerated. The elements of " bad " would not play the rôle suggested here if they were perceived by the mind merely as things unavoidable and inferior. Consequently a conscience to any satisfactory extent could not operate. To secure this a distinct awareness of the two moral poles has to prevail resulting in a tension of bipolarity between two unspecified (non-conceptual) but still clearly distinguished main elements representing " good " and " bad " in general.

12. All processes of the mind, however well attained their particular goal, include a number of by-products. In addition the degree of perfection in endopsychic performances varies

greatly in various individuals. Such by-products are bound to be large particularly in view of the bipolarities (and multi-polarities) existing in all the component processes of the psyche.

It is, therefore, inevitable that the bipolarity of moral attitudes, charged so intensely with polar tension, should result in the creation of some untoward elements. Prejudice is one of these products. It is associated with the intolerance of the " bad " in human beings, the subject included. The very enthusiasm for the " good ", as well as the enjoyment of one's capacity for self-restraint, belongs to the category of sentiments that include some passion of prejudice. The existence of the process on which conscience is based at the same time makes prejudice possible. The educational influences furthering the growth of ethical sense not only encourage the " good " and discourage the " bad ", but implicitly maintain a polar tension with all its potential sequelæ.

13. It appears that suppression by outside influence of " illusionistic " tendencies may result in mental products that suggest a failure in the repression of instincts on the deeper levels. In a number of people the forcible neglect of their ethical thirst facilitates the development of psychoneurosis proper. In a vast number of individuals the outcome of such suppression is a biased outlook in mundane spheres of life. They may become fanatics of political convictions to a degree that makes them uncompromising and even apparently illogical in particular questions of social life. There is in some of these individuals a definite paranoiac trend with regard to a problem towards which their particular bias manifests itself. For these people their principle may mean more than a means for the attainment of actual peace, contentedness, and order within their environment. They may entirely ignore the beneficial aims for the sake of which this particular principle was advocated by the authentic founders and authoritative exponents. They are also lacking in the elements of prudent diplomacy with which the more sane adherents of the same principle proceed in social life. One cannot fail to be reminded of the uncompromising claims of religious dogmas and laws where intransigent validity is upheld, however painful may be the sacrifice involved for the subject or for his fellowmen.

This outcome of religious repression may be surprising in view of the bias generally exhibited in the past by people who rigidly adhered to their denominational ideology and rituals. Nevertheless it is a fact that bias and narrow-mindedness are not privileges of the zealous believer. In both instances the phenomenon is due to the unsuccessful repression of the freedom of the mind. In the case of the religious fanatic it is the obstruction of the free expansion of his intellect and critical faculty that produces the aggressiveness of his ideological bias. And in the alternative case of suppressed " illusionism " there is a restriction of the mind that is comparable to the former type. Undoubtedly the religious tendency likewise aims at the expansion of the psychic spheres, through projecting on to God and the after-life the perfection and power unattainable to the mortal subject.

Surely there are individuals who have no desire to any perceptible extent for revealed religion, for reliance on God, and for immortality. Likewise, the number of those whose structure of personality apparently gains by being freed from the fear of God and the idea of after-life, is very substantial. But a certain type and extent of quasi-religious illusionistic function appears to be indispensable for the vast majority of people if they are to enjoy a fair degree of peace of mind.

The result of suppression of religion cannot be equal in all individual circumstances. In the presence to a substantial degree of scientific accomplishment, which preferably includes the fundamentals of modern psychology, the gradual severance with theistic notions may have no untoward results. There is something to fill the gap satisfactorily, whilst, at the same time, the mind is more free for the experience of happiness and for unfettered productivity. If, however, culturally backward groups are suddenly freed of religious traditions, the outcome must be undesirable from an ideal point of view. An analogy from pharmaco-physiology may illustrate the phenomenon.

There are drugs specifically capable of influencing the vegetative-autonomic system. It has been realized that the result of their application is not independent of the balance of tone prevailing in this system previous to the medication. Therefore, the amount necessary for a certain effect varies with the pre-existent balance and tone within the system, and so does the quality of the reaction. We may compare with this the case where religious forces are suppressed, whether through political pressure or forceful propaganda in the name of Science. The pre-existent mental status in that group will determine the success of the repression and the quality of its secondary products.

14. The "soul" of the individual in a specified ethnographic group differs from the individual "soul" of another national region. Two different groups dwelling in two distant regions of the globe may subscribe, for instance, to the same religious denomination, but deep down this general identity includes differences in the minute composition of the religious pattern existing within the minds.

The Roman Catholicism of two individuals in two different countries, for instance, is in the deeper psychological sense not quite identical. And a similar divergence might hold true of two Socialists or Conservatives, who hail from different ethnical soils. The impact of a dogma or idea on the subconscious psyche of various individuals must result in a variety of repercussions and interpretations. We should be reminded of the Rorschach tests where undefined figures (blots) are differently interpreted by various individuals. Likewise an idea, however well defined in terms of word-expression, contains much that is not defined or that permits of a further elaboration or alternative interpretation. This additional element is provided by the specific psyche of the individual or ethnical group. Thus the social or political manifestations of Roman Catholicism, of Socialism, or Conservatism (in its various senses) may at times show local differences, unexpected by those who believe in the literal sense of such notions.[1]

Even more interesting is the existence of similar differences in the reactions displayed by various freethinkers and "materialists". Only some of these people justify the anticipatory picture which people have about their personality. Not a few freethinkers betray conspicuously prejudiced reactions toward particular questions. In the recent clash between sane humanity and psychopathic brutality not all freethinkers sided with Logos and Ethos.

Persons known to their environment as freethinkers, but whose minds have become prone to mass-prejudice owing to unsuccessful repression of infantile elements—both libidinal and religious—have proved to be a particular danger to peace and justice. Their otherwise scientific ideology recommends them to the masses, and all that they say and advocate, even if clear nonsense or obvious prejudice, may thus receive an authoritative backing.

The repression of religious elements is a problem deserving more examination than afforded to it so far. Scientists capable

[1] Cf. Ch. IIIc, 2.

of dealing with this phenomenon may, in many instances, be indifferent to it, because of a specific scotoma they themselves have in this respect. In the field of medical psychology, Stekel and Jung enriched the literature with useful observations on the psychological rôle of religion. In the wider field of social behaviour much knowledge might be gained by psychologists focusing their attention on this special point.

# CHAPTER XV

## INTERNATIONAL ORGANIZATIONS

*This work does not deal in detail with international difficulties.—The prospect of substantial improvement through international bodies, at present, appears remote.—Only the belief and hope in such future results may have a beneficial effect on the minds of people at large.—It is doubtful whether a happier frame of mind would leave the individual fit enough for times of emergency.—The complicated problem of small nations with powerful neighbours.—Violence and revolutions.—The dual aspect of such phenomena from the viewpoint of the party in power.—Prejudice plays a great rôle in the behaviour of both the revolutionary party and the one defending the* status quo.*—How manifestations of discontent or attempts at reforms are frequently dealt with.*

1. This work does not deal explicitly with the discords in the international world. It merely registers the repercussions of these events in the life of national communities and the mental spheres of the individual ; but the author is reluctant to go further in this work. It ought to be clear to the student of human affairs that ethnic peculiarities of the mass psyche are deep-rooted irrational forces, not justifying much optimism. Moreover, the absence of genuine democratic tradition in most parts of the world is hard to replace adequately by a forceful short-term policy.

2. The coming era of the U.N.O. offers comparatively little prospect—almost none—for a deeper change in mentality all over the world. Indispensable though this great organization will be for the immediate future the critically minded sociologist must not over-estimate its potentialities. Prevention of wars, control of atomic energy, a certain improvement in the distribution of raw materials are tasks extensive and great enough to render this organization a vital factor for mankind. The full securing of these aims even for decades may, however, leave

untouched spheres of social life that breed disharmony, aggressiveness, and the desire for archaic aims. An ideological propaganda through the medium of print and wireless is not a force capable of competition with deep-rooted ethnic peculiarities, particularly if ideological prejudice is presented as daily food to the citizen. The few idealists existing all over the world feel glad to read and hear about a more refined atmosphere on a specific spot on earth. They may respond by letters to the newspapers or by books they write voicing their agreement and hopes. Unsophisticated people may think—as they have done more than once—that the world of harmony is in the making. Official circles of various countries may support their distinguished citizens in making mellifluous utterances when addressing the world abroad. This, however, must not lull into complacency any sociologist who wishes to base his writings on reliable assumptions.

3. Fortunately, wishing is a potent factor in creating pleasant hypotheses ; and in particular, the desire to get rid of deficiencies and sufferings creates a confident belief in future improvements. Thus, in many unsophisticated minds a hope in an extensive power of U.N.O. will decrease tension and make for more spontaneity in living. A child, because it is ignorant of all the difficulties that beset the adult world, is able to live with greater spontaneity than grown-up people do. A hypothesis, if not obviously contradicted by experience or theoretical but established knowledge, may be as strong a factor as any picture of reality. It seems, however, that because of the extent to which trends of contemporary history do contradict the optimistic hypothesis, the sum-total of aggressiveness within human groups is unlikely to decrease.

Reforms and expectations of improvement will have, therefore, to confine themselves to intra-national spheres. In spite of turbulent waves reaching a country from the general international tension, gradual progress in internal harmony is a feasible thing.

Unfortunately it is not quite certain that a happier and more peaceable frame of mind would leave the individual fit enough for wars brought on by unavoidable emergency. It is the dormant restlessness, resentment, and destructiveness that counteract the natural reluctance to sacrifice one's comfort and risk one's life. Idealism and the realization of emergency are complementary factors, but hardly capable of rendering superfluous the contribution by the afore-mentioned volcanic elements of the mind. The idea of a preventive war or that of armed intervention in aid of a smaller nation or group brutalized by a superior power, is not popular enough amongst the masses of average people, and would hardly animate them to sacrifice their comforts and lives. It still appears to be the case that the masses of average people present an easily manageable material with which to wage a war, if they are to any extent enslaved both by external administration and a surplus of mental difficulties. For this reason a type of human being approaching the ideal, as imagined by psychologists, might not be sufficiently interested even in defensive wars. Obviously this indifference might prove a questionable virtue, were the desire for peace and international justice, at a certain period of history, only a unilateral sentiment not appreciated by a powerful would-be aggressor.

4. This leads us to the problem of the small nations. In theory it ought to matter really very little to which state-organization a certain geographical region or group of people belongs. Sovereignty of nations, small or large, is a thing of no absolute significance in itself. If large state-organizations would be concerned solely with securing their people's happiness, then small groups would in all likelihood prefer to belong to a " bloc ". But as the case is sovereignty has meant power over others, and has been employed frequently for political pressure, for obliteration of the souls of small nations and for various degrees of exploitation. It is, however, more than probable that the rigid adherence of small nations to their sovereignty is not only the result of fear of oppression but an independent archaic tendency shared by all types of nations.

5. It has been pointed out that the existence of small nations constitutes an allurement to aggression by big powers. On the other hand, it has been suggested that the very existence of small countries ought to be considered by big neighbours an opportunity for developing in themselves the virtuous art of self-restraint. The advice is surely more of a religious sermon than social psychology. The facts of history do not testify favourably to the capacity of large powers to refrain from temptations of conquest or coercion when an opportunity—or some economic necessity—arises. We should not advise, for instance, an artificial

increase in the number of small sovereignties merely to give larger countries the benefit of practising the art of self-restraint. The fundamental danger lies in the very notion of archaic sovereignty, whether attached to a small or big country. The other fundamental wrong lies in the idea of power wielded *at the cost* of minorities. It is of a certain advantage that small independent nations are scattered among the large state-organizations. Each representing a peculiar soil for political conceptions, the opportunity for the creation of large homogeneous blocks is rendered less easy. Such a division of the world into large political-ideological blocs would be a danger rather than a blessing in view of the fact that the equality in well-being of human groups is not yet the aim of all foreign politics.

6. There can, therefore, be no short-term plan for an effective international social psychology. Diplomacy in the traditional sense will continue to struggle with problems that emerge because of economic inequalities and psychological differences between nations. These two factors prevent any real agreement on a basic social ideology.

7. Violence of all degrees has played throughout history a great part in the pursuit of large-scale changes in national and communal affairs. Mass demonstrations of a menacing character, political murder, bloody revolutions, civil and aggressive wars, account for not a few reforms and results that have received the sanction of posterity. The cynical saying is only too true that a revolution, if successful, becomes a legal factor, whereas it remains a crime if it has been defeated. It is a fact that comparatively little has been achieved through peaceful measures; therefore, the outright condemnation of "idealistic violence" may appear a trifle unrealistic to those who feel that their lives in the broader sense are not satisfactorily safeguarded. It appears that those who are in superior power and possession will have first to prove to the world that they themselves are able to give, to yield, and to accept limitation without being forced by threat of war or economic attacks; then the world might settle down at least to the belief in peaceful measures and try out the principle.

8. Revolutions and political murders are the work of passion that is based on prejudice in the psychological sense. The cause

or claim, which is the conceptional label of the passionate attitude, may be anything from pure justice to fully-blown delusion. The emotional forces arrayed behind the slogan are to the least degree stimulated by the objective aspect of the problem. It is possible that a cool examination of the political or economic plight of a wronged minority precedes the decision to violent activities ; but these could not be carried out without employing mental forces that are in essence pre-existent prejudice in a dormant form.

The reception of the revolutionary action by the attacked party, and also its perception by the neutral or distant observers, is likewise coloured by irrational emotions and particular prejudices.

In general, murder by a professional gangster or manslaughter in the heat of an argument causes but a short-lived public indignation. After a day or two most people feel no substantial interest in the tragedy, except for individuals whose mind has been prepossessed by a death-wish against someone. The indifference equally refers to the fate of the victim and to the crime of the assailant. This is satisfactory as long as society employs officials and a press to watch the interest of the community. It is better if the average citizen forgets the murder and continues to feel and think in terms of his ordinary life.

The assault becomes an object of protracted interest when forces of prejudice keep it alive. This is the case when racial, national, or religious feelings in the observers are aroused through a violent act by an individual member of a different group. Though there may be in a certain case no reason whatsoever to assume that the motives of the violent act are national or religious, a large number of people will react to the news with prejudiced passion and call for a " holy war ". And if the motive of revolutions or violent acts is avowedly political, religious, or national, then it is only possible for a very few observers not to have their vision clouded by irrational elements.

9. As a rule there is not much indignation if a psychotic behaves violently. Nor, in fact, does the violence motivated by prejudice deserve a different reaction, apart from the legal and expedient counter-measure to be taken. The fully-fledged psychotic can be charged with no responsibility whatever. On this point psychiatry and law are in agreement. The revolutionary, on the other hand, does *not* usually expect mercy if he is defeated.

In several instances the political murderer and the revolutionist, standing up against the existing order, wish to take the risks of their actions. It is up to the party attacked by them to defend itself and to protect, with all the available legal means, what is generally (or by those in office) deemed to be the right cause. It is fair to deal with both the act of violence and its sentimental motives according to their individual merits. That is to say, sabotage or murder, if not committed in self-defence or personal desperation, remains legally a crime; the alleged motive ought to be looked on with the eyes of a psychologist, that is, either with true sympathy or with pity because of its psychopathological nature, as the case may be. This is the only course justifiable by logic and fairness.

In practice, however, such events are handled differently. Attempts at revolutionary changes as well as political murders are not infrequently examined from the angle of existing political or economic interests. This is the natural consequence of the fact that there does not yet exist a society where that which is common is more dynamic than the interests of particular groups. This problem of *community* does not refer to mere emotional fellow-feeling, but to the phenomenon of community in concrete as well as in ideological spheres. In the absence of such circumstances separatist ideologies are likely to develop, enforced by elements of prejudice.

On several occasions the passion of prejudice in a certain group has been used by another party for its own ends, for precipitating developments of a desired kind. Not rarely the prejudiced attitudes are even fostered from a hidden background, by *agents provocateurs*, for the incitement of that group, or its victims, to excessive manifestations that are likely to lead to the ruin of one or both parties. By such tactics also a principle or aim that in itself is justifiable and even approvable might be made to appear utterly disreputable. From the success or failure alone of a revolutionary movement it is hardly possible to judge its intrinsic value; support or opposition of it may or may not indicate a sound judgment on the problem. Elements other than objective weighing up are contained in mass attitudes, and frequently also in the deliberate policies of leading bodies. A psychologically exact attitude is not yet the foundation of all approaches in dealing with the revolutionary aims or grievances of a group.

# CHAPTER XVI

## CLOSING WORDS

*Prejudice is the pivotal element in almost all social anomalies.—Conceptual and emotional factors in judgment.—All impressions have an additional symbolic significance for the mind.—The stimulation of complexes.—There is no possibility of eliminating these irrational elements from the psyche.—Being psychoanalysed or psychoanalytically trained is no sufficient protection against the impact of these factors.—The peculiarities that have been characteristic of members of analytical schools are the results of their particular repressions.—All rigid systems, whether psychological or politico-social, go together with an amount of repression.—The up-to-date psychologist ought to deal with the* repressed aspect *in all systems; this refers also to such ideal movements as socialism.—The planned environmental influence ought to aim at an optimal effect.—Simplicity of life may mean to the modern man something more valuable than to the individual of primitive epochs.*

1. THE writer thinks that the pivotal element in the innumerable manifestations of social difficulties is the mental phenomenon called prejudice. Having in mind the psychological discussion of this many-sided problem in the various chapters of this work the reader will have recognized that actually the notion of prejudice cannot be confined to the customary sense of the word. Processes of the kind that lead to ordinary mass-prejudice may be operative in the course of all the judgments and reactions of the subject.

2. In every judgment there is a conceptual and an emotional element. We expect a logically appropriate relationship to exist between the two components. Both the quality and the amount of the emotional counterpart should conform to the conceptual content of the whole mental element. But everyday experience shows that the quantitative factor in the emotional accompaniment is frequently larger than is logically justified.

In a minority of cases also the quality of the emotional response associated with an event, impression, or thought appears different from what we should ordinarily expect. A statement or incident may evoke in a particular person resentment, disgust, or vague anxiety, whereas others present are not affected in the same way.

This latter possibility can be accounted for by the assumption that the statement or incident has for the person in question a symbolic meaning of its own, in addition to, or in excess of, the literal one ; and the unexpected emotional reaction is appropriate to this parallel meaning. In fact there is no external impression without its simultaneous symbolic meaning for the *subconscious*. This is the reason for the employment by language of many words in a figurative sense besides its literal one. The large-scale transformation of concrete impressions by the dream is explained by the same phenomenon. In all cases the objective event evokes in the subject not only emotional response of a certain quality, but at the same time it stimulates symbolic associations in the psychic depths, and for this reason the original impression implies something different from, or much more than, its conscious content. Owing to an efficient intrapsychic regulation these secondary meanings stimulate only subconscious processes, without being allowed to interfere substantially with the conscious emotional sphere and associated behaviour. But in a number of instances concrete events are responded to in a way not easily accountable by common sense. It must be realized that such an extraordinary apperception of an impression can only occur in a mind where there is at the time a pre-existent pathological element capable of being stimulated too easily. (Cf. Appendix II, p. 249.) We realize that such a state of affairs is fundamentally similar to intra-mental circumstances making for the formation of well-defined prejudice. In the latter case, too, an external element, be it a person, or the mention of an idea, unpleasantly stimulates a burdensome intra-mental element, and becomes the object of the resentment and aggressive hatred respectively. A person who is exceptionally sensitive to a popular or vulgar melody, or to the sight of a cheap piece of art, is one instance of this phenomenon. All those with a more average mental composition may be moved only to ridicule these things or will ignore them.

3. A great number of people become irritable, and display cynicism betraying some uneasiness, when psychoanalytical

explanations of human phenomena are attempted in their presence. We see, then, clearly that *stimulation of a complex* within their mind has occurred.

Much more frequent are the instances where there is only obviously overdone passion associated with a judgment or objection, though basically the quality of the emotional reaction conforms to that of average persons in a similar situation. This superfluity of zeal springs from sources other than the recent impression that has brought it out. In such cases there are two component reactions ; one referring to the recent impression and the other to a pre-existent subconscious element. It is as if we have opened the gate to chase out the dog and cannot prevent the impetuous little boy from running out too.

4. Such additional and irrelevant emotional reactions operate in all human relationships. All the apparently unnecessary passion in discussion of various kinds is attributable to the presence of subconscious tensions that avail themselves, for the sake of abreaction, of various concrete incidents. In a large number of persons the *ad hoc* association between a recent and objective event on the one hand and a pre-existent intra-mental process on the other takes place too easily. The impression created by an incident of no apparent importance is shifted on to a track where it lets loose a process of an independent content. Thus an additional amount of zeal or passionate opposition is produced.

5. It is hard to see how these phenomena of ordinary life could be eliminated. The individual's psyche can never be free from such emotionally charged subconscious elements. No human being can ever live his life without a wealth of intra-mental processes, without a number of serious conflicts, without having to bear in himself, at any time, problems incapable of immediate or satisfactory solution. It appears possible, however, that through the knowledge of the phenomenon under discussion any person may, from time to time, be able to check himself. Theoretically one could assume that being analysed should constitute a particularly potent corrective against too much bias or superfluity of zeal. Indeed, in face of certain human problems that excite average people's mind the analysed psychologist's reaction may be exceptional. The news of various crimes and sexual perversions

is hardly able to evoke in him the passion so characteristic of a large number of people.

6. But it would be unfair—unfair to the non-analysed person—to ignore in this connection the almost unintelligible passion with which certain psychological circles meet " heretics ". One could justifiably contrast this intolerance on professional matters with their undubitable calm over other human phenomena.

7. For a considerable period I thought that repressed religious sentiments, to which so few psycho-analysts dare consciously subscribe, are responsible for this specific psychoanalytic intolerance. I have suggested that the system of their psychology is for many of them religion and dogma. Any violation of the system by others therefore evokes passionate resentment. I still maintain the validity of this explanation ; but I have come to realize that the problem is actually of wider scope. To be a psychoanalyst in the classical sense implies a transformation of the mind's function from the average into something artificial. However true our assumptions are as to the working of subconsciousness, it remains artificial to make this knowledge a dominant content of our consciousness, and a factor directing our apperception and thinking. Much of what is " normal " in belief and judgment for other people has to be, if not repressed, at least held in check by the psychoanalyst. This transformation of the outlook, and practically of the whole personality, appears to me exceptionally great in the case of those who are convinced (who have been " made " convinced) of the absoluteness of their particular school, whatever it may be. These psychologists have acquired, as a matter of fact, repressions peculiar to their professional group. Broadened as their outlook is in some directions it has been narrowed down on other planes of mental functioning. This obviously makes them prone to some kind of illogical reaction. The fact of having been analysed and being practising analysts has blocked many channels of psycho-neurotic abreaction customary in the case of average people ; consequently, their attitude towards their system becomes the main point at which their specific repressions and symptom formations can manifest themselves. Undoubtedly there are among medical men, physicists, and even philosophers individuals and groups with differing opinions, but they can still meet each

other and discuss problems within their domain. This has been much less the case with psychoanalysts.

8. A number of medical men and laymen interested in medicine have left their bodies to universities to be used in the course of pathological research. A few exceptional figures of medical history have become famous by submitting to experiments involving serious risks to themselves. Surely the members of various psychological bodies should have no objection if an author dares to draw conclusions from phenomena manifested within their circles. The science of social psychology has much to be thankful for to observations made on specific groups created for the furtherance of different aims. The group atmosphere in factories, in armies, in collective settlements, at schools and universities offers information on a number of specific social problems. And so I think that the circles of various psychological schools, if permeated by some rigid discipline of mind, should likewise be fit to offer valuable material for study to the all-round social psychologist.

9. The particular group phenomenon just discussed is only one instance of massive repression and its sequelæ. Where fundamental mental tendencies are repressed there is bound to result some surprising secondary product. Rigidity of outlook or overstressed rationalism, if dictated and backed by a group that is conceived as an influential part of society, appears to produce a type of " mass prejudice ". In the particular instance under discussion it is of no great social significance ; but its lesson seems to me very valuable.

10. I have advocated throughout this work a large-scale education of the thinking and feeling of people. I have assumed that environmental factors both of a material and of a spiritual nature can substantially influence and improve the subconscious of the members of a social group. I shall find general agreement with my thesis that a more genuine security afforded to the individual is bound to decrease the proneness to undesirable social phenomena. I ought to find a good deal of agreement with my suggestion that the environmental factor (approval or disapproval) is capable of deciding the course of prejudice in

a desirable or deplorable direction. But one fact seems to remain particularly obvious ; as obvious as it has been at all times to unsophisticated people ; it is the paramount significance of elementary emotional tendencies. Thus there will hardly ever be a society in which religion, or some equivalent of it, can be suppressed without producing dangerous or ridiculous results. Persons who prove an exception will always be in a minority. There will never be a society in which the vast majority of people will be able to exist happily without some measure of wilful blindness in the course of everyday life. Similarly, some measure of individuality, of tastes and modes, some degree of emotional freedom, even if not in conformity with strict logic, will ever remain a necessity for the members of a healthy human society. Accordingly, no planned social process that neglects these facts can ever result in a fairly reasonable world, a world that affords really human values. I am sure from a close observation of various contemporary individuals that those who believe in a too mechanical administration of human affairs are, as a rule, lacking in humane warmth and are not dependable where human tragedies call for appropriate action.

11. *In every rigidity, political or scientific, there is an element of unhealthy repression.* And individuals who feel at ease only within an excessively rigid system, whether it be a social or a scientific one, do so perhaps because their own fundamental psychoaffective structure is not stable enough for the enjoyment of more freedom. A person who expects every duty toward the needy, the weak, the sick to be performed by the impersonal State, feels so because he himself is poor in emotional qualities or fettered by inhibitions, thus unable to give himself to others.

12. These psychological facts have to be faced courageously by our contemporaries, though they are unpleasant. My explanation implies the presence of some weakness in the rigid political attitude of many who claim to stand for a system " of the best possible make ". I feel that in each period of cultural history the psychoanalyst of society has to discover the factor which is the *repressed element* in life. Should, for instance, there be the task of analysing socialistic tendencies, it would be the duty of the contemporary scientist to examine both aspects, those which are obviously beneficial and those which could be considered as

psychoneurotic sequelæ due to the suppression of non-socialistic tendencies. It is impossible to create, particularly within short periods, a new atmosphere without some measure of unhealthy repression. This is why I suggest that the best service psychologists can do to progressive social principles is a multi-dimensional and far-seeing research. The best and most approvable case may only lose in the long run by our ignoring its *repressive aspects*.

The suggestion of interfering with the automatism of mental processes refers thus *only* to environmental influences that are likely to ameliorate life ; and this ought to be measured by the concepts of a " humane " social psychology. The consistent pursuit of a one-sided system is a prudent political measure, but certainly not a process of scientific eugenics. No one of the so numerous and intransigent advocates of one-sided social programmes would like to be operated on by a surgeon who, in his own field of activity, is as biased as his patient is in the capacity of politician or civil servant. An environmental pressure, were it justifiable, should be, in fact, capable of furthering an intra-mental development that is felt fundamentally desirable by the deeper levels of the subject's mind.

There is no question of giving a compulsory direction to human wishing and striving that does not conform to the elementary tendencies of the average personality. But we are right in taking it for granted that peace and ease and friendship, and the emotional satisfactions ensuing from uncomplicated human relationships, are the essential aims of the human personality. All other individual aims and tendencies we may consider as reactive, and as attempts at compensation for the lack of these elementary satisfactions.

13. A firm public opinion that genuinely condemns aggression, genuinely frowns upon petty competition in inter-human affairs, would actually express the opinion of the deepest elementary layers of the human mind. It appears, indeed, that after the vicissitudes in the history of social structure and modes of thinking the vast majority of human beings wish to return to elementary peace and ease, to a quasi-idyllic form of life which has at all periods been conceived as desirable by a few thinkers at least. The individual of to-day is much more suited to appreciate and to live this type of life, because of the very disappointments suffered by society from the trial of various complicated modes

of existence. The joy a town dweller derives from a holiday in the country is more refined than the contentment of the people who live there. In an analogous way the human personality of modern times, in possession of up-to-date technical knowledge and of the modern outlook on human nature, should be more deeply attached to fundamental, elementary modes of human inter-relationship than were probably the members of a more primitive society in the past.

14. A person who wishes to retire into a life of simplicity after he individually has failed in various experiments of our customary competitive life, is as a rule not genuinely fond of this simplicity. His new attitude is rather that of an invalid who praises his arm-chair merely because he cannot walk and run. More often than not, after a period of retirement from competitive life, the individual forgets his past disappointment, and the attractions of customary life prompt him to return to it.

This would not be the case with respect to a reformed, more natural outlook of mankind as envisaged here. The modern man's subconscious craving for elementary modes of life is too well founded to be only a temporary attitude of tiredness. The picture of a complex and intricate world is constantly present in our minds through our very knowledge of modern science and its implications. The actual and potential sufferings associated with modern life serve as a constant warning against making complexity itself the desirable principle and aim of existence. Thus, by way of a corrective balance, the attractions of elementary simplicity are constantly kept alive within the mind. Moreover, it is a general human characteristic that the sudden realization of a possible loss renders the possession of a thing more valuable. This is why we may assume that the modern man's mind craves more genuinely for simplicity than it could have been the case in the less developed periods of human history.

If environmental influences of a tangible and spiritual nature should ever force the individual largely to abandon secondary *a*-social attitudes, this environmental pressure would only too readily be met half-way by what I suggest to be the elementary nucleus of the individual human personality.

# APPENDIX I

## THE MYSTICAL ROOT OF ANTI-JEWISH SENTIMENT

*Militant prejudice manifests itself in a large variety of fields.—The discussion of specific instances is not advisable.—Anti-Semitism is a certain exception.—It is fundamentally a religious complex.—The crucifixion and the Jews, as seen by the N.T., and later by religious prejudice.—The old Jewish sources of literature present a different picture.—All the essentials of modern ethics were already in vogue before N.T. times.—The "oral tradition" carried out various expositions to qualify crude features of the O.T.—Why it was impossible for the orthodox Jews of old to believe in a Christ who was the Son of God and died.—Dogmatic questions are no longer of interest; Christology was never part of Jewish theology.—Acknowledgment by orthodox Jewish theology of the human significance of all who are not devoted to idolatry and to immorality on principle.—Anti-Semitism prefers to speak of Jews collectively.—This is an anachronism.—The value of the advice to Jews to remain inconspicuous.—Various pretexts for anti-Jewish attitudes.—Instances of unrecognized deep-seated bias.—The much criticized extermination of the Heathens.—The problem of anti-Semitism as it stands to-day.—The disappearance of Christianity would be a definite loss to mankind in our epoch, and probably for a long time afterwards.—The lesson to be learned by social psychology from the history of religious anti-Semitism is the psychology of conversion by force in all spheres of life.—Such measures cannot result in a healthy spirit within human society.*

1. Resentful and militant prejudice is a universal phenomenon. It may enter any field of individual and social life. No period has made this fact clearer than the present one with all its national, political, and social complications. Certainly for the world at large these manifestations are at least as important, if not more so, than racial and religious prejudice in the sense known in the past. In those periods they were deemed the main instances of social paranoia; yet it is certain that all spheres of social and individual life may be permeated by this anomaly. What appears to be an almost tragic inability of various nations to come to some understanding is due, apart from tangible economic interests,

to the element of ethnical prejudice. There is no need to discuss particular instances [1]; in fact the sensitiveness prevailing at present in all parts of the political world might advise against the inclusion of such instances in a scientific work.

The phenomenon of anti-Semitism is fit to be an exception. It contains features from which various things can be learned about the whole problem.[2] Moreover, because of the universality and age of this phenomenon its discussion is free of the risks referred to above.

It has been a widespread social phenomenon in all Christian countries for centuries; and the symbolic significance of the Jew is a mental element of which very few individuals have been entirely free. Anti-Semitism has been, in the first instance, an indispensable programme of religious zeal; in addition it has been employed by individuals and parties in power for achieving economic gains. In periods when crude violence, such as robbing and mass murder, was not in accordance with the general trend, this prejudice has at least been of great interest for people, with a considerable influence on cultural life. Its significance for the present cannot be understood without the knowledge of some historical details relating to it. Here the religio-mystical aspect of the problem is the object of discussion; the one ensuing from the competitive complex requires no individual treatment.

2. It should not be doubted that the anti-Jewish attitude is fundamentally a religious complex.[3] The thirst for a " religious truth " as well as the tendency to fight the " devilish element ", is a psychic force of considerable significance in a vast majority

[1] Kimball Young's excellent *Handbook of Social Psychology* contains interesting fact material and its interpretation.

[2] The " political " application of anti-Semitism illustrates most graphically the operation of similar forces in general. In fact, there is no difference between the planned employment of anti-Semitism and that of other types of irrational mass-sentiment fostered by influential bodies for certain ends. The reader may, therefore, be interested in a well-documented article, " Anti-Semitism," by Lucien Wolf; it appeared first in the eleventh edition of the *Encyclopædia Brittanica* (pp. 134–146), and is now included in *Essays in Jewish History*, edited by the historian Cecil Roth (1934).

The careful reader of this article ought to compare its content with present events in the general political field; he will then see how little the overt shape of phenomena betrays of their background. This realization explains the failure of so many well-meant attempts to create a peaceful atmosphere through logical discussion of controversial points, as well as repeated declarations of good will. For this reason alone the article by Lucien Wolf merits the attention of the serious student of social problems. The fact that it has been written more than thirty-five years ago makes possible the examination of its content in a spirit that is free of passion rooted in recent impressions. The illustrative value of the article is thus enhanced.

[3] " Complex " means here a mental element of some structure and dynamic significance.

of people, however near or distant their manifested attitude to churches and their rituals may be.

As the historical events in the genesis of the Christian Church stand, the idea of the Jew has become a notion closely related to the idea of anti-Christianity. But in point of fact what is generally considered to-day as the essence of Christian ethics—as distinct from the specific dogmas of the church—has been widely believed among Jews before the New Testament was written.[1] The theological counterpart of these ethical principles, the belief in immortality (as well as the revival of the dead) was likewise a Jewish dogma long before Jesus.[2] Nevertheless, no amount of apologetic literature has ever succeeded in making this historical fact common knowledge, since statements to the contrary were used to accompany the persecution of Jews.

It makes very little difference, of course, at which period of history the principles of justice, loving-kindness, and brotherhood originated; or, which historical personalities are, rightly or wrongly, associated by tradition and legend with these tenets. What really matters is the extent to which people translate them into action. But for the problem of organized prejudice the deliberate ignoring of the facts has been of practical significance. Irrational hatred and the zeal of mysticism had to be associated with a concept of popular appeal. The idea that Jews were in ideology and behaviour the embodiment of anti-Christianity was a suitable concept to be associated with the elementary passion for persecution.

3. Those who have carefully read the discussions relating to prejudice will guess that the general cultural and social conditions in those ages were responsible for the accumulation of impassionate prejudices; this is likewise the case to-day. There was, in fact, very little psychoaffective freedom and gratification, and a great deal of apprehension with regard to the fellowmen's intentions. The authority of a few privileged people had to be acknowledged, but the resentment related to this fact could not

[1] T. H. Huxley, in his *Lectures and Essays*, writes: "Again, all that is best in the ethics of the modern world, in so far as it has not grown out of Greek thought, or Barbarian manhood, is the direct development of the ethics of old Israel. There is no code of legislation, ancient or modern, at once so just and so merciful, so tender to the weak and poor, as the Jewish law; and if the Gospels are to be trusted, Jesus of Nazareth himself declared that he taught nothing but that which lay implicitly, or explicitly, in the religious and ethical system of his people."

[2] Cf. Eccles. 12, 7, and the history of the Sadducees, who, in opposing the existing religious tradition, also denied the resurrection of the dead, a cardinal dogma of the Pharisee and the Talmud in general.

be entirely suppressed. There was no hope in science and social progress, and the adherence to law and social morals was for the majority of people an irksome burden. It was well-nigh inevitable that prejudice and aggression should follow; and the comparative crudeness of religious conceptions did the rest.

4. For the same end another scotoma had been cultivated. The New Testament contains very few details about the social and cultural life of the Jews. In the main it concerns itself with the teachings and messianic rôle of Jesus as well as the crucifixion and resurrection. Obviously the rôle ascribed in these books to the Jews is one suitable for the purpose the authors had in view.

On the other hand there is a large Talmudical literature reflecting the life of the Jewish people, both in Palestine and Babylon [1] during the first five centuries. It includes some traditional material of the pre-Christian era as well. This picture presents a highly developed cultural life, with refined ideas on human ethics; and it does not, of course, ignore the existing evil in social life. The inevitable admixture of contemporary *naïvetés* and crudities in conception, racial and religious bias of thought, and the overwhelming rôle of scholastic discussions, frequently of a type strange to the modern mind, have not clouded this essentially favourable impression for the dispassionate scholar of all ages.

Until the nineteenth century the vast majority of Jews all over the world lived and thought in accordance with the Codices compiled by their spiritual leaders from the Talmudic literature. The uninitiated cannot imagine the large number of "duties" and the austerity of the moral atmosphere that characterize these Codices; at the same time, however, they encourage happy life within the lawful boundaries. In addition, a number of popular works on religious philosophy had been produced in the course of centuries; every person of some education studied them seriously, particularly after the daily service. There were no books of secular science, fiction, or newspapers; thus, this religious-philosophical literature was the staple food of the

[1] After the destruction of the "First Temple" (586 B.C.), a considerable proportion of the Jewish people was deported to Babylon. Not all returned after the official end of the *exile*. Following the destruction of the "Second Temple" (and the final end of the Jewish national state) in A.D. 70, the centres of national life and learning had increasingly been transferred to Babylon, whereas Palestine with Jerusalem played only a secondary rôle. Since 63 B.C. the actual rulers of Judea and Jerusalem were the Romans.

people. Many of these works show the influence of classical Greek philosophy (particularly Aristotle) and contemporary Arabic culture. We may compare this literature with the interesting talks transmitted over the wireless by the B.B.C. on religious outlook. For the average person of to-day the Jewish popular literature referred to would appear to be rather heavy going, apart from the fact that large parts of its scholastic-religious content would be beyond understanding. In spite of the bloody persecutions and severe restrictions which the Jews had to suffer during the Middle Ages, the authors of these works had not lost sight of the concept of a universal humanity.

Yet to the masses of ignorant and uninformed people a different picture of the Jew was constantly presented, and to no small extent even by priests in their sermons ; it was in part arrived at from the episodes in the New Testament and from certain episodes in the historical books of the Old Testament. The Jews themselves, on the other hand, did not regard the literal meaning of their Bible in all parts as authoritative ; the Rabbis of the Talmud had a peculiar way of interpreting various sentences and stories that appeared crude to them.[1] In essence, thus, they boldly renounced several parts of their Bible, for which parts, however, even centuries later aggressive prejudice used to blame them.

5. The impression created, and in all probability intentionally created, represented the Jews as a crowd of peculiar people, hopelessly out of date, uncanny, and the embodiment of forces hostile to peace and progress.

The story of the crucifixion had become a central element of Christian sentiment ; its appeal to both the conscious and the subconscious needs no particular explanation for the student of

[1] Jewish theology referred these interpretations to an " oral tradition ", which they believed to be as old and authoritative as the Mosaic law itself. Thus, the much-quoted " an eye for an eye " becomes in these expositions and canonic codes a principle of financial compensation. The death sentence, so frequently threatened by Mosaic law, was rendered well-nigh impossible through the number of formal conditions required by the " oral tradition ". Its occurrence once in seven years was considered a horrifying event ; another author of the Mishnah speaks of a " murderous High Court " should such a sentence be passed once in seventy years. Two other experts of law recommended that all permissible formal and objective arguments should be used to make the passing of a death sentence practically impossible. To this a fifth author objects only for the sake of protecting society from murderous criminals. The tendency to dispense with the death sentence is thus obvious. Cf. Mishnah Makkoth 1, 10. (See Appendix III.)

Post-Talmudic authors have employed similar re-interpretations to qualify conceptions found in the Talmud if they appeared to them crude in the light of unquestionably refined precepts of the same Talmud.

modern psychology. Only a large scale research, carried out by men with the necessary detachment of mind, could show the rôle played by the popular interpretation of the crucifixion in creating anti-Jewish attitude throughout history. This interpretation by prejudice runs : " The Jews wanted the Son of God to be killed *because* he was good and preached the advent of the Heavenly Kingdom. All Jews, whenever and wherever they may exist, are guilty of this supreme crime."

The writer remembers how his fellow pupils in the grammar school, after receiving religious instruction, were frequently unable to speak a friendly word to him—incidentally one of the top students of the form. It took them, as a rule, a whole day to overcome the sentiment of embarrassment evoked in them through the vivid description of the life of Jesus by their religious instructor.[1] Likewise, a few of my best friends at that time felt unable to acknowledge me during the Easter-week. One or two of them have become, nevertheless, broadminded individuals ; the others are up to the present " reactionaries ", though otherwise quite average human beings. To most readers, brought up in a liberal spirit, all this may appear incredible. But it is always useful to illustrate a psychological phenomenon both by its most marked manifestations and its " sublimal " forms. Cf. (16).

6. Little do people know that the existence, the rôle, and tragic fate of Jesus was largely unknown to contemporary Jews. If some of the historical notes contained in the Talmud do refer to Jesus of Nazareth—there is a great deal of confusion and anachronism in these notes—they only show that to the Jews of that time the life and end of this remarkable personality, and true idealist, implied no more than one of the various incidents in revolutionary times.

Few people are unbiased enough to realize that, even after Christianity had begun its victorious course amongst the nations, it was very difficult for orthodox Jews to believe in the Trinity, in the dogma of incarnation, as well as in a Son of God who had to die to save the believers. These notions were something incomprehensible for them. Moreover, their tradition prophesied a Messiah who would abolish in a literal sense all aggression, wars, and human suffering. Manifested opposition to the new doctrine referred solely to attempts at converting Jews. Cf. (9).

[1] This took place thirty-five years ago, in a country other than Great Britain.

7. All these things have no longer any significance to the Jews of to-day. As in general the interest in dogmatic questions is extremely small amongst Jews to-day. The number of those who merely need some religion, as well as occasional religious services, for psychological reasons, and on the other hand the number of full and partial agnostics, is very large amongst them. Each of them finds it unfair to be considered an anti-Christ. They are totally uninterested in the historical or dogmatic aspect of Christianity, as were in fact even their more orthodox ancestors if left alone by those who wanted to convert them. To say that they do not share the general principles and ideas of an enlightened society would be an untrue statement.

8. For Christian theology the life-story of Jesus, as described by the books of the New Testament, is sacred in all its details. It appears that the crucifixion, and the rôle ascribed by these books to the Jewish dignitaries in Jerusalem of that time, occupy in this theology a place as important as the remarkable teachings and parables of Jesus. It would be somewhat unfair of the Jews to ask Christian authorities to ignore the story of the crucifixion and its theological implications, for the sole purpose of diminishing irrational Jew-hatred. Orthodox Jewish theology would find it likewise impossible to give up its own specific beliefs. It is only fortunate for the Jews that their official theology (Halacha) is not burdened by tradition with any element relating to the life and crucifixion of Jesus. A rabbi can be considered the greatest authority in Jewish theology though he knows no word about Jesus, the New Testament, and the dogmas of the Christian faith.

9. Jewish theology of olden times has carried out an adjustment in which the science of social history might take an interest. It was impossible for the ancient Jews to deny the racial character of Mosaic religion ; nor was it possible for them to ignore the Biblical tradition that the descendants of the twelve tribes were a people specially chosen by God for the care of a very complex ritual and legislation. On the other hand, the prophets introduced the idea of general humanity. Later authors pointed out that the Bible begins with the creation of a general *Adam* [1] and not with a Jewish ancestor. Therefore, the rabbis of old invented a dogmatic principle that all non-Jews must, by the command of God, adhere

[1] Cf. Genesis Ch. V ; see the edition by Dr. J. H. Hertz.

only to a few laws, which (if stripped of religious colouring) may be considered to-day as the elements of civilized conduct. They persuaded themselves that Noah after the deluge received from God a number of commands for the world at large; such as a satisfactory legal order; conjugal and family morality, with the exclusion of incest; the prohibition of eating parts of animals not yet killed; and the prohibition of idolatry.[1] All who adhere to these principles as God's commands are sure to participate in the after-life.[2] So it was possible for the orthodox Jews of old to extend general human acknowledgment to those outside the fold.

10. The principle of "extra ecclesiam nulla salus"[3] would, thus, not interfere with the social adaptation in a Christian country of the most orthodox rabbi. For him the decision of authoritative sources has decreed that Christianity is monotheistic; and, apart from born Jews, those who adhere to it are not condemnable on religious ground.[4] The discriminating laws referring to heathens no longer apply, since idolatry coupled with a cult of sexual immorality, characteristic of ancient heathens, no longer exists.[5] Moreover, the whole of the civil laws of the country in which a Jew happened to live, was declared binding religious law (Talmud).[6] But common sense had made its decisions independently of and prior to learned theological definitions; nowadays very few people know of them or are even interested in such scholastic details. Human intelligence and humane feeling have always been stronger factors in social attitudes than written concepts, which frequently express only what common sense and practice have already decided.

For the small number of strictly orthodox Jews the tendencies to projection and moral condemnation centre, even in the present, on a heathen ideology of long past centuries, to which various features of an insensible and even inhuman character were ascribed by Talmudic authors.[7] With the particular elements of

[1] Tr. Sandedrin, *56*.
[2] Tr. Sanhedrin, *105*, and Code of Maimonides, Ml'chim, *10*, 9.
[3] Outside the Church there is no salvation for the soul.
[4] R'M'A., *107*; Sh'ch J.D., *151*; R'N. end Tr. A.Z.
[5] Tosf. Jomtov, Tr. A.Z., II, 2; Bes Jos. Ch. M., 266; Encyclopædia by J. Lamporonti.
[6] Based on Talmud Tr. Gittin, 10.
[7] This holds good in so far as a stimulation of this process by traditional religious concepts is concerned. It is obvious that personal experiences are an additional source of a tendency to project the "bad" on to others. It cannot be doubted that voluntary

Christian theology they are not concerned at all, since, as explained above, the original system of orthodox Jewish theology (Halacha) and the acknowledged old codes contain no explicit discussions on it. It was only later, in the ages of religious persecution, when Christian rulers and bishops forced learned rabbis to take part in theological disputes, with a view to converting them to the Christian faith, that they began to know what the tenets of Christian theology were. There are a few works from these times containing the apologetic material elaborated by some of these authors. But these works are read only by the very few professionals of Hebrew philosophical literature; they are no part of the religious canon of orthodoxy, and they have remained without interest for, and influence on, the average masses and their rabbis.

Thus it was only the tendency to projection on the part of their environment which has attributed to the Jew the significance of an anti-Christ.

11. Anti-Semitism prefers to speak in terms of "*the Jews*", as if they constituted a well-knit body all over the world. I think this results from the collective expression "the Jews" used in the New Testament; more accurately from the idea of the Jews as collectively representing anti-Christianity. In fact, there

isolation and unfair treatment on the part of their environment made the Jews fear the average Christian. It was difficult for the average Jew to distinguish between the specific anti-Jewish prejudice of people and their general human character.

There is a slight paranoid trend in many Jews manifesting itself in a fear of prejudice where there is none, or where there is only a non-specific lack of kindness towards a fellow-being. This fear has diminished greatly since the first decades of the nineteenth century. But the experiences in the years 1933–1945 will, for a long period, prevent any progress in this direction. Many Jews cannot rid themselves of the idea that the mass slaughter of almost six millions of their brothers and the economic ruin of another million has been a legacy of the prejudiced attitudes of the Middle Ages. The fact that other sections of mankind—though to a lesser degree—have suffered together with them cannot entirely cloud the idea that their race has received a selective treatment by contemporary German brutality. But in all fairness they ought to realize that there were very large numbers of Christians who sympathized with them and tried to help them as far as it was possible; and at the height of persecution there were, perhaps, not many people conscious of their Christian faith who gave their approval or even a helping hand in the extermination of Jews.

Traditional anti-Semitism was only in part responsible for the fact that far too little help was given to contemporary Jews in their mortal danger. The competitive complex, as well as other customary factors in politics, frequently played its rôle in causing large groups of human beings to suffer even though they were not Jews. There have been, in the past and the present, instances enough where groups of Christians have behaved cruelly towards each other. The cool and almost merciless attitude shown to various degrees by practically all countries, when in 1939 refuge was sought from oppression by the mass of European Jews, was certainly in the main prompted by *non-specific social motives*. Sooner or later this will be realized, even though at present the average Jew is unable to feel so because of his personal experiences.

existed—at least for decades before 1939—no firm bond amongst Jews, apart from the one created by their knowledge and personal experiences of anti-Semitism. Their religious unity implies hardly more than this factor does in the Christian world. And since they have no supreme religious authority, each community being autonomous, the organizing power of religion amongst Jews is even less.[1] Each congregation is autonomous. The religious leader is no more than a teacher ; he is not an ordained clergyman, but a learned *primus inter pares*. His influence is thus rather of a personal than of a mystical character. More often than not his sermons and activities are the object of free criticism ; and I am told it is in most cases not a constructive one. Apart from matters of charity and the basic elements of service there is, so it appears, little unanimity during discussions on communal administrative matters of the congregation. Jews are rather individualistic if amongst themselves ; this being a *reactive character trait* conditioned in them in response to their traditional social difficulties. For all these reasons the uncanny unity of the Jews is but a delusional bogy of prejudice, to be utilized for the notion of an " international secret Jewish plot ".

12. The average Jew attends his religious service from the same psychological motives that prompt people all over the world to practise their faith. The general colouring of his religious sentiments is the same as that all over the monotheistic world. The vast majority of Jews, as people in general in countries with European civilization, have rather loose ties with outmoded dogmatic thinking ; no amount of sentimental attachment to formal tradition can prevent the far-reaching influence of the progressive environmental process. In fact a considerable proportion have been champions of modernism to a degree that has earned them blame from quarters of reactionary bias. There is nowadays very little specific in the thought and reactions of the average Jewish individual as compared with the members of his progressive environment.

In the case of Eastern Jews who have not changed entirely their traditional externals—which often happens because of inertia, but in the case of many to safeguard their adherence to religious orthodoxy—it is obvious that such peculiar features

[1] It has been realized by experts that religious prejudice and social oppression from which the Jews have suffered, have greatly been responsible for their comparative unity and race-consciousness. Admittedly, not all ethnical groups respond to oppression or discrimination with increased vitality.

in the externals of behaviour are likely to attract attention. But in many cases the impression created by this group of Jews is causing irritability only because of pre-existing prejudice. However peculiar such a Jew may appear, I feel that the same impression would be perceived with more tolerance by observers were they to believe that this conspicuity is characteristic of any other exotic race, in particular one of Christian faith.

A particular bias against the Jewish business man prevails by tradition ; not against the individual who is apparently liked by those who are his customers by free choice, but against the concept in itself. I feel that the central element of this prejudice is a vague realization by people that the goods necessary for life ought to be made available without profit ; or, that the dependence on money for livelihood and a fair amount of pleasure is an anomaly. The element of envy ranks only second, even though it is intrinsically associated with the subject's weighing up of his own position. [Cf. Ch. XIII. 1.] According to this conception the resentment of the "Jewish exploiter" is a projection in the fullest sense, a condemnation of our traditional economic system. This state of economic affairs is one with which we will have to put up as long as we know of no better system that would genuinely appeal to the vast majority of people. But the realization of having relatively to like a necessity does not eliminate from the psyche the resentment against the pains involved in the acceptance of the system.

Clearly, particular features of the Jewish person, in so far as they are different from those of the average citizen, make for the process of symbolic externalization. The additional element of religious hatred, even though suppressed, acts as a sensitizing factor.

In the case of a dealer or manufacturer who is *not* singled out by local prejudice, and who does not appear strange by nationality or race, the resentment referred to is more or less suppressed ; this occurs particularly when the owner or the manager of the business appears impressive to the customer. But we know from psychoneuroses that a mental conflict or a dynamic complex does not lead to symptoms in all the circumstances that would seem logically appropriate for such a manifestation. There is always a selective limitation with regard to the field—and period—where a deep-lying pathogenic complex manifests itself in the shape of symptoms.

In addition to all this it is a fact that, particularly in past decades, the small Jewish business man—if he was an average specimen of a human being—at times displayed features of behaviour in his dealings that appeared odd and were the object of ridicule or resentment. Only very few learned persons have been able to realize that the abnormal status of a member of a foreign race, particularly if an immigrant and not in possession of sufficient education, is likely to develop reactive character-traits of a petty or even objectionable colouring; and it is also true that people in general may resent comparatively small vices much more than crimes on a large scale or essential badness. We have referred to this illogical phenomenon in the course of previous discussions; indeed, it is hard to understand it fully, even though one may have grasped the periphery of its psychological background. (Cf. more in Appendix II.)

There is no doubt that the Jews in choosing to remain a religious or ethnical entity have been facing a task of appalling magnitude. There appears no prospect of their difficulties entirely disappearing within a future period we can foresee. The secret of solving the problem cannot lie in the further cultural and ethical improvement of the individual Jew. It is impossible for a racial group, participating in all that modernism implies, to free itself of the average vices of average human beings. Besides there are instances enough in history where groups of absolutely harmless Jews, hermits as it were, lacking all mundane interest and devoting themselves only to mystical studies and a life comparable to that of the early Christians (cf. the Essenes), have been maligned, attacked, and even brutally murdered. The author feels unable to do more than analytically describe the facts as they appear to him.

13. As a community Jews can do little at present against anti-Semitism. Not being a nation in the customary sense they have acquired little of the refined modes of collective diplomacy applicable to their self-defence. The Zionist movement has gained in recent years more popularity amongst Jews than formerly; but it has no influence on the factors responsible for anti-Semitism. It is not competent to deal with questions other than that of the settlement of Jews in Palestine. It has enabled millions of Jews to be conscious of their national tradition without being attached to religious orthodoxy; and it has restored to Jews the love of the soil and manual work. Anything more needed for the modernization of Jews can only be achieved by further patient efforts at social development. A substantial

decrease in prejudice against them is an essential condition for the success of this process.

14. It has been advised by various sources—Jewish and non-Jewish—that Jews should avoid publicity, and should be very careful about the law and social customs, more than average people of their environment. This sounds all very well; for individuals of exceptional wisdom or those who are by nature inconspicuous this course is certainly commendable. Few persons, however, can realize that such a continuous self-restraint is not practicable if people are to live an average human life. There are limits for enduring emotional restrictions. And it is assumed that many Jews are racially "temperamentful". (I feel sure that this is to a considerable extent a reactive restlessness.) Apart from the practical difficulty in following the advice mentioned it amounts to a practical affirmation of the biased attitude. If there should be human equality allowance ought to be made for groups to have their share in the deficiencies of human behaviour. Vices are largely socially conditioned; the particular temptations of various occupations must not be forgotten; in a number of individuals criminal impulses are based on a functional deficiency of the brain. (See Ch. IIIA, 6.)

15. Objective statistics should be able to show the factual aspects of this problem. It could be ascertained, for instance, how great is the proportion of Jewish business men who break "the regulations" as compared with those in other groups of a similar educational and economical background. Or how great is the proportion of Jewish alcoholics who make themselves nuisances. It could be established by a poll and objective information how great a proportion of Jewish medical men is considered to be well-trained, conscientious, and humane; or, what is the proportion of the exceptionally valuable as well as the average Jewish individuals in various occupational groups. In the past small statistics of this kind were attempted with respect to criminality and drunkenness.

Whatever the results of such an inquiry they would prove hardly anything for the problem of prejudice.[1] It is independent,

[1] *This chapter is not an apology on behalf of the personal Jews. Moreover I do not regard as prejudice the preference in choosing friends from one's own narrower circle; certainly not as a prejudice-paranoia described in this work. Naturally, such a preference leads to a certain*

to a substantial degree, of the actualities; it only utilizes facts, mostly exaggerating them, in its own support.

There were regions and periods in the social history of the Jews when these objects of religious prejudice certainly were equal, or even superior, in cultural standards to those who were their attackers. There are various regions of the earth where it would be possible even at present to arouse people's passions by reviving the notorious charge of ritual murder (religious cannibalism),[1] unless the authorities took a firm stand against it. The independent element of prejudice-paranoia cannot be doubted to constitute the central element in anti-Jewish attitudes.

During the lifetime of the writer anti-Jewish mass propaganda has been conducted under a variety of slogans. The Jews were condemned, collectively, as capitalists; as socialists or communists; as a race interested only in business; as a group filling the grammar schools and universities; as people who are not patriotic; as a section of the community that concerns itself with national politics, though a strange element in it; on the frontier of two hostile countries they were classed as sympathizing with the other party; and finally as "inferior parasites" in general who are not fit to live in a Christian country.[2]

*avoidance of members of other groups, and this may resemble an irrational dislike. But such an element need not be present. There are a vast number of people whose faculty of adjustment is limited, and who, therefore, are unable to feel at ease in the company of heterogeneous persons. This is, admittedly, a certain weakness, analogous to the limitations of a fastidious individual who can only enjoy a small variety of foodstuffs. Hence there might be people who dislike mixing with Jews, merely because they need, for their ease, the feeling that their friends are Christians. Certainly, there are likewise Jews who behave similarly; even though in most cases a measure of traditional fear is a contributory factor. It is well known how happy the simple average Jew is if he finds that his casual acquaintance, a Christian, "has been genuinely friendly to him."* Cf. p. 154.

[1] This was written in May, 1945; subsequent events sadly confirmed the writer's psychological assessment. In the period between June, 1945, and June, 1946, there were such riots in three European countries.

Since June, 1946, further bloody pogroms, and numerous less fatal attacks on Jews have taken place. This warfare against the remnants of a much tried racial group is organized, or supported, by political parties, frequently with the help of the above-mentioned irrational charge. Sheer aggressiveness, lust for robbery, and degenerated religious passion join hands in sponsoring and carrying out these attacks.

[2] There are numerous gentiles who emphatically declare their appreciation of Jews who happen to be excellent scholars, or are otherwise well educated. Likewise, there are many white people who are ready to suppress their colour-prejudice in favour of some excellent individuals of the coloured races. This attitude is hardly a clumsy disguise of primitive prejudice. The true measure of sanity is the amount of natural recognition afforded to the masses of average persons of foreign groups. This logically satisfactory attitude can be put to the test when a member of such a foreign or tabooed group becomes unpleasant, troublesome, or a law-breaker. Then the subject ought to compare the quality of his indignation with that felt towards a criminal who does not belong to any resented group.

16. The reader, if himself free of this bias, might think that in our epoch the religious source of prejudice is on the wane. But this is not the fact. A large proportion of well-educated people, men of science included, are sensitive in this respect. It is apparently very difficult for them to rid themselves of such mental elements acquired in youth. I adduce a few illustrative instances. They concern individuals and not large groups and demonstrate what we may call *minor symptoms*, but they are characteristic.

A professional man distinguished by a number of academic degrees, and in the first instance by an exceptionally tolerant character, was convinced that a person who believed in loving-kindness and justice for all men did so because he was a believer in Christ, the Son of God. It had never occurred to him earlier that there might exist millions of people who held the same principles though having a non-Christian tradition.

17. The counterpart of such an attitude on the Jewish side is illustrated by the following episode which the writer had the opportunity of witnessing. At a party of a few Jewish persons a great figure of the Church of England, who had died at that time, was discussed. One of those present suggested that the eminent clergyman in question, who during his life had distinguished himself in the cause of social improvement and general enlightenment, could not genuinely have believed in the dogma that Jesus was the Son of God as well as in all the accessories of this dogma. This statement was endorsed by one or two members of the party. These people were of average intelligence, and appreciative of enlightenment and ethics, no matter what their source or origin. On the religious side, so it appeared, they belonged to the orthodox minority who knew no compromise with respect to the dogmatic tenets of their faith.

It was obvious that they thought it incompatible to be, on the one hand, a distinguished writer, educationalist, and socialist, and on the other hand a believer in Christian dogmas. This conception originated, doubtlessly, in religious bias ; it is clearly contradicted by actual experience. We cannot deny that a few distinguished individuals have been capable of dividing their mind between the large and impressive field of modern science and the traditional dogmas of their religion ; and they have been genuinely attached to both spheres. Their mind's capacity has been large enough to carry the results of the two outlooks, without any apparent disharmony in their personality.

The ideas of the virgin birth and incarnation may seem strange to Jews brought up on lines of abstract monotheism. For the unbiased outsider, however, there is surely nothing incomprehensible in this belief, provided the rules of empirical science are not applicable to religious spheres. There are dogmatic beliefs in Jewish orthodoxy which, in the opinion of outsiders, require as much unconditional acceptance as do the aforementioned dogmas of Christianity. Thus, for instance, orthodox Jews have to believe that on the occasion of the *revelation* not only the ten commandments have been promulgated, but also all the details of the Jewish ritual and social legislation as contained in the vast Talmudic literature of much later times. It needs no particular mention that the biblical record of revelation itself implies the putting aside of empirical thinking and the acceptance with devotion of miraculous stories.

Returning to both instances, it has to be realized that the desire for enlightenment and social improvement is an ancient human tendency. If to-day these problems are receiving more attention, and on a much larger scale than two and three thousand years ago, it is only because of the progress made since in general scientific outlook. With the passing of time, it has become inevitable that society takes notice of the implications of accumulated knowledge, whether based on satisfying or disappointing experiences.

18. A woman (45 years old, writer and socialist) who described herself as an agnostic, on the eve of Christmas brought to a friendly family, who were orthodox Jews, a branch of the Christmas tree with a candle on it. She well knew that Jews in general do not celebrate the birthday of Jesus. On the next day she admitted feeling hurt because the candle had not been ceremoniously lit. Her analysis revealed a strong leaning towards Roman Catholic mysticism, though she was the child of Protestant parents. She had in herself something of the missionary spirit and would have liked to convert those whom she liked to Christian mysticism.

19. A man, 55 years of age, well read, fond of classical music, and editor of a modern periodical, was present in 1939 at a party where the growing intolerance against Jews in Germany was the topic of conversation. He said : " All this is very regrettable ;

but one should not forget that, according to the books of the Old Testament, the Jews cruelly exterminated the heathen population of Palestine when they took possession of the country." [1] Provided that the biblical accounts are reliable, that is, free of exaggerations peculiar to the early historical records of the nations—the event referred to had taken place approximately three thousand years ago. The man ignored this fact; and this suggests that an irrational complex was at the back of his statement. I wish to add that he was an atheist—as he thought from his early manhood—and consciously free of religious prejudice.

20. I am quoting in English the translation of a few sentences related in the course of a psychoanalysis by a past patient of mine: "I am a Roman Catholic; my father was very cross if we bought anything in Jewish shops. But we children hadn't enough money at our disposal to go to expensive stores, and had to buy our goods where we thought they were cheaper. My father was a passionate lover of a series of leaflets edited by Father Coughlin, and in his conversations he frequently attacked Jews as being mean." On the next occasion she related: "My father had a very good business and apparently earned a lot of money. I know for a fact that he was a twister, his deliveries were short of weight. So he must have made a great deal of profit . . ."

21. It happened during the last war. A few enlightened Christians invited a small number of Jews to discuss ways of combating anti-Semitism. After a number of various points were mentioned, the chairman, a person of distinguished position and higher education said: "Of course, we Christians cannot forget the share of the Jews in the death of Jesus."

22. Here the problem of anti-Jewish prejudice stands to this time. Many things have changed since the French revolution, since the

[1] This story is one of the numerous parts in the O.T. that have undergone a refining exposition by Jewish theology, as mentioned above (231). A traditional legend states that actually three alternatives were open to the inhabitants of Palestine at the time the Jews took possession of the land. They were free to leave with a view to settling somewhere else; or, they were invited to give up idolatry and immoral customs, without becoming Jews, and continue living in peace in their native land; and only those who chose armed resistance to these proposals were exterminated in battle. The qualifying tendency of this exposition is clear. Cf. in the commentary by Nachmanides, Deut. 20, 10.

advent of scientific thinking and the acknowledgment of human equality. Jews have been admitted, in various degrees, as partakers of the average social life. Their life on the whole is regulated by what takes place in general in society. Christians have the opportunity of knowing individual Jews, their personal views, their family life, their standard in elementary or higher scholastic education. It would be hard to say that fundamental differences in general human characteristics prevail. But, besides this inevitable realization by common sense, there lurks in many minds another picture of the Jews, as a body of uncanny, peculiar, mean, and anti-Christian people. Religious forces coloured by prejudice permeate the thinking of persons who themselves would very definitely deny the existence of such an element in themselves.

23. There are certainly a large number of people in whom the religious element of anti-Jewish sentiment is practically non-existent. There are a large number of people who, though conscious of their being religious Christians, have hardly any of this mystical prejudice in themselves, for the simple reason that they have no proneness to prejudice paranoia. There were, in the darkest periods, high dignitaries of the Church who stood in friendly scientific intercourse with learned rabbis ; and others, in past and present, who afforded protection to whole congregations when threatened by fanatical mobs. Thus it is certain that Christian mentality, even if ensuing from a firm belief of traditional concepts and dogmas, may be compatible with the absence of anti-Semitism, at least in the practical spheres of life. There are certainly many who from sheer competitiveness and general aggressiveness feel it appropriate to attack the Jews in public, because the fact of racial differences gives them an opportunity for letting loose elementary forces, but they are not really prejudiced themselves. I think there is some hope for the decrease of prejudice based on religious forces ; not by propaganda carried out by the few who are free from this illness, but by comprehensive changes in the social process.

24. The writer, though himself very doubtful of the truth of any religious conception, would definitely consider it a tragedy were organized Christianity suddenly to disappear. He is convinced that further social progress cannot come from religion, but only

from the secular sciences utilized by a humane social programme. At the same time it appears inadvisable to trust the management of the world to people who are entirely indifferent to religion, or are even cynical in their attitude towards it.[1] The greatest part of charity called for in times of emergency, as well as the friendly care of those who are weak in the competitive struggle of general life, has come so far from social layers more or less associated with ethical and religious movements. We cannot yet be very much impressed by the practical self-sacrifice of those who are merely educated and free of superstition and prejudice. Comparatively few members of this modern group seem interested in, or really capable of, carrying out the great task that confronts us in view of the large suffering of humanity. This being their deficiency, it at least justifies doubt in their capacity to manage, unaided by others, the affairs of society in times of so called peace. Further evolution may change this impression ; but to-day a vast number of free-thinkers are not yet free of a surplus of coolness in their personality. I think this is the case because they actually repress their religious tendencies, and with this goes a certain measure of obstruction in the emotional spheres in general. But manifest attitudes and reactions are functions of these mental layers. Were the people referred to really free of suppressed religion—or had they the courage of accepting the existence of this thirst in themselves, though without belief, they should be fully capable of the sympathy possessed by their manifestly religious fellowmen. It is not individually but as a group that they may fail in their social task (cf. end of Ch. VII, p. 139).

[1] In this connection I wish to quote from memory a sentence contained in the work of a German author who held a University chair : " A believing Christian cannot be a genuine anti-Semite ; a genuine German anti-Semite must not have anything to do with Christianity. . . ." (I can remember neither the name of the author nor the title of his book, which was published as far back as 1900.)

In a similar spirit was couched a resolution by a German students' union in approximately 1928. It stated : " We wish to have nothing to do with a Jew whether he be Professor Einstein or Jesus of Nazareth."

Hans Blüher wrote : " In the opinion of the Nationalists (Voelkische) in the broadest sense, Christianity is a strange element, an importation ; moreover, it is of Jewish origin and mould. When it will be thrown off (Abschüttelung), the ancient religion of Light and Virtue is bound to reappear ; only then it may be possible to revolt successfully against the oppressors of the nation both within and without. . . . We know to-day that our ancestors were a nation of a first-class culture ; the Christian mission by Kaiser Karl (Charlemagne) robbed, forcibly, the nation of its sacraments."

In the opinion of this author, Luther made good the crime committed by this ruler. Blüher also thinks that the idea of world democracy implies Judaism. Anyone who is in favour of a strong state ruled by an upper stratum, which is rooted in the native soil and led by a Christian King, has to be anti-Semitic. (Cf. *Klärung*, a symposium on the Jewish problem, Verlag Tradition, Berlin, 1932. It is, admittedly, difficult to follow and translate clearly the hazy discussions of this author once popular in Germany.)

25. It is necessary to inquire whether anything of importance might be learned from the facts presented in this chapter, for the problems of co-operation and toleration in general. The psychology of projection and aggressive prejudice has been discussed extensively in previous chapters, and here merely a comprehensive instance has been added for its illustration. The condemnation, persecution, and burning of heretics did not confine itself to Jewish victims ; the inner history of the Christian Church and that of the various religious wars provide ample instances. In the persecution of all kinds of reformists one of the deeper psychological motives was, in all probability, the fear of freedom ; the atheistic element as well as a general tendency to revolt against established authority is a *complex* which, though suppressed, is present in all believers and law-abiding people. The desire for religious reform and more freedom of thought obviously stimulates the anarchy complex in general ; intolerance is one of the defence mechanisms of the mind coping with this complex, and militant prejudice a welcome mode of " abreacting ". The persecution of non-Christians in Christian countries was in essence the same phenomenon, only it referred rather to the " externalization " of the devilish element in the human being.

The main thing that might be learned from this history of religious anti-Semitism is, so the writer thinks, *the psychology of the tendency to enforce uniformity of feeling and thinking.* It cannot be doubted that the idea of a universal religion, preferably one which appeals even to the simplest individual, represents a progress from the racial and complex systems of religion. A similar uniformity, or more accurately a unanimity, in general human relationships has been an aim sponsored by all enlightened leaders of society in the past and present. Nevertheless, it is a fact that the history of mankind has produced a variety of ethnic traditions and human types. For this reason, any forcible uniformity is at least as undesirable as the existing divergence of thought and cultural pattern.

Anti-Jewish sentiment, and particularly its practical manifestations, are an instance of an attempt at the forcible conversion of people to a uniform pattern. Such tendencies in the larger international fields are likely to prove disastrous ; this is easy to realize. Both psychology and concrete history prove that a massive repression of tendencies, carried out in favour of a new social pattern, might result in the creation of volcanic forces, if there is no genuine desire in psychic depths for such a change (cf. Ch. XI).

As much as *unanimity* represents the most desirable ideal in human relationships, *enforced uniformity* is bound to hamper the genuine development towards this aim. For the very reason that enforced uniformity creates tendencies that are the opposite of happy unanimity, such a sweeping programme in cultural, religious, or political spheres cannot dispense with *unfounded statements, a certain distortion of history, intellectual scotomas, and the fostering of prejudice.*

On the rational level of the mind, a person who feels superior in knowledge or insight to some of his fellowmen is, first of all, glad about his own progress. In the main, he feels some pity towards others, but also an earnest desire to teach them. Intolerance and fear ought not to be the reaction, if logic remains the guiding force. It is the impact of subconscious emotional forces that, in many cases, brings about the irrational attitude towards those deemed to be less progressive. The same applies to groups and nations in their relationships to each other. The writer thinks that the discussion in this chapter aptly illustrates this problem.

# APPENDIX II

## PROBLEMS OF PSYCHOPATHOLOGY RELATED TO THE PREVIOUS CHAPTERS

*Symbolic stimulation.—Paranoia and allied conditions.—The stranger, and the novelty.—The ethnic psyche, and ethnic prejudice.—The libido; instincts, tendencies, and energy.—The libido and social behaviour.*

### Symbolic Elements and their Stimulation

1. There is sufficient reason for assuming that objects, persons, and actions in dreams refer, in a symbolical way, to elements of the mind other than those suggested by the literal meaning of the motive in question. It is equally probable that psychoneurotic symptoms, and, even more, delusional formations in schizophrenia and paranoia are expressions of a similar category. It is also a fact that the phraseology of all languages employs the metaphor. These observations not only suggest that all impressions *may* be perceived by the psyche metaphorically, as it were, but it is justifiable to infer that secondary meanings are regularly evoked, largely in the subconscious, in addition to the literal and conscious one. Since these secondary elements are habitually produced, they have, presumably, a rôle within the psychoaffective mechanism. They satisfy, so we may divine, a corresponding need of the mind; as if the intra-psychic elaboration of the impressions we receive is not limited to the act of intelligent perception, but is to play more than one rôle in assuaging psychoaffective hunger. All this, however, does not lie within the scope of our inquiry here. The question of main interest in this work is, what are the conditions conducive to an undesirable intensity of these symbolic perceptions accompanying concrete impressions and conscious ideas.

2. It is obvious that the symbolic stimulation of "complexes" in the wake of concrete impressions only occurs where there is some instability of the psyche, whether habitual or temporary. If a complex, or the tendency to externalize a moral conflict,

requires very little to stir it up, then a comparatively indifferent event, through one of its secondary meanings, may be capable of supplying the additional force necessary for an overt psychoneurotic manifestation. One has almost to believe that the intrinsic readiness for an outburst invites the very creation of a secondary meaning appropriate for the psychoneurotic manifestation. We are reminded of the case of epileptics whose fits are successfully suppressed through constant use of luminal, but who at certain times feel uneasy and tense until an epileptic attack relieves them of this condition. Accordingly, it is not so much the external event, with its symbolic meaning, that is the primary agent in eliciting irrational manifestations, but rather an intrinsic need to be stirred in this way. In this connection the student will remember that a similar intrinsic need for paranoiac delusions has been postulated by *Kraepelin* and *Bleuler*.

3. The multiplicity of meaning attached to a concrete impression may be observed by the subject even consciously. The experience of a storm bending and breaking off the branches of trees evokes, as a rule, ideas that are outside the concrete implications of such an event. There are persons who, on such occasions, feel that the apparent stability of conditions in life may be disturbed by powers beyond the control of the human being. In addition, there may be a feeling of admiration for the forces of Nature; or alternatively a distinct fear of them, in accordance with the personal make-up of the subject, or the state of his mind at the moment. The howl of the wind, as well as the creaking noise of trees and the rustle of leaves stirred by the storm, has given rise to a variety of metaphors in poetry and fiction; and these ideas are consciously present in many individuals watching a storm. The cleansing aspect of such a phenomenon, or, on the other hand, its quality of raising the dust of the earth have been very prominent in stimulating metaphorical concepts. In this conscious process the *intrinsic* desire of the psyche for such meditations is obvious; and this fact may support the hypothesis advanced above with regard to the subconscious category of symbolic ideation.

4. In Appendix I mention was made of the tendency of many people to display passionate indignation at small improprieties, even though they may easily forget crimes, provided they

themselves or their friends have not been the object of attack.

Admittedly, in the case of a small business man with an excess of competitive or profiteering zeal, there are always a large number of people who may feel themselves directly affected. But it cannot be overlooked that the masses of average people readily fall in with such moral indignation even if they themselves are entirely unaffected. Perhaps this is so because they feel that each of them might easily encounter the same undesirable situation; their anger is anticipatory. On the other hand, violent assault and murder are comparatively infrequent forms of attack on human life; the average person does not really think himself a potential victim.

The writer feels, however, that this paradoxical phenomenon may have additional, deeper reasons. The one is that since people in reality *envy* the profiteer or the successfully competitive individual, their moral indignation contains a large element of insincere externalization.[1] This cannot be the case where serious crimes are in question. Very few persons need to overcome in themselves the tendency to commit a real murder; even though they may revel in, or have to combat, such phantasies.

The other point of significance is the symbolic process at work in such exaggerated indignation. A comparatively small vice may imply for the subconsciousness the additional meaning of a serious crime.[2] In this case the indignation is passionate because unrecognized criminal or serious sexual complexes have been

[1] Passionate indignation at any offence or misconduct is hardly ever free from the admixture of envy. Some people say openly: "I am annoyed with myself for being unable to be anything but honest." In fact, the transformation of desire for condemnable tendencies into their rejection constitutes a substantial part of morality. There may be, from the outset, a firm aversion to a particular vice, but this does not exclude the presence of a certain measure of desire for its adoption, or an interest in the offender. This amoral component has to be rejected and transformed into the negative of a wish, since genuine indifference is in most cases only a hypothesis. Clearly, any incident that perceptibly illustrates the possibility of offending or misbehaving is apt to stimulate a conflict in the onlooker's psyche, and to signalize the need for metamorphosis of a component tendency.

It is natural that such a process of transformation cannot be always fully successful. Hence, in most individuals some measure of the tabooed wish stimulated by an impression remains essentially unchanged, even though suppressed. This fact amounts to the frustration of the desire; and in the wake of this phenomenon some envy of the less scrupulous emerges. The emotional charge of this *a*-moral element is contributing to the passion of moral indignation manifested by the same person. No doubt, the indignant individual is genuinely perturbed if an offending fellowman demonstrates that it *is* possible to break the law or a conventional rule in order to satisfy an impulse. Apart from his concern for general morality, such an impression may stimulate a conflict in him and necessitate the process of transformation of a component tendency, for which fact the offender is responsible.

[2] This possibility does not exclude the subconscious interpretation referred to on p. 237.

stimulated. On the other hand, an actual serious crime above all implies to the average mind its full, real significance, and there is no place for the roundabout stimulation of secondary meanings. But the writer thinks that the irrational stimulation of affective behaviour cannot occur unless the process involves spheres of symbolic and repressed elements. The symbolic meaning of a trivial vice, of loud behaviour, or a strange accent used in the course of a business may cause a commotion in the receptive subject, particularly if there is in him a measure of suspicion or resentment towards the other person ; and this is frequently so in the case of an individual who takes people's money and makes a profit at the cost of their daily needs. On the other hand, a serious crime or an encounter with essential badness impresses the conscious mind of the subject by its actual meaning so strongly that the aspect of symbolic stimulation by such an event remains insignificant to the average psyche. We know, of course, that in a person whose mind is burdened with a " death complex " the reaction to news of a crime or even to a play of such a colouring is violent enough. But our discussion is concerned with average people who do not display such violent reaction in the presence of serious crimes, whereas they are passionately indignant at the real or imagined impropriety of a small business man.

## The Literal and the Symbolic Meaning of Neurotic Complaints

1. There are further problems relating to the phenomenon of symbolic meaning ; and some of them have an immediate significance for psychotherapy. It was pointed out above that the dynamic charge of secondary meanings is not always sufficiently strong to compete with the literal, conscious concept referring to an impression. The subject under analysis habitually insists on the main or sole significance of the conscious version ; it is part of our analytical work to redirect his attention towards what we deem the more important meaning. But on many occasions we ought to admit that the literal form of an obsession or the conscious picture of a concrete impression that allegedly worries the patient indeed merits our full attention.

There is a patient who suffers from depression, which he attributes to a loss of prestige in the firm for whom he works ; as the case is, he is certainly right in assuming that his position there will never be the same as it was previously. A closer examination of his case shows, however, that his breakdown has been precipitated through unsatisfactory conditions in his marriage. His wife is of an unresponsive type and unintelligent. It is clear that for this reason he feels the setback in his job a greater tragedy than probably he would were his personal affairs more satisfying. As long as his occupational activities were a source of pleasure for him, he could suppress his wishes for the death of his wife. In the new circumstances, however, he is no longer able to do so efficiently and he becomes ill, in the main troubled by fear of his work and by suicidal ideas. In the course of his analysis he soon learns to discern between what is justifiable resentment against his employer and what is but displaced from his wife. In brief, he recognizes the symbolic significance of the office and the employer. Nevertheless, we cannot deny that on the whole his occupation *is* of great significance for him. We must realize that, in view of the unsatisfactory emotional circumstances in his marriage, an improved position in the firm might be capable of restoring his self-confidence and desire to live. Moreover, it is in the nature of things that it is easier to imagine an improvement of conditions in one's occupational field than to believe that a cool and unintelligent wife might ever change into a more desirable type. This latter anomaly cannot be eliminated unless death interferes ; but the anticipation of this outcome creates psycho-neurotic potentials. Thus, the student will realize that in the case under discussion, however certain might be the symbolic, secondary significance of the job, the latter in its concrete sense has, in fact, attained supreme significance for the life of the patient. The *symbolic meaning* of the office and employer has reinforced the *concrete significance* of this domain of life ; and for all practical purposes this problem has become the main object of interest both for the patient and the doctor dealing with the case.

In this instance it is comparatively easy to understand the superior significance of the conscious element, as contrasted with its symbolic meaning, because, in point of fact, the problem of emphasis might also be conceived from a different angle. We might simply assume that in view of the unsatisfactory home conditions the subject has concentrated all his interest on the business, and deficiencies there are bound to affect him to a substantial extent. The phenomenon of displacement might be excluded from the discussion of the case if we were prepared to ignore psychoanalytical experience and believe that depression with anxiety attacks and suicidal ideas may be *entirely* accounted for by a loss of prestige in business. The psychoanalyst, however, knows that the patient in question produced during his analysis a large number of phantasies in which his wife was dead and he himself was free to go out with a special type of prostitute which in his day-dreams he always desired to meet.

2. There are, however, other instances where the details of the case are different, and where it is indeed difficult to describe the deeper conflict in terms of the conscious form of the complaint. There we have to realize that the literal meaning of an impression may be reinforced from the symbolic spheres and become, for all practical purposes and for a time, the central object of our therapeutic work. Attempts by the analyst to turn the patient's attention entirely to the deeper-lying elements, or to conscious conflicts that he wishes to ignore, must result in a delay or failure to progress.

A man sought treatment because he worried too much if his old mother or father had a cold. The analysis of his dreams suggested incestuous experiences with his sister as well as homosexual scenes with his brother. The patient admitted that this had really been the case. Nevertheless, his analysis continued without practical result as long as the analyst concentrated his efforts on this material. Only when a different line was taken and the attitudes of the patient towards his parents were discussed extensively, did he begin to feel better. This implies that the sexual complexes and the associated sense of guilt have lent their psychoenergetic charge to the problem of the parents. After this question had received sufficient attention, the patient readily submitted to the analysis of the sexual problems and his working capacity was entirely restored.

Since father and mother imply sexual partners, and the average child finds this thought embarrassing, the memory of the tabooed incestual experience could easily enter into association with the idea of the parents. Thus, it was possible that some of the psychoaffective charge referring to the incestuous complex was displaced on to the spheres of ideas referring to the parents. This explanation, however, does not yet fully illustrate the thesis under discussion ; it shows, in fact, no more than the phenomenon of displacement, through which a comparatively trivial or peculiar concept by way of some association becomes invested by an emotional charge due to another element.

The reader's attention is, however, directed to the symbolic meaning of a cold, or for that matter of any other physical ailment. Its literal significance is an abnormality with the implication of possible danger to life. Hence, it is a frequent symbol in dreams of what we consider to be *complexes* in repression, capable of creating a sense of guilt or anxiety. Thus, we shall understand that the symbolic, secondary meaning of the idea that the parents are ill is really capable of carrying the affective charge of the incestuous tendencies; and this cathexis may intensify the legitimate concern of the patient at the minor ailments of his aged parents. Dynamically, this meant that this person was in reality more concerned about his parents than average people would be under objectively similar circumstances. After his readjustment his response became less exaggerated. Hence, in the first phase of his analysis the whole question of the parents had first to be dealt with along lines of conscious knowledge; that is by discussing the medical aspect of illnesses as well as the personal relationship of the patient to his parents and family life altogether. Only then was the way opened to a fuller discussion of the incestuous complexes and their rôle in the psychoneurotic complaints.

These remarks must not, however, be misunderstood by the tyro in psychotherapy as advice to enforce a certain order in the course of the analysis. In cases like the one described, the insistence of the free associations on the conscious element actually makes it imperative to deal with it to a sufficient extent, whilst not ignoring the free associations referring to psychoanalytical complexes proper. Our explanation renders intelligible the insistence with which such apparently trifling, non-psychoanalytical elements reappear; and it also shows why it is wise to yield to the wishes of such a patient, instead of simply referring to the factor of *resistance* in the recognition of deeper processes.

## Paranoia and Allied Conditions

1. The view is held in this work that *prejudice is the paranoia of the non-psychotic person.* This thesis requires further examination in the light of current notions in psychiatry. In the course of the discussions in Ch. III reference has been made to the type of eccentric " prophets " of religious, medical, and social systems, and the writer has classed these phenomena as mild paranoias. In official psychiatry they are described under the heading of " fanatic psychopaths ". From the monograph by *Schneider* on the subject it is nevertheless obvious that the close relationship between this group of psychopaths and genuine paranoia has

been recognized. This author accepts the statement by *Ziehe*r that " the point of difference is not so much one of diagnosis as one of prognosis ". Schneider only adds that the expression " paranoid attitude " implies first of all an element " of reference to the self ", and only in the second place the presence of an over-valued, quasi-delusional, concept. Nevertheless, in his chapter on the *depressive psychopath* the same author recognizes that the term " paranoid " may well be applied to the delusional tendency itself.

2. Here we are not concerned with questions of psychiatric terminology or classification, only in so far as applicable to social psychology. It can hardly be denied that Kraepelin's " geniune paranoia " on the one hand, and the condition represented by the fanatical eccentric on the other, are closely related. In both instances there is a logically coherent system of belief, clearly constituting a component of the personality. This can be said neither of the delusions in schizophrenia nor of those in mania and melancholia, and even less of the type manifested in the organic reaction psychoses (g.p. of the insane, etc.).

It is obvious that if two phenomena appear more or less different, even though they have much in common, they imply different things. If a number of persons develop paranoia, another group appears as fanatical psychopaths, and a third, admittedly larger, group manifests one of the current prejudices, then we must keep in mind that we are dealing with three distinct manifestations. Nevertheless, these three types of psychopathological phenomenon are so strikingly similar that we are entitled to classify them together, and even assume a fundamental identity of the underlying processes. The three-faced manifestation of this presumably common process is merely the consequence of differences in the fundamental structure of the personality, resulting thus in some differences in response to the identical intramental difficulty.

In all the three instances the personality is coherent, with a fair—at times even keen—intellect ; and there is no sign of a metabolical or otherwise organic psychotic process. The delusional system is in these three instances logically coherent, circumscribed, insistent, and to various degrees militant and aggressive in tendency. These beliefs appear to be variations or imitations of other firm beliefs that are recognized as normal or justifiable. The element of reference to the *self* is clearly present in prejudice ;

only the person refers the danger or anomaly to be fought against to his group or to humanity at large, himself included. In the case of fanatics and " prophets " on the one hand and the prejudiced " normal " on the other, it is obvious that we deal with *social attitudes*. The timid, or the over-cautious brand of psychopath represent other types of a deficient social function ; in a number of cases the subject accounts for his behaviour and isolation by blaming " the world at large ", the cool and selfish nature of his fellow-beings. There are also *depressive psychopaths* who are embittered, irritable, and nagging, persons who are " always dissatisfied and hurt " (Aschaffenburg).

It appears obvious that the psychopathological types referred to here display diseased social attitudes. It would not be right to say that the unsatisfactory attitude is merely a secondary feature of a distinct psychopathological condition ; the truth is rather that the inability for average coexistence and co-operation is the central feature and essence in these conditions. And it is suggested that we view the manifestations of paranoia from the same angle. Whether such a patient is a megalomaniac, or suffering in the main from persecutory delusions, he manifests in a distorted form current social attitudes. Many a man wishes to be great and powerful ; and the number of persons who feel deprived, by mishap or injustice, of a higher rôle allegedly due to them is very large. There has never been any doubt that paranoia is, as it were, a malignant degeneration of such sentiments. The prejudiced person represents a different picture in so far that his delusion emphasizes not so much injustice to his individual self, but anomalous conditions endangering society, and that he is prepared to share the position of superiority with a large community, to the exclusion of an inferior group.

## The Stranger and the New Phenomenon

1. In Chapter II reference was made to the fact that the presence of a stranger, or for that matter the mention of a new concept, may evoke in the subject a measure of uneasiness and even lead to the display of passionate antagonism. The notions of *neophobia* and *xenophobia* are surely not new to the reader of this book. These reactions are, in the opinion of the writer, attributable partly to the stimulation of the competitive complex, and partly to the *ad hoc* symbolic significance of the " strange ", representing some repressed elements in the subconscious. Obviously, the reaction

of irritability to the appearance of a stranger or to new concepts is only one, admittedly very frequent, type of response to such an environmental stimulus. We know that new ideas have a strong appeal to many people, and that the stranger may, at least in the beginning, be received with a definitely positive attitude. In such cases the subject apparently expects from the new phenomenon, and in particular from the new type of fellowmen, a fulfilment of some of his desires or a compensation for his frustrations. In another context (*Man and his Fellowmen*, Ch. xx) the writer has discussed the phenomenon in connection with resentment the subject may feel towards his relatives and confederates (cf. also Ch. V in this work). Here it is intended to view the problem from the wider aspect of psychoaffective dynamics in general.

2. Emotional hunger makes a person disposed to expect from various new things, be it a person or situation, some fulfilment of his desires, or at least the enrichment of his day-dreams. This anticipatory attitude cannot occur, however, if the subject's mind to some extent fears emotional experiences; this phenomenon is a frequent defence mechanism employed in the service of instinctual repression. In this case, only members of one's own group (co-nationals or co-religionists)—preferably those known to the subject—may be capable of relaxing the anti-emotional defences, whereas the appearance of the stranger on the scene is reacted to with intensification of these psychopathological potentials. We have, therefore, to realize that the endopsychic interpretation of the "new" or the "stranger" depends on pre-existent conditions within the mind; the ensuing response varies because of the variety in the basic psychoaffective tone, which is the ground of repercussion. A subject who is afraid of the free course of his emotional function may react to the presence of the stranger with uneasiness, projection, and manifest prejudice; because, for him, the new impression becomes a symbol of tabooed tendencies in repression. It is well known that persons of a cheerful and social character, who enjoy life without much moral conflict—because they probably feel that they need *not* fear excesses on their part—are comparatively immune from neophobia and irrational prejudice. For them the stranger, or a new concept, in average circumstances does *not* represent a dreaded tendency, and does not automatically suggest an encroachment on the precarious stability of their moral processes. Likewise, people who drink moderately though regularly, and also persons who

are not very strict [1] with themselves in sexual morals, seem to be less disposed to aggressive prejudice. These latter types deal with their moral difficulties in a manner that makes other indirect solutions well-nigh superfluous for them ; whereas the "jovials" have by nature no considerable difficulties in their deep moral processes. The reader is reminded of the concept according to which it is the subjective perception of mental elements rather than their quality and quantity that is responsible for reactive processes. The jovial type (largely belonging in the pyknic category) apparently does not suffer from such an accentuated apperception of their deeper mental processes.

3. Returning to the main trend of our discussion, we shall have to realize that intolerance in general, and that towards strangers in particular, may be the result of the fear of sexuality. Friendly interest for one's fellow-being on the one hand, and libidinal interest (both hetero- and homophile) on the other, are as it were on the same affective keyboard ; and some person's psyche anticipates that vibrations at one end of the scale might cause a repercussion at the other end. This apprehensive anticipation may be justified in some individuals, or with regard to some situations in the life of many ; but in most instances, the defensive attitude of the emotional function is rooted in psychoneurotic potentials. To a substantial extent the reactive products of such psychoneurotic elements are tending towards externalization, and it is easy to imagine how all this paves the way to intolerance. That a stranger evokes this defensive intolerance more readily than a homologous type of individual is intelligible, because of the endopsychic symbolical significance attached to the *new* and *different*. Representing as it were the foreign mental element in repression, the stranger or the heterogeneous concept unfavourably stimulates the tabooed complexes, and amongst these there are sexual tendencies to a large extent. The writer has the impression that intra-mental attempts by average "normals" to neutralize homosexual complexes is, in many instances, responsible for intolerant or prejudiced attitudes.

The extent of potential aggressiveness in the subject is one of the factors deciding whether a stranger, or fellowman in general, stimulates positive libidinal friendly attitudes, or alternatively mobilizes defences in the form of intolerance. The reader is reminded of the fact that pre-existent psychoaffective constella-

[1] That is, persons who do not dwell on their lax morals.

tions are responsible for the particular character of reactions ; in the instance under discussion, likewise, such a pre-existent, affective potential is responsible for the interpretation in either way of the *new* and *strange*. The more resentment and *primary aggressiveness* (cf. Ch. XI) exists in the subject, the more likely is his psyche to identify the stranger with tabooed and " dangerous " tendencies in himself.

## The Ethnic Psyche and Ethnic Prejudice

1. In the preceding chapters the concept of the ethnic psyche has been referred to in various contexts. However indubitable the fact that group differences with regard to the character of mass phenomena exist, the clear delineation of the notion of a " group mind " encounters logical difficulties (cf. R. H. Thouless, *Gen. and Social Psychology*, Ch. xvi, 5). There is, obviously, no psyche other than that of the individual, provided we do not have in mind the notion of a metaphysical soul ; because the latter concept could, without difficulty, be applied also to a separate group-soul. The existence and function of the metaphysical soul is obviously outside the scope of this work. Accordingly, that which appears to be the *group mind* can only be a certain aspect or mode of functioning of the individual psyche. There are a number of psychic processes that operate only when the individual reacts as a member of a group ; or, there are aspects of the individual's psyche that refer to his membership of a group. We may also say that certain mental processes assume a more or less modified character and content if the individual is clearly aware of his being a component of a " crowd ". In this way it is possible that the members of such a group feel and do certain things, even though when they are not aware of their group, and think of themselves as private individuals, the same feelings, ideas, and impulses apparently do not exist in them.

2. There are a number of tendencies and beliefs that the individual projects on to his group, as if not wishing to attribute them to himself. Such are, for instance, in primitive societies various superstitious concepts of which the member of the group prefers to think in terms of extrinsic magical forces and processes ; in some instances, the priests and temples, as well as the chieftains, are invested by popular belief with these qualities and characteristics. From these group-phenomena we are able to infer the

structure of what is referred to as *group mind* and *group spirit* in general. As a rule, the individual ignores these elements in himself and lets them become dynamic only within a manifested group, as if shifting the responsibility and credit for them to the " spirit " of the group, and conceiving himself as being influenced by these allegedly extrinsic elements.

The significance of this displacement is obvious. A belief appears to the individual more weighty if conceived as characteristic of the group (race, nation, religious community, and any party or team). Group pride and a contempt for the outsider is a loftier attitude if attributed to a community than if conceived of as an individual sentiment. Likewise, hatred or prejudiced belief felt and manifested by the individual becomes for him more significant and more justifiable if he is able to associate it with his group.

3. Through mutual agreement and tradition within the group, the concepts of humanity, nationalism, tolerance, as well as the extent of repression and refinement of elementary tendencies, assume a local colouring ; and the individual member of the group reinforces his own spontaneous sentiments and complexes by the acceptance of extrinsic patterns of behaviour and reaction. The resulting tendencies and complexes, however, may become a burden to the less sophisticated and comparatively unadulterated layers of the psyche ; there ensues a conflict between the elementary social sense (cf. Ch. I) and the acquired complexes, and this tension stimulates projection, intolerance, and prejudice. It is in the nature of things that in such societies the administrative and social pressure on the individual subject is rather crude, and the psyche derives little satisfaction from the environmental atmosphere (cf. on this problem Ch. VIII, (3), (7)). Indignation at the poverty of soothing impressions and the crudeness of existing conditions in turn intensifies the irrational hatred, and this hatred employs the pathways of projective resentment. This is, in brief, the genetic development of what the writer calls ethnic prejudice.

4. The reader is justified in asking : what are the factors that in relatively progressive societies have led to a comparative refinement of the communal atmosphere, and in others to the preservation and cultivation of primitive superstition ? The writer admits

that it is difficult to locate exactly the point at which in some of the instances the course of events turned in the direction of progress. Nevertheless, it appears possible to add a few thoughts to the previous discussion.

There were phases in all the progressive societies of to-day when spirited leaders, ahead of their contemporaries in enlightenment, and at the same time respected by them, have stimulated in their environment the forceful suppression of individual savagery, and achieved in their country the creation of a refined social hypothesis (cf. on this notion Ch. XII). That is to say, the masses of individuals were persuaded that the communal spirit—embodied in law, religion, and the opinion of its best members—is much higher than the average character of individual behaviour. Thus, the subconscious of the individuals, appreciative of this higher standard, even though incapable of entirely adhering to it, became accustomed to a dichotomy of moral concepts. Projecting largely on to the communal aspect of life all that is noble and humane, the individual members created an extraneous factor, and then submitted to its influence. The persons capable of further contributing to the refinement of the social spirit tried to make themselves heard. But only where the concept of personal freedom was a fairly dynamic factor, appreciated at least as legitimate principle, did the influence of such idealists become an element of the public spirit. Where the masses feel that an idealist, aiming at some change of the existing order, automatically becomes a person of less social significance, his theories and efforts are reacted to with contempt and even hostility.

Why the sense of personal freedom and significance has been more, or less, developed in certain regions, is not easy for me to answer.

Much depended on the personal preferences of the ruling circles. But the writer feels that he has to come back to the concept of a *racial nucleus* in the individual. This includes a larger or smaller capacity of the material brain for broadmindedness, which implies differences in efficient repression and in the capacity for the creation of higher compensatory interests. It is certain that geophysical (climatic) factors are largely responsible for racial differences. But it is equally true that fortuitous factors in history have directed the streams of cultural influence coming from the ancient Greeks, Romans, and Judeo-Christians towards some regions more purely and forcefully than towards others. Notwithstanding this fact, other dynamic phenomena that have been created within nations and groups in a rather planned manner, by ruling cliques for the defence of their interests, have resulted in a lowering of the repressive and sublimating capacity of the masses. Instinctively, as well as from tradition, such rulers knew that it is easier to keep in dependence, and employ for aggressive wars, people who are not refined, or not appreciative of the significance of the human personality.

If in a country that has been conspicuous for technical and scientific achievement, the politicians and philosophers have adored power—beyond appreciating its defensive value—and writers and theologians have given a kindred self-conceited colouring to their teachings, then in spite of all intellectual progress, the deeper unsophisticated mental spheres have been bound to revolt against the violation of their needs ; and this, as we know, may lead to projection. And if, in addition, there has been a ready pattern of national self-aggrandisement, the tendency of externalization has found a preformed pathway towards aggressive prejudice. This element has subsequently been transformed into a quasi-supernatural ethnic factor to which every worthy son of the nation must submit to be guided by it in all his individual behaviour.

## The Libido

1. The reference to the libido in Ch. XII calls for an explicit discussion of this Freudian notion.[1] In so far as it applies to phenomena whose sexual significance is indubitable, this term requires no further elaboration. The necessity for this only arises when the object of discussion is the group of those deeper mental processes which only orthodox psychoanalysis assumes to be of libidinal character. This doctrine holds the libido responsible for all psychoneuroses, that is, its faulty development and unsuccessful repression ; the latter taking place in the main through the influence of the " castration fear " and its functional parallels, such as the fear of losing the love of the mother or of society, or the fear of disapproval by the subject's super-ego. It is assumed that both the libido and its disturbances in question are beyond the conscious recognition by the subject. The world of dreams does lend itself as a proof, provided the various objects and events of which the dream picture consists are interpreted in accordance with the symbolic system laid down in the *Introductory Lectures* and the *Dream Interpretation* by Freud. In addition, the frequently

[1] The meaning attached to this word by *Jung* is outside the scope of our discussion.

obvious erotic character of what is called the transference attitude of the analysand may be taken as some evidence that his deeper mental processes are, to a large extent, libidinal. This is all the more possible as the transference emotion apparently plays a substantial rôle in bringing about therapeutic success.

Clearly, the symbolic interpretation of dreams cannot be an unequivocal proof. The intensity of the transference emotion on the other hand, certainly suggests the extensive rôle of libidinal processes in the psychoaffective mechanism. It seems, indeed, that this is the only point regarding the libido we are able to establish indubitably. If in the course of the psychoanalysis of an obsessional woman, with no apparent interest in life other than that of her illness, a vehement libidinal tendency towards the analyst emerges, and this under circumstances that, by common sense, do not justify such a feeling, then we must believe in the existence of dormant libidinal currents. I have in mind patients who not only received no encouragement whatsoever for such a sentiment, but who thought their analyst an unattractive and impolite person. Cases of young women falling in this sham-love with old male analysts are well-known ; or, of women who thought themselves frigid and were averse to intercourse, but clearly felt that the case would be different were the analyst or his son their partner. Even more indicative of the existence of repressed but dynamic libidinal tendencies are instances of homoerotic transference in both sexes emerging to the surprise of the subjects.

2. There is no cogent reason for denying the possibility that " unconscious libido " exists even to an extent that is beyond recognition in the course of a psychoanalysis ; mere interpretations are, of course, no recognition in the sense I have in view here, but bare assumptions based on a ready-made theory. But, equally, there is no immediate proof for the existence of an unconscious libido that is not manifested in an unequivocal manner.

Nevertheless, the writer feels that we might take seriously even the unprovable hypotheses of an author such as Freud, because his statements in a number of other aspects have proved to be right, or at least fruitful. It is therefore suggested that we assume that unconscious libido occupies a considerable place in the psychoaffective mechanism both normal and pathological, whilst at the same time realizing that, perhaps to an even greater extent, other forces are also operative behind what we call the integrated personality. Freud himself accepted the existence of "ego-tendencies", and in his latter works he frequently, and with emphasis, referred to the rôle of subconscious aggressiveness, originally postulated by Stekel. There appears, however, no sufficient reason for limiting the extent of the non-libidinal mental spheres to these particular elements. In the present work reference is made to a number of other distinct forces; they, too, may safely be called *complexes*. The rôle of innate collective elements in the sense of Jung must not be forgotten in this context.

3. Even if we assume thus that the libidinal processes constitute but a sector of the whole psychoaffective life, it might still be true that psychoneuroses proper develop where a disturbance of libidinal repression prevails. It would be logically permissible to assume that non-specific aggressiveness (that is, with the exclusion of the sexual, Oedipal hatred), the competitive and possessive complex, jealousy and striving for power and prestige, are of paramount significance; and that of no lesser significance for mental balance is the extent to which the subject tolerates the variety of polar tensions within his psyche, as well as the particular mode of his reacting to this aspect of his mental functioning (cf. Ch. XII). This notwithstanding, one could still believe that psychoneuroses in the narrower sense are the consequence of libidinal difficulties as assumed by orthodox psychoanalysis. Clearly, even if we were to take this stand, it would be unjustifiable to limit the scope of *our* inquiries in social psychology and social pathology to the mechanism allegedly at the root of the psychoneuroses. In this case, of course, we could not simply assume, as is however done in general, that mental phenomena of pathological nature are only distortions of processes occurring in the average normal.[1]

However, there are sufficient reasons to doubt that the psychological background of the personality is actually as simple as it is made to appear by the Freudian theory of psychoneuroses and the application of this doctrine to the normal functioning of the mind. There are, undoubtedly, cases where treatment on Adlerian lines has freed a patient in a few sessions of a phobia that had troubled him previously for years. Where, however, the treatment by an Individual-psychologist extends over several months, I am unable to ignore the contribution by the Freudian

[1] Cf. Bleuler, *Psychiatry*.

*transference.* One may speak to a patient in terms of power and inferiority complex, and his psyche understands all this in terms of libido. But, as mentioned, the more clearly such a cure has been brought about by explanations and logical interpretations rather than by mere encouragement or a long period of analysis, the more the central rôle of the libido in both the neurosis and its cure appears equivocal. Should we, however, choose to say that in such cases the therapist has, in fact, indirectly restored the balance of the libido, then we were already admitting the complex nature of psychoaffective happenings.

4. There is one thing that appears to be a peculiarity of libidinal tendencies, certainly much more than of other tendencies discussed in this work. It is the amorphous character of the libidinal drive ; its objects and objectives are not so well-defined and exclusive as those of the other tendencies referred to. The desire for power, possession, and prestige can be satisfied only in concrete fields and in distinct ways. Envy and jealousy, too, refer to the environmental atmosphere of the subject. The feeling of human inadequacy in all respects has no meaning at all without the concrete human environment. Libido, on the other hand, may be definitely narcissistic ; and what is even more characteristic, it can be satisfied to a very large extent subconsciously. The writer feels that, in spite of the justifiably critical attitude towards psychological hypotheses, there should be no doubt about this latter fact. Illustrative instances are sons devoting their lives to their mothers, and daughters to their fathers ; and likewise, brothers and sisters, or friends, living together, with the exclusion of manifested sexual desire towards strangers or the objects of their fixation. And even if, from time to time, the vague idea of a libidinal tendency towards these objects of fixation does enter consciousness, during the overwhelmingly larger part of this community of life the libidinal satisfaction remains an unrealized process ; yet indubitably it takes place.[1]

A more or less unconscious satisfaction of the libido with not well specified objects occurs, in all probability, in people who, as a rule, live an active sexual life, but through exceptional circumstances have for a substantial period to be without it. In this case, the libido is satisfied with the help of memories as well as the concrete presence of various persons in the subject's environment : the conscious character of this process may, in some individuals,

[1] This is a veiled but manifest satisfaction of the libido through emotional ties, not " unconscious libido " (p. 263).

be limited to a vague realization lasting only for a few seconds, whereas in the main the process remains, for obvious reasons, unrecognized by them. The libidinal current does not cease if circumstances interrupt active sexual life.

5. We should find it intelligible that critics of Freud deemed his "pansexualism" unacceptable, and could not agree with him that the libido is the central agent in psychoaffective life. There was, admittedly, a risk that the significance of tendencies other than those of the libido might be overlooked, and that consequently a rather monotonous psychology, doomed to remain sterile, be created; and in addition it appeared that a hedonistic philosophy of life might be advocated under the disguise of a scientific doctrine. Unfortunately, Freud—admittedly the founder of psychoanalysis—used to refer to his own theories and hypotheses very frequently as "findings and results of *psychoanalysis*"; but the scientific world and the general public was expected to believe that this orthodox psychoanalysis is a well established scientific domain comparable with physiology. In fact, even to this day there is very little of the large amount of theoretical discussions that may be justifiably considered as firmly established. Happily, these few component parts of Freudian psychology proved to be of supreme practical significance.

The writer feels that decades of sustained criticism and discussion have by now secured a better sense of proportion; and we may perhaps venture the acceptance of the substantial rôle of the libido within the psyche. It appears more satisfactory to conceive of the elementary processes of the psyche in terms of a fundamental, comprehensive form of energy-current, rather than to adhere exclusively to a psychology based on a number of instincts. Unfortunately, the libido alone cannot account for human psychology. But we know that both the value and weaknesses of the instinct-psychology, mainly represented by McDougall, have become apparent to those who tried to develop further our domain with an eye on the large accumulation of newer observations. The initiated student will remember the attempt by Jung to modify the concept of libido with a view to building on it a general psychology. The writer, however, wishes to deal here with the notion in its original Freudian application, but without discarding the simultaneous validity of Jung's concept (cf. his *Psychology of the Unconscious*, Part II, Chs. I and II. See also the comment by Freud in *Narcissism*, Ch. I).

6. One must not overlook the distinct difference between what is assumed to be the libidinal energy and its manifestations on the one hand, and what are tendencies of various kinds on the other. It is hardly possible to attribute, for instance, to the tendency of competition or aggression a specific kind of energy. The writer has in various contexts tried to show that these, as well as a number of *a*-social tendencies, are capable of being understood as manifestations of the instinct of self-preservation. Tendencies, so the writer thinks, cannot be conceived of otherwise than as representatives of *ideas* and the associated impulses for their materialization. It is indispensable that psychoaffective energy be utilized in the course of these events ; but there is probably nothing specific in this energy, nor is this current of energy a characteristic factor in the structure of the particular tendency. The tendency and impulse of aggression are in so far different from the general category of tendencies that there is a mental tension due to a mutual opposition of goals, which fact implies the aim of eliminating entirely or partly the " counterpart " ; the latter is in most instances conceived as a concrete object ; cf. Ch. XI.

The libidinal tendency aims in essence at a pleasurable satisfaction of a psychosomatic kind, through a specific stimulation of the subject's body-structure. On the mature genital level, the presence of a partner-object is an essential prerequisite. In the absence of such a concrete partner, the psyche has recourse to the image of such an object ; and in the narcissistic process the image of the *self* plays this rôle. But even in this latter case, the satisfaction consists in the libidinal stimulation of the subject's *soma*.[1] Moreover, we have no cogent reason for denying the possibility that a non-conscious process of this kind also exists. In the case of coitus, masturbation, or thrilling sensation at the sight or thought of a partner, one ought to distinguish between the conscious libidinal sensation and the subsequent satisfaction of the deeper psychic spheres ; the latter is never a conscious process, even though its reality is obvious in cases where it is deficient and results in symptoms. The specific stimulation of the *soma* cannot be well imagined without assuming that some energy receives a specific character in the course of the process. The whole process takes place through the *sexual instinct*, which is a vital disposition comparable to the mating instinct of animals. But in the human being this disposition is, to a large extent, also in the service of the

[1] Cf. in Ch. V (5) of *Foundation of Dream-Interpretation* by the writer : " The affect lies at the meeting point of *soma* and *psyche*."

psyche, aiming at a specific—that is libidinal— satisfaction of the mental aspect of the personality. That is to say, this instinct is responsible for the libidinal desire, the transformation of some energy into a sexual one, the specific stimulation of the *soma*, and in the case of external action for the genital process.

The reason for speaking in the case of libido of an *instinct*, and not merely of a libidinal *tendency*, ought to be obvious. Above all, we have to keep in our minds the association of the pleasure-libido with the forces of procreation ; secondly, there is in the psycho-sexual satisfaction no *idea* striving for its materialization. In so far as the procreative aspect of sex is concerned, an idea aiming at its concrete materialization is indubitably present. Yet, the writer is dealing here with the psychoaffective significance of the libido. The absence of a central idea is the very reason inducing the writer to conceive of the libidinal process in terms of energy ; the specific transformation and current of this energy appear to be the essence of the process. Moreover, there is sufficient reason for believing that libidinal currents are present continually within the subject ; and this implies the continuous transformation of energy into a libidinal one, though to an ever-changing extent. Incidentally, we realize that the much mooted question of *sublimation* may thus refer to two possibilities ; the one is the deflection of specific libidinal energy—or tendency ; the other the prevention of the creation of such a specific energy.

7. In view of the substantial rôle we attribute to the libido, it must be intelligible that factors disturbing its currents may really lead to psychoneuroses. In this work, however, we are primarily concerned with another problem. It has been suggested that a new element to be introduced into the subconscious of the masses has to be capable of appealing to the subconscious libido. Certainly, it must not disturb the libidinal satisfactions if its acceptance by the mind were not to be opposed from the outset. But, in fact, much more is required for the end in view. The reader of Ch. XII will remember that a number of potent factors may stand in the way of a suggestion being received into the psychic mechanism. Therefore, it has to be capable of positively contributing to the pleasure-giving mental potentials, and above all to the processes concerned with the reduction of endopsychic tension. The writer believes that these relieving mechanisms have an intrinsic connection with the libidinal processes ; hence, he

assumes that the new element ought to be capable of aiding the intra-mental libidinal satisfaction if it is to do the work assigned to it.

8. All this is obviously pure theoretical speculation. May be that at some future period, perhaps before long, we shall have to recast our concept and realize that the libidinal satisfaction is but a component sphere of another, more comprehensive process concerned with relieving psychoaffective tension and granting pleasurable satisfaction. But the writer feels that to-day we have no real reason for departing from the hypothesis that libidinal satisfaction is the elementary pleasure *par excellence* in so far that in it there is no " idea " seeking materialization nor a biological need of the type of hunger, evacuation, etc. The desire for a concrete partner is not exactly an " idea " striving for fulfilment comparable to the content of other tendencies ; this feature of the libidinal force belongs to the procreative function, and on the higher level of sex, to the desire for personal love. Clearly, in the latter process there is a tendency with a goal that goes beyond a temporary satisfaction on a merely intra-mental plane of happening ; the aim is the possession of an extrinsic object and a partner to whom the subject likewise may give himself. This is no longer an *elementary libidinal process*.

The strong appeal of the *infantile* and *comical*, as well as of scenes on the stage and screen where human beings are caught by embarrassment and involved in painful situations, ought not to be attributed directly to a libidinal satisfaction by referring, for instance, to the attraction of nudity, to sadism, etc.[1] There is, however, a fairly logical hypothesis to bring into relationship the afore-mentioned pleasure-stimuli with libidinal satisfaction. We may assume that the public opportunity of enjoying infantile likings, as well as malicious sentiments, relieves some of the moral inhibitions weighing on the psyche, and this in turn facilitates some measure of endopsychic libidinal freedom. In the case of public performances the individual is allowed—with consent of his fellowmen—to enjoy infantilism, comically coloured mishaps of human creatures, and also scenes of downright violence and murder ; thus, the unconscious is in a position to realize that the strictness of ethical and legal principles is not to be taken in its fullest sense. And this may, as it were, encourage the psyche to

[1] The student is advised to read Ch. XI, 1–8, in *General and Social Psychology*, by R. H. Thouless.

relax, to some extent and temporarily, the reins of inhibition that limit the freedom of intra-mental libidinal currents.

The writer is aware of the fact that his explanation is not free of weaknesses. Moreover, he wishes to admit that in the discussion of the *libido* in general he does not feel to be on safe ground. He thinks that a more satisfactory concept on the appeal to the masses of the *infantile* and *cruel* might at the same time be capable of throwing more light on the whole process of satisfaction, as well as indicate the actual place the libido proper occupies within the psychoaffective mechanism. The rather uncritical fashion of average psychoanalytical presentations, and the attraction the notion of libido has for scientists and laymen alike, make a clearer vision difficult for the time being.

9. There now remains the task of trying to correlate the notion of the libidinal energy and processes with the notion of instincts and tendencies as well as mental " factors " of a distinct function.

Instincts, as McDougall has described them, are innate dispositions of vitally important specific activities. Such are, for instance, the impulse to seek food and eat it when hunger signalizes a need for it ; the activities of defence either by escape or pugnacity ; the parental love and care for the offspring ; the desire and capacity to share life with others, etc. These activities are of a complicate character, as if carried out according to a well-thought-out plan and with the help of acquired knowledge. In their essence, however, they occur through impulses of inborn nature. It is obvious that an expenditure of energy is involved in all these performances ; but it would be far-fetched to assume a specific energy peculiar to each of them. On the other hand, the impulse at the root of each of these performances is a markedly specific force of the cerebro-psyche. We have to realize that it is not only the impulse but to an extent also the pattern of the instinctive behaviour that is innate ; but, clearly, in the human being this pattern of performance is much less stereotyped than in animals and is influenced by experience and learning. In fact, man's food seeking or defence instinct, for instance, is comparable with that in animals only in regard to its essence, but certainly not to its pattern of execution. We refer in these instances to *instincts*, because we feel with certainty that in their essential character and innate deep-rootedness there is an identity with similar performances of animals. However, we could well speak in the case of human instincts of tendencies. We also realize that in other, numerous modes of human aiming and striving we may speak only of tendencies but not of instincts. All the ways and modes of manifesting, defending, and attempting to enhance the significance of the individual amidst his fellowmen are *tendencies* in the narrower sense.

Neither human " instincts " nor " tendencies " can be conceived in terms of a specific energy process in the sense described above with respect to the libido. In the case of the latter, we assume a specific impulse aiming, as suggested, at the specific stimulation, for the sake of pleasure, of extensive somatic structures ; in the course of this process specific energy is transformed into libidinal one. And whereas we assume the continuity of the libidinal current, none of the other instincts and tendencies are at work uninterruptedly ; their operation have a close bearing on certain situations and well-defined aims.

It could be argued that vanity, for instance, is a tendency, a constant mental aspect, always ready to manifest itself. But in such an instance we deal with a " characteristic of the personality " ; one could speak of a " factor ", which is the dynamic force behind the tendency to display vanity, which, however, occurs in the form of individual actions on certain occasions. In so far as the factor of vanity is stimulated by the feeling of inadequacy,[1] it is obvious that a continuous supply of energy is employed for keeping the element of vanity, this secondary product, alive, that is, ready for manifestation. We cannot, however, say that specific energy is involved ; it is rather the associated idea (" I have to impress people," etc.) that is well-defined and thus specific. But this has obviously no resemblance to what we assume to be the continuity of the libidinal current.

From a broader angle, however, it must be admitted that the factor of vanity on the one hand, and the force aiming at libidinal satisfaction on the other, are similar in so far that in both instances there is a constant wish as well as a constant dynamism concerned with its fulfilment. The same may be said, for instance, of the tendency in an enterprising person to produce and attain results ; no doubt, this factor is never entirely at rest in his mind, even though it recedes into the background at frequent moments when the attention is focused on other wish-fulfilments or urgent tasks.

No wonder that Jung speaks of libido when he means life energy in the broader sense, in its functional aspect. The process of life is certainly continuous ; and since in the human being

[1] Cf. Ch. Ic.

its material aspect is inseparable from the psychoaffective events, these have likewise an unbroken course. It is permissible to say that the psychoaffective events aim at mental satisfaction in a general sense; and in this respect the sum-total of energy involved is indeed comparable to the libido proper, the operation of which we consider to be the wish and satisfaction *par excellence.*

10. These discussions should not merit a place in this work were it not for certain practical aspects involved. The postulate that new social elements to be introduced into the subconscious ought to appeal to the libido has already been mentioned. The reasons for this necessity also account for the fact that it is imperative to treat the libido in the course of psychotherapy.

We need to add a few words about "tendencies" and "mental factors" as objects of individual and social psychotherapy. The fact that they are largely distinct from the libido and its processes makes it intelligible that they might be diseased in themselves and in need of the special attention of the therapist and social psychologist. Obviously these tendencies and factors have two aspects; the one is their specific structure and function; the other, their contribution to general psychoaffective satisfaction and balance.[1] From the latter aspect there follows the possibility that the fair proportion of the various dynamic mental factors may be disturbed; or that alternatively in some instances there may be a need to stimulate the better development of a particular tendency or factor, the cultivation of which has been neglected by the subject in the previous phases of his life, for the sake of one-sided interest and direction of aims. Playful relaxation, for instance, may become at certain periods of a businessman's or scientist's life necessary, even though earlier in his life there was apparently no need for this. A contemplative dealing with one's problems—by way of psychological concepts—may become indispensable for another person at a certain phase of his life, even though he was previously quite successful in all he did, without the slightest measure of such a mental discipline. More, or less, *pugnacity* may be desirable for a third person, after a breakdown made necessary an analysis which in its turn indicated such a course for the future life of the patient. Even more frequently there is an urgent need of giving up competitiveness or high aiming in favour of a more indifferent attitude towards personal position. The writer hopes that these brief references

[1] Cf. the notion of *affect-ego* in *Man and his Fellowmen*, Ch. VIII.

are sufficiently intelligible so as to enable the student to elaborate further details for himself.

Returning to the main theme of this part it is suggested that the libido stimulates energy-processes that permeate the whole psychosomatic organization. This, however, does not mean that, for instance, inquisitiveness is in essence a derivative of sexual curiosity, or that the parent's affection for their children is fundamentally a libidinal sentiment. Here the writer has to part with the orthodox psychoanalytical theory of the libido.

### *The Social Sense and the Libido*

11. Frequent reference is made in this work to the social sense and the faculty of co-operation. In the course of our discussion we have taken the presence of these mental factors for granted, and have mainly dealt with the pathology of their function. It nevertheless appears advisable to examine more closely the essence of what appears to be the innate social sense. Obviously the vital *necessity* for co-operation in the life of the human individual is a potent environmental force in the creation of a corresponding *desire* for it. Objectively the individual requires, for most of his needs, the co-operation of his fellowmen ; moreover, he has to adjust himself to their joint existence on the stage of life. Hence the satisfaction derived from the operation of the social sense is not unexplainable, not elementary. The human mind is capable of enjoying its achievements, but also the functioning of the faculties employed for this end. What is recognized by the psyche as an expedient and indispensable constant function may even become desirable ; a compliance with such tendencies becomes associated with a feeling of satisfaction.

In the ultimate result there is a desire for human companionship ; and this propensity may justifiably be regarded as a distinct emotional tendency, that is, as one which, to a great extent, is independent of concrete utilitarian goals. The condition is similar to that existing in respect of the sexual instinct. In this sphere it is difficult to ignore that procreation is the paramount goal : the anatomy and physiology of the genital organs make this realization cogent. Nevertheless, it is equally certain that, in the human being, sex has also another, i.e. purely psychoaffective significance. If nothing else, then the difficulty of suppressing the sexual desire on the part of a person who already has children must bring this truth home. In an analogous way there is a double aspect in what we call the social sense. Even though the desire for companionship develops from a vital necessity, the result is a mental tendency of an independent emotional character. In practical life it is this emotional aspect of the social propensity that is largely conducive to and helpful in voluntary and expedient adjustment ; just as in the other sphere mentioned the libidinal drive is largely responsible for the performance of human fertilization.

The parallel between the two types of function, the social and the sexual, is all the more fitting, since there is even a direct link between the two spheres of human life. It is indubitable that libidinal attraction and revulsion enter *all* human relationships. In view of the complex nature of human sexuality—owing to the regulative and repressive processes—the social sense and will for co-operation cannot remain free from complication by the libidinal currents and idea-patterns prevailing in the subject. Both kinds of influence, furtherance and inhibition of the general social function by the libidinal processes, play their substantial part. We know that also the reverse process takes place. The competitive struggle for power between man and woman has been responsible for many difficulties in marriage and sexual life. There are cases of impotence and frigidity in the psychoaffective background of which disturbances of the social sense play a substantial rôle, reinforcing or activating the strictly libidinal sources of maldevelopment. As is well known Adlerian psychology attributes the sole causal responsibility for impotence or homosexuality to non-sexual forces. The fact that the adherents of this school also attain good therapeutic results speaks in favour of their theory. It is necessary, however, to point out that any psychologist who treats a patient for a considerable time stimulates the mysterious process of *transference* ; and through the revival of the analysand's life-story, the mobilization of subconscious emotional forces as well as complexes in the Freudian sense is inevitable. Thus the therapeutic success of an Individual-psychologist illustrates only to a limited extent the rôle of non-sexual anomalies in various psychoneuroses. But earlier in this section reference has been made to cases where appeal to the conscious and its logical faculty has been able to remove psychoneurotic complaints. In these instances, as well as in the successes of the non-dogmatic Stekelian method, the rôle of non-sexual, social complexes in mental dynamics is clearly illustrated. So much the writer wishes to say as to the facts.

He also feels that there is a possibility of extending the discussion to the field of remedy. Any person who is capable of coping with his sexuality—both intra-mentally and in practical life—more naturally and under less pressure than is the rule in most people, has a definite advantage also regarding his social faculty, compared with his fellowmen, who are less mature and less healthy in the former respect. The difference between better or worse here is solely a matter of deep psychic functioning. This comprehensive formula would be capable of elaboration, taking up a volume for itself. The writer has to add that, admittedly, in practice not every type of personality is fit to attain a sufficient balance of his libido. Those who are fortunate in being very happily married,[1] and at the same time are sufficiently broad-minded to recognize in themselves, on occasions, the impact of sexual attraction and revulsion, are very few. The vast majority of people have to manage life without becoming entirely mature, and without ever having had the benefit of emotional maturation through a successful psychonalysis. Hence in most people there will always be some volcanic material that interferes with their faculty of social adaptation. Happily there are persons in large numbers who are, by nature or particularly favourable educational circumstances, totally fit for a life of successful co-operation. But the vast majority of people will find it difficult to understand why they cannot co-operate with certain persons or on certain occasions, and also why other persons behave so strangely and irrationally as they do.

There can never be a world without sexual repression, and no human beings without some degree of sense of guilt and without some amount of inhibition. But it is a fact that a more reasonable education on these matters, and in many cases a shorter or longer psychoanalysis in youth—or as soon as some difficulties are felt—would be capable of improving a person's capacity to deal with the vicissitudes of his libido, conscious and unconscious. In the wake of this the function of co-operation is bound to improve to a degree it could not develop under less reasonable conditions. It has to be stressed, however, that no sexual education can be of any appreciable value as long as the human individual is not more free in social position than he is at present. The careful reader of this work will understand why. A slave is afraid of the very shadows of his *subconscious;* whereas a free personality may be capable of a more balanced subconscious judgment of the complicated processes of the

[1] Happy marriage is due largely to psychoaffective health.

mind. Here lies the secret, here the way of social improvement.

12. The intricacies of the libido—as well as the complexity of the psyche in general—account for the almost confusing multiformity shown by the co-operative faculty in various persons and in various circumstances. There are some who can get on very well in a small circle, but are inefficient within a large team. Most individuals, however, are at their best if members of a large group or organization. Obviously the impression of the size of the group is one factor that accounts for their improved subjective and objective condition. The reader is referred to what is said about the tendency of submission. Admittedly some individuals feel "significant" if in a small party; but many others feel "stronger" if members of a large organization.

Another factor is the motley multitude of impressions reaching the senses of the individual who is in a factory, large office, or armed group. This aspect has, in the opinion of the writer, close bearing on the libidinal spheres of the psyche. There are personalities whose mind needs such varied stimulation, because of the immature or not fully harmonious state of their love-capacity. There are individuals whose capacity for work and co-operation gains through their contact with people who, consciously and subconsciously, stimulate their libido; but there is an equally large number of individuals whose work—and even subjective ease—suffers through the same environmental factor. In exceptional cases the libidinal spheres do attain fair gratification solely from a monogamic love-relationship and the additional enjoyment derived from social intercourse with a few close friends. This is, however, a very rare condition. Similar to this human ideal, but in essence pathological, is the case of the person who is *unable* to maintain relationship with more people than the members of his closest family and his immediate associates at work.

The number of persons who get on well with their family but hardly ever with strangers is fairly large. Even more numerous are those with whom the opposite is the case. Naturally family ties are permanent, and can be a great mental burden (cf. Ch. V). In addition to this reason, we have to take into consideration the complicating influence of the sexual relationship. Undoubtedly there are personality types who develop hatred towards their conjugal-sexual partner, whereas they do not hate others without serious reason. It appears as if the sexual relationship has poisoned the inter-human atmosphere. Individual psychoanalyses may show that such persons—as in fact many others—have an antisexual complex; their own and their partner's yielding to the sexual urge is considered by their subconsciousness as something mean, poisonous, interfering with the anagogic tendencies.[1] Apart from this latter reason adult sexual life is frequently an attack on infantile fixations. From this angle the unfavourable reaction to normal sexual activity is comparable to the sense of guilt associated with fraud or adultery. Another possibility is the distinct identification of one's wife, the mother of one's children, with one's own mother or sister, and this may intensify the general antisexual tendency. Adler would say that such an identification is secondary, a protest against conjugal obligations.

Here we have drawn attention to the association of the co-operative faculty with the spheres of the libido (or pleasure principle, if we prefer this term). The careful reader of the various chapters must, however, have realized that all the discussions deal in essence with the disturbances of the social function. From the negative aspects it is easy to draw conclusions as to the nature of the conditions making for efficient functioning of the co-operative faculty.

The reader is also reminded that paranoia in the broader sense, as implied in this work, is a psychosis of the social-moral faculty. In the opinion of the writer these conditions are primarily psychotic disturbances of the social sense.

## Narcissistic Libido and Primary Aggressiveness

1. Freud has stated that the infantile narcissistic libido is to some extent re-employed later in the libidinal cathexis of the ideal-ego. This thesis is borne out by manifest phenomena. The passion and display of self-sufficiency with which people at large advocate their ideals, as well as the associated aggressiveness towards real or imaginary outsiders, appear childish; this behaviour matches neither the higher notion of ethics nor intelligent principles in general. Admittedly, were ideals not charged with enthusiasm they would be less capable of influencing life. Comparatively few persons are able to have ideals which are unequivocally firm as well as fruitful in practice, and at the

[1] Psychic processes concerned with the spiritual aspect of the personality.

same time to be free of intolerance and irrational self-sufficiency.

It thus appears that primary narcissism and elementary aggressiveness are not only similar in respect to genetic independence, but later in life they become interlinked in the super-ego. I do not mean here the aggressiveness towards the *self* in the form of the strict super-ego, described by Freud, but the self-sufficiency associated with the " idealism " of so many people, which induces them to contemn and assault those deemed to be different and therefore inferior.

2. The turn of objective aggression towards the *self* may obviously be compared to what is called the narcissistic libidinal cathexis, through which a surplus of extraverted libido is disposed of. But we have to realize that this secondary narcissism is only possible because of the existence of a primary fundamental narcissistic cathexis. It is even assumed that the capacity to direct libido to objects is secondary in genetic development to that of the narcissistic form.[1] It can safely be said that if it were not for the narcissistic libidinal cathexis, the object libido could never function. In more general terms the appreciation of the self enables the subject to appreciate others.[2]

The writer thinks that the primary disturbance in psychosis is a deficiency in the feeling of the *self* (narcissistic libido), and this is followed by a partial or total loss of sense for external realities and environmental persons. This conception is in a certain opposition to the theory of paranoia by Freud, who stated that in the psychosis the object libido suffers and is greatly replaced by regressive narcissistic libido.

3. There is an apparent resemblance between the competitive tendency and fear on the one hand, and ideological intolerance on the other. From the discussion in Chapter II it can be seen that ideological intolerance is, to an extent, the result of the feeling of personal inadequacy (cf. (5), (6)), apart from the rôle played by the tendency of externalization which results from the difficulty of the moral process. The accentuated competitive restlessness springs, likewise, from fear related to the individual's inadequacy. Thus, the afore-mentioned analogy is true even in the deeper sense.

[1] Cf. Freud on Narcissism (*Zur Einführung des Narzissmus*).
[2] Leviticus *19*, 18, 34, may be interpreted in similar terms.

On the other hand, it is probable that accentuated awareness of human inadequacy goes hand in hand with a disturbance of narcissistic libido. It is perhaps right to assume that the feeling of inadequacy is one of the consequences resulting from the unsatisfactory course of narcissistic libido. That is, the endopsychic libidinal disharmony makes the personality unduly sensible of its actual weaknesses. Obviously there is no average human being in whom the narcissistic feeling of the *self* is entirely undisturbed ; and, equally, it is impossible for a human being to ignore entirely the fact of human inadequacy. The impact of environmental influences does not fail to bring home to the individual his vulnerability and the limitations of his powers. If for no other reason, from this source alone there is bound to result some interference with the current of narcissistic libido.

These brief remarks, together with the pertinent discussions in Chapters I, II, III, make intelligible that the orthodox psychology of the libido had to fail in the full explanation of human phenomena. The optimism with which increased sexual freedom has been advocated as the main line of subjective relief for the individual of our era, appears obviously illogical, since the endopsychic libidinal processes are governed to a large extent by non-libidinal factors.

## An Interesting Phenomenon

1. There are men—their number is large—whose libidinal desire and sexual potency derives a substantial stimulation from their thinking of another man who was, or might be, associating with the female who is their sexual partner. This phenomenon has been referred to by *Stekel* as a manifestation of the homosexual tendency. His explanation, in its broader sense, is indubitable in the light of numerous clinical cases. It appears, however, possible to go deeper into the problem and discover other processes that may account for the development of such a libidinal pattern.

The one possibility is that an early love-attachment of the child or adolescent had as its object a married woman, such as the mother, a married nurse, or a married sister ; the position is similar in the case of an elder sister, or any other girl, who is being courted by her young man during the period of the subject's attachment to her. In such a situation the existence of the competitor-man becomes, to varying extents, part of the picture relating to the beloved woman. In those individuals in whose psyche such early love has left a lasting impression, this Oedipal constellation, as it may be called, is capable of resulting in the love-condition under discussion. The significance of the early competitor becomes rather complex for the child's or youth's mind. Since he has to reconcile himself to sharing his love-object with this adult man, the competitor becomes, as it were, part of the beloved female person. Through putting up with the facts he cannot alter, the young lover attains some peace of mind required for the enjoyment of his love ; the inborn homosexual component, as well as the process of identification, makes this prudent adjustment more easy. It is clear that in the wake of this process further mental elements may develop, of which the personality avails itself in later life. One of such products may be the introduction of a homoerotic object-image in the course of a heterosexual love life.

2. Another soil from which the libidinal pattern referred to may develop is a peculiarity of the subject's ego-image. The feeling of personal inadequacy common to all people might include a particular emphasis on deficiencies of the subject's manliness. Such a man may feel having a sufficiently strong libidinal urge and capacity for love making, but at the same time be troubled by doubts as to the masculine impression he creates in general. For the sake of compensation there is, as it were, a certain hunger for the image of other men acting as libidinal stimulus. One could speak of a desire for identification with these other men in respect of their sexual activities and the strong impression they create in the eyes of women. But it appears more accurate to conceive of the process referred to as *an attempt at supplementing the ego-image of the male individual, in particular regarding his sexual activities.*

It should be added that the feeling of inadequacy regarding the subject's manly attributes as presumably seen by his female partner need not be based on objective deficiencies of a comparable extent. Here, as in other respects, the subjective complex may be more, or less, incongruent with the impression received by the fellowmen. However, as pointed out earlier in this work, it is in the main the degree of intrapsychic awareness of the subject's " complexes " and deficiencies, and not their objective extent, that decides the creation of compensatory elements.

In females the subject's comparison of herself with other women is a much more constant and conscious process than in men. This phenomenon is rooted in the social fact that in love-life the female is the sought after and the chosen partner ; consequently the feeling of competition, that is, of being superior, equal, or inferior in comparison with other females in her environment, belongs to the normal course of the psychosexual process in the average woman. Hence, the conspicuous interest of women in each other's sex appeal must be considered as much more " normal " than the similar phenomenon in men. Certainly this characteristic of women interferes to a far lesser degree with their libidinal economy and dynamics than is the case with men. An important difference is, of course, the necessity of an erection in man *before* the sexual act has started, and inhibitory factors may interfere with the libidinal course from the outset. In the female, on the other hand, there may be time for the accumulation of libidinal tension after the love play has started. On the whole, however, it appears true that not many females have to resort to the image of another female in order to facilitate the libidinal current, whereas this is indubitably the case with a comparatively large number of men.

# APPENDIX III

## PARTICULAR PROBLEMS OF ETHICS

*Capital punishment.—Sexual abnormalities and the law.—The traitor's punishment.—By-products of being exceptionally ethical.—Social psychology of uncompromising pacifism.—Degree of responsibility (free will) in the offender.*

### DEATH PENALTY

1. IN our epoch, after so much bloodshed—both by fighting soldiers and political murderers of defenceless millions—the problem of retributive killing has attracted the interest of the wider public, and the voice of those who on principle oppose the death penalty, appears to become louder. The problem is, of course, not new.[1] For the social psychologist the question has two distinct aspects, each of which ought to be examined separately. The one is the aim of deterring prospective killers; the other is the ethical principle proclaiming the absolute inviolability of human life. Taking up the latter position, there appears no justification whatsoever for retaliating murder with another death. Should it be even no more than probable that such an absolute ethical law exists—whether by virtue of an extra-human legislation, or arrived at through subjective recognition by a comparatively few outstanding minds—indeed no other principle of social expediency ought to be allowed to interfere. In view of the sacredness of human life in such a sense there must not be retributive death whether from juridical vengeance or with the aim of acting as a deterrent. Should a gangster state once more decree the extermination of innocent individuals or masses, it would be the absolute duty of those who believe in such a sacred principle to refrain from all violent counter-measures, and remain content with saving a limited number of those in mortal danger. Obviously, in the presence of such a state of affairs, oppression and extermination would go on—appetite grows with the eating. And if not for the determination of those who combine idealism with realism—

[1] Cf. p. 231 footnote.

above all for the sake of their own families' future—we might witness the coming into being of a world of slavery and political cannibalism which might last for decades or perhaps for centuries. Admittedly by such overclean aloofness a comparatively small group would be in the position of having its sensitiveness satisfied—provided they were allowed to enjoy, for a sufficiently long time, their own personal freedom which is the prerequisite of such sublime pleasures. It is obvious that every human being has the right to as much sensitiveness and unperturbed frame of mind as his mental make-up requires, if he can afford it and his own pleasures do not greatly interfere with the elementary interests of organized society.

2. It should, however, not be overlooked that many people's exceptional horror of the death penalty is not simply identical with an exceptional degree of humanity and kindness; moreover, their attitude obviously does not safeguard collective efforts and sacrifices for the sake of oppressed or defenceless millions who might be helped only by such measures as the threat of capital punishment, and defensive or preventive war.

It is desirable, of course, that people should feel pleasure at their virtuous conduct, and revulsion at the idea of what they deem to be wrong. It is these sentiments towards the *good* and *bad* that safeguard in people at large the automatic choice of the right course of action in social life. Were, on the other hand, the decision of rejecting the wrong for the sake of the good on most occasions associated with the displeasure of sacrifice, clearly the victory of the "good" were unlikely, as far as the behaviour of average people is concerned. Admittedly the individual cannot be expected to live a life of average virtuousness at the price of a constant strain. Thus the pleasure-displeasure factor in prompting the ethically preferable behaviour is a normal and indispensable force.

This fact, however, is responsible for much unsatisfactory application of people's moral sense. The simplest instance is the overlooking of vices in those whose benevolence is gainful to the subject. Thus a biased, though well-intentioned, person may actively support an essentially *a*-social individual in maintaining his good reputation and influence, which may be detrimental to a large section of society.

Nevertheless it remains an unalterable fact that the structure of the moral ego of each individual is such as to be a source of satisfaction if complied with. Hence it may happen that the components of the moral pattern are selected and developed from subjective preference, and thus from reasons other than a pure social sense. Accordingly the fear of one's own death and the reluctance to sacrifice one's life, if the need be, for a common purpose, is a substantial root of some people's opposition to the death sentence. Another root, which in the experience of the writer is fairly frequent, results from the unrealized death wishes of the subject against close relatives, together with the reactive counter-wish for their continued health. In addition there is in the subject's mind the idea of the possible death sentence should he actively cause the death of such a relative. In other words, the idea of *jus talionis* brings about the association of the death wish with the death fear. In a personality type characterized by general ethical inclination the complex described may produce uncompromising antagonism to the death penalty as well as to defensive wars. Summarizing, the fear of one's own death, of a possible violent premature death, is the main spring of objection to the death penalty in persons whose minds are otherwise too ethically inclined. Their particular make-up implies that several of the reactive products of their psyche result in some ethical principle. It is easy to see the psychological relationship between such formations and prejudice proper as the latter has been conceived by the writer. The practical and moral difference between the two types of reactive belief must not lead to our overlooking the fact that, to some extent, the deeper background of both phenomena has definitely at least one common root. This fact might explain the irrational colouring of ethical principles in some cases. In several instances such an individual does not even see that his principle, if it is to be carried out at all costs and under all circumstances, might involve more actual cruelty than kindness, and be much more selfish than altruistic in character.

3. These paragraphs have been written and added to the main work in October, 1946. Only a few weeks earlier the newspapers published a large number of letters about the Nuremberg executions; a substantial number of readers—and a few leader writers, too—appealed for clemency for persons who in all deliberateness, on a large scale, and without any real necessity, have destroyed the lives of millions, and discarded on principle most of the tenets of social justice which mankind has been in

the habit of considering paramount for at least three thousand years. The reasons put forward for these appeals were various: political, juridical, and by most writers "ethical".

All thinking persons are justified in having their opinion; and in a country with a free press also the right of trying to convey their ideas to the wider public. What has been most conspicuous in the majority of these writings is the utter ignoring of the fact that the condemned men were the planners and organizers of wholesale murder and suffering, quite apart from what has been termed their responsibility for a chain of aggressive wars. Incidentally the juridical argument for clemency was that there has been no pre-existent law against aggressive war, and all that goes with it. In the opinion of the writer this argument is unreasonable. Laws are made for the protection of society, and not for the sake of themselves. It is the objectionable act that is punishable, and not the offence against the written law; this is true with the exception of offences of an administrative nature. In the latter case the objectionable character of the act is only given through the existing law. We *must not*, however, say that mass-torture, disruption of family life, as well as aggressive wars prepared by a powerful lying propaganda, *agents provocateurs*, fifth columnists, etc., are not punishable crimes because there has been no pre-existent international law explicitly forbidding these things.

In the case of what I call an administrative offence the culprit might rightly say that, had he known that his act offends against a certain rule, he would certainly have abstained from it. This may be considered an acceptable argument; even though in most instances we may doubt the sincerity of such an assertion. But the very offence in question is, in most cases, such as not to hurt deeply our social sense and humane sentiments. We realize their limited significance. The state of affairs was quite different in the case of the German leaders. Only an illogical and biased mind can really say that their criminal regime would *not* have existed *if* international law had expressly forbidden political slander, the training of criminal fifth columnists, the breaking of agreements, the systematic provocation of frontier incidents, mass robbery and torture by a state-power, racial persecution, etc.

4. There has been also an argument about creating a precedent. This, too, seems unrealistic. Should a regime of brutal tyranny

ever again attain sufficient power and institute a rule of selfish brutality, indeed, the wielder of such a power would *not* care whether the present criminals have been executed or not. This reference to a precedent may strike one as somewhat naïve or merely academic. On the other hand, should the condemned political criminals have been reprieved at Nuremberg—from whatever reasons, whether political prudency or humanitarian sentiments—it would have been most clearly demonstrated that there is no great risk in being a political gangster and multiple murderer; moreover, many, too many, could not have interpreted this act otherwise than as international sympathy with the greatest enemies of mankind in history. True, the substantial number of sensitive people—whom we described above—would have had their satisfaction. But what about the others? There is the large number of people with marked aggressive disposition; a substantial number of would-be mis-leaders and demagogues; the host of small and big Jew baiters still in existence; the large variety of leftish and rightish fanatics. Their existence is at least as much worthy of consideration as the psyche of hyper-sensitive "ethicals". It is not certain whether the death penalty carried out on the Nuremberg criminals will very much improve the world. It is certain, however, that had they been reprieved much, perhaps very much, harm would have been done both for the present and future.

5. In the same period in which the afore-mentioned newspaper discussion took place, a few common murderers were executed. There has been no, or comparatively negligible, interest in their cases. An irony of fate, one could say. But in the opinion of the writer the reason for this paradoxical behaviour is much more tragic than would be generally assumed. The facts seem to confirm one of the main themes of this work, i.e. that large-scale aggression and success in any crime whatsoever is an attractive phenomenon for the deeper layers of people's mind. The small murderer who, in the writer's opinion, is almost always either a mental defective or a criminal psychopath—or even less, a mere victim of temporary passion, does not attract much attention. He has had no army and Government at his disposal, no political successes, no loot with which to bribe his underlings, not even interesting uniforms to thrill the cinema public. Amongst the elements most dynamic in the deeper psyche of many practically well-behaved people, is some admiration for powerful brutality

and the success attained by it. This statement will be doubted by many readers, for obvious reasons. We know the rôle of repression in all human opinions. But, in fact, the phenomenon of Nuremberg, in all its aspects, appears to confirm the main themes of this work.

6. The case of ethical opposition to the death penalty for deliberate political gangstership and murder has been put to me by a logical person who is well informed on depth-psychology and by no means of an unkind disposition. He said: "We have to sympathize with the opponents of the death penalty. Knowing that their motive is partly ethical, but to a large extent rooted in subconscious personal fear,[1] their aversion merits the same consideration as the pains or psychoneurotic complaints of any sufferer. Should society ever be able to afford the absolute abolition of the death penalty it would be a social crime to continue with this archaic penal measure, if for no other reason than for the sake of those who feel very uneasy about it. But as long as conditions are not ideal enough, and particularly in view of the German regime in the recent past, and its influence on extremists, the absolute abolition, at present, seems to be unadvisable. Thus, the large group of ethical opponents have to bear their discomfort for the sake of the common good. On the whole it might be said that the ideal attitude in this question would be the practical imposition of the death sentence in severe cases of murder or mass murder, yet with the feeling of a strong sentimental protest both on the part of the public and of the judges."

The present writer cannot help seeing both the logic and broad-minded humanity in this statement. He wishes to add that on the whole he himself is not in favour of the death sentence or even of long-term imprisonment in most cases where such sentences are actually carried out. He cannot fail to have sympathy with the judges who have to follow the intentions of the existing legal system, even though they may feel that there is, in view of modern psychiatric knowledge, no possibility of an absolutely just penal code.[2]

[1] The free associations of persons in analysis may clearly illustrate this statement. The writer has had the opportunity of observing this causal connection in two of his patients during and after the Nuremberg trials.

[2] It is, however, possible that a deficient valuation of the individual's life may contribute to a penal code punishing premeditated murder merely by imprisonment for a number of years.

7. Many people may share with the writer the impression that it strikes one as not very courageous and dignified if an imposing police force and armed prison staff are employed to deal with a single individual who has happened to offend against the law, and was caught and " disarmed ". This is so even in the cases of premeditated murder. Such a person dominated by some impulse or passionate motive has lost his clear vision and self-control, and through committing the crime has exposed himself to severe legal retribution, for the sake of a satisfaction that can on no account be adequate to his subsequent suffering. The writer feels that even in such indubitably serious cases the impression created by the large legal apparatus is not quite free of a somewhat ridiculous or cowardly feature in so far as an overpowered individual—who through his offence has at any rate excommunicated himself from the society of average people—faces the infinitely stronger force of state justice.

This fact cannot be easily altered ; perhaps the feeling of having become insignificantly weak in face of such state power and public condemnation, is part of the intended punishment. But those representing the firm and all-powerful justice ought to be aware that as individuals or as representatives of their fellow-individuals, they are in essence exploiting an unequal relationship. They do not act by means of abstract justice or scientific truth but by superior physical force.

8. Quite different is the case of a political group or Governmental regime that makes oppression and extermination part of its legal policy, whether such a policy is exercised as a routine or only on individual occasions. Those responsible for such acts of crime are different from the common murderer. They do not act under the force of an ordinary passionate motive that is difficult to resist. They are fully able to pretend decency and abstain from crime as long as they are not in power. They act criminally only when backed by authority and in a position that surrounds them with a halo of legality. Then they can reckon upon the sympathy and approval of large masses, inside and outside their country, and they themselves may entirely overlook that their aggressive and murderous actions are morally worse than common murder. Power and decorum secure public support and admiration for whatever actions, as long as this crowd of yes-men feel themselves to be outside the group of likely victims. A social and political science that does not realize

these facts will never be able to contribute, in the slightest degree, to the amelioration of the world's archaic organization and customs. Those who at all times and most clearly did realize this mass-psychological phenomenon, were the aggressors and large-scale criminals amidst various nations.[1]

In the case of such political criminals a penal code might be appropriate that is different from that which is valid for common offenders, murderers included. The common murderer offends against the law of human society. He, for varying reasons, feels impelled to act in spite of the accepted legal order, and in full knowledge of the exceptionality of his actions. Criminal political groups on the other hand deliberately and on a large scale create a new legal and administrative atmosphere. They do not sincerely believe in the common law and common humanity. They—one might say—put themselves definitely outside the customary conceptions of a humane law. Therefore one might argue that except for some mystical religious conceptions on justice and forgiveness, or alternatively, for the sake of the sensitiveness of the world at large, such criminals of the "political" brand deserve no better justice than that instituted by themselves, or at least a sterner justice than average (of course, no torture is envisaged). This has nothing to do with common vengeance as some reader might at first think. Vengeance in the ordinary sense would only operate if a common murderer, who was lacking in sufficient self-control, were being killed by relatives of the victim ; or it is legal vengeance if such an offender is condemned to death by a court and executed.

But, as we said, the common criminal concerns himself solely with attaining his private aims ; he does not wish to reform and to brutalize the legal and political system of the world. If caught and tried he is certainly entitled to the most humane penal justice. Otherwise it would be crude vengeance and not cultured justice with which our courts and judges were concerned. Both

[1] Fairness requires that we acknowledge any good quality a criminal individual may have. The same attitude was taken by some towards the criminals who created the concentration camps, gas chambers, as well as a policy and law of utter immorality. They have been praised for their courage (?), military skill, and political efficiency. The wisdom of and moral justification for such an attitude if displayed in public by persons of position or by newspapers may be questioned. The result is inevitably that sympathy is created for the criminals, and this increases in psychic depths the aggressive potentials and stimulates the savage liking for cruelty. Anyone who doubts this does not keep in touch with modern psychological research. By abstaining from the partial praise of mass murderers and antisocial criminals, no harm is done to them. Rather than to risk the evil consequences of such avoidable fairness towards criminals of this category, it would be less harmful for society if they were given *in secrecy* all physical comfort possible for lifetime.

parties, the human offender and the peaceful public, deserve that no brutality but justice and even kindness should rule the atmosphere of the courts and prisons. This has to be so because the prisoner in the hands of a state authority has become a weak pitiable creature.

9. It is obvious that in the opinion of the writer the concern for social good and the well-being of the individual citizens is the main principle by which administrative as well as penal measures ought to be measured. Other factors, such as patriotic sentiment or religious-ethical principles of traditional origin, however valuable for social life, must not increase the severity of the penal code of a truly enlightened state organization. Retribution for such questionable offences must not be other than a disagreement voiced by that part of society adhering to an ideology sinned against by the person in question. Thus, for instance, continued interference with the most private life of the adult homosexual—whether his condition be constitutional or acquired—in our period of modern psychiatry, expresses utter reluctance to accept a surprising truth.[1] Not only are thus comparatively, or in fact entirely, innocent people persecuted, but society's sense of justice is wasted on an insignificant problem at the expense of other more worthy and urgent tasks.

## The Case of Sexual Abnormalities

1. It is true that some cases of "sexual perversion" are curable by psychoanalysis. It appears that *homosexuality* has a somewhat better prognosis than the other types. *Stekel* and his pupils have achieved success in a considerable number of cases by a technique that has brought practical cure in less than six months. In view of these experiences Stekel in his publications denied the inborn and unalterable character of homosexuality, even though he had to admit that only patients with a strong desire to change have a fair prognosis. He also had to admit that the treatment of this condition requires great skill, much experience, and considerable efforts on the part of the psychotherapist.[2]

The writer wishes to point out that Stekel's optimism has admittedly encouraged a number of affected persons and therapists

[1] Cf. K. Walker and E. B. Strauss: *Sexual Disorder in the Male*, Hamish Hamilton Medical Books.

[2] Cf. W. Stekel: "Is die Homosexualität heilbar?" *Nervenarzt*, 1929, 6.

alike to turn to psychoanalysis ; but we have come to realize that only a comparatively small number of such persons are really fitted for cure. Those patients who did come to treatment felt unhappy in their condition ; and this is a fair sign that psychoanalysis may be successful. It is very probable that the majority of homosexuals do not belong in this category. The fact that they are utterly indifferent to the idea of treatment, and quite happy in their condition, is in general an indication of their being unfitted for treatment. Only very few of these change their outlook and seek treatment after a strong disappointment or serious clash with the legal authorities on account of their sexual activities. We can say no more than that these few exceptional cases were only apparently genuine unalterable homosexuals.

I feel that through stressing too much the psychogenesis of this condition we may contribute to the outmoded and unfair prejudice to which these persons are exposed. It is *not* true that mere consent to submit to treatment would be sufficient for its success, and that those who do not submit are " wicked ". Only the feeling of a genuine desire, that is to say, a subjectively felt conflict on account of the condition is a prognostically encouraging sign. In other cases, we may still be justified to undertake treatment if we are insistently asked ; but both analyst and analysand must be aware of the prevailing therapeutic limitations.

Moreover, the number of psychotherapists with sufficient experience in this particular field is too small yet, and the expenses of the treatment may be considerable. Orthodox psychoanalysis of this condition may last, so far as I know, for years ; and even the Stekelian technique requires on the average 100–150 sessions. Picture the position of homosexuals who live in places where there are no suitable psychoanalysts, and of those who could not afford more than the fees of out-patient departments even if they lived, let us say, in London. I cannot imagine the successful psychotherapeutic treatment of a firmly established homosexuality in a mental hospital, or in a psychiatric out-patient department within the time limit available. Thus the vast majority of homosexuals cannot even be charged with not seeking treatment.

2. Two years ago I signed, jointly with Mrs. H. Stekel, a letter published in xxxxx, in which we denied that Dr. Stekel had

believed in the unchangeable nature of homosexuality, as a previous letter-writer had mistakenly stated. Following this we received a number of letters from homosexuals who asked for advice as to treatment. Among all of them there was only *one* who could have had the treatment ; firstly, because he moved to a place where an experienced analyst lived, and secondly, because he was in the position to pay at least a moderate fee for his prolonged treatment. All the others lived in small towns, and in addition were without means.

Realizing the disservice we might have done to a number of people I wrote another letter pointing out the difficulties of treatment for the large number of homosexuals ; unfortunately the Editor did not find the publication of this corrective necessary. Since then *I* feel that we should not have written the first letter at all.

In continuing to interfere with homosexual practices of adults amongst themselves, the legal representatives of society implicitly declare that they are determined to employ severe measures in the service of a principle that is based merely on emotional revulsion. The non-homosexuals are in the vast majority ; their power is infinitely greater than that of the " perverts ". Thus they can say : " We do not wish to tolerate the idea that homosexuality is being desired and practised, because this idea is to us revolting. Even though psychiatrists know that these perversions are inborn or at least deep-rooted ; even though psychoanalysts are at pains to explain that strong revulsion has something to do with repressed wishes ; even though it has to be realized that successful treatment of these ' perverts ' is comparatively rare and a difficult matter ; and even though there is no logical reason for being intolerant of these people as long as they create no public exhibition or interfere with minors . . . we are determined to prosecute them."

It is true that people at large cannot tolerate mice and rats and insects, not only because these creatures are harmful, but also because they evoke revulsion ; consequently people find it legitimate and even a command of human culture to kill these animals. Apparently something similar is being felt towards and done to homosexuals. Let us not forget that interference with homosexuality is comparable to preventing an average human being from marrying and having a sexual life. To punish a homosexual is a measure similar to punishing a person for having heterosexual intercourse within or without marriage. The power of an overwhelming majority is strong ; when they wish they are in the position to act in accordance with their emotional tendencies and the ensuing mistaken conceptions. The least a social psychologist should do, in view of such a state of affairs, is to throw an objective light on it.

3. The reader, desirous of being undogmatically humane, as well as scientifically objective, will realize that the problem discussed here merits in itself inclusion in a work on Social Psychology. Beyond its own significance, and the peace of a considerable number of harmless and even valuable citizens, the discussion of this question may illustrate the phenomenon of emotional intolerance, and its capacity for interfering with the lives of a large section of people. In essence, the components of this particular problem are similar to that of organized prejudice. Unfortunately the problem of the homosexual is made more difficult by the fact that religious and secular law have sanctioned the associated revulsion felt by people. To the best knowledge of the author the source of the prevailing legislation is the canon law, based on a paragraph in the Old Testament. Great as the ethical significance and deep humane wisdom of the Bible are, it is difficult to deny that its underlying psychology is not quite modern. Certainly, if the author of the Pentateuch had known that there are persons with inborn homosexuality, which is beyond their volition, he would not have branded such an act as a horrible crime. Having shown so much sympathy with the poor, the weak, and the oppressed he might rather have extended his sympathy to those who are unable to live a happy family life.

Returning to the more general angle of the problem the writer advises the student to devote some thought to the fact that *complexes* may create prejudices, as well as prejudice-like ethical and legal concepts. The other associated question of importance is the degree to which an individual—or group of people—might be, in fairness, limited in or deprived of their emotional satisfaction, spontaneity, and average ease of life by a differently disposed majority. No doubt we find our horror of dirt, slovenliness, or crude language legitimate and even praiseworthy, and on this account we interfere complacently with the ease and spontaneity of a number of people by condemning, ridiculing, and ostracizing them. Obviously it is not easy to establish the limits between what is fair or indispensable interference and what is unnecessary cruelty.

## The Traitor's Punishment

1. For the broadminded social psychologist a sentence of death on what is called a traitor to his country may appear rather outmoded. What should it matter to a nation of millions if one or a few of its members prefer to behave like a spiteful child or a resentful relative, particularly if the harm done to the native country by such psychopaths—that is what they as a rule are—prove to be insignificant in the perspective of contemporary large-scale events. It is fully justifiable to guard against any future attack to the detriment of the national community, as long as sovereign national economies exist ; any measure undertaken in the pursuance of this defence may be considered reasonable. But to kill a person, or even to imprison him for years, because of his anti-national intentions, expressed in words or writing, or even in actions, appears somewhat unreasonable if no substantial damage has been done by him. How, indeed, can we compare that which such traitors in most instances do, with the effect of books and speeches inciting people against innocent or average human groups in the name of prejudice and through slanderous lies. Such hatred propaganda always attains its aim ; it interferes with the peace of a larger or smaller number of citizens, through brutalizing many or a few would-be aggressors. Nevertheless this type of " political " activity goes on all over the world, and it might be difficult to eliminate entirely without interfering too greatly with the precious right of free expression in general. But it must be realized that, in the light of this fact, the offence of treachery in most cases is a child's play ; even if the traitor succeeds in transmitting to the " enemy " some information the harm is frequently not such as to interfere perceptibly with the life of individuals or the state-administration. It is perfectly true that a state affords the individual the advantages associated with citizenship on the condition that the individual adheres to a certain approved conduct. But the disappointing behaviour of a few persons does not seem to justify severe retribution such as a sentence of death or lifelong imprisonment ; expulsion ought to be the only measure logically justifiable, should there be no reason to detain such a traitor in order to prevent practical harm for the country in the future.[1]

[1] The right of the state to " own " his citizen is generally taken for granted, even though the extent of this claim varies with conceptions regarding the significance of the individual. In a really free society, however, every person would be at liberty to leave his country and settle wherever he may find it fit, but only very few would feel impelled to do so.

## By-Products of Being Exceptionally Ethical

1. A sense of justice, altruism, hatred of base aggressiveness as well as an attitude of tolerance are mental elements not unopposed within the minds of those who may practically be considered decent persons. The disapproved tendencies, which are suppressed on moral grounds, are bound to manifest their influence in some form and on some occasion. The more such decent people approach ethical perfection in the humanly possible sense, the more they may have to cope with particular repressions and the more they have to dispense with affective spontaneity of the kind peculiar to those of a less scrupulous disposition. Admittedly decent personalities do greatly enjoy their ethical outlook and behaviour [1]; and this compensates for the loss of affective spontaneity. But, in fact, ethical pleasure on the one hand, and the giving vent to primitive tendencies on the other are in essence different processes; thus, in the average decent person there cannot be an absolute replacement of the one alternative by the other. In proportion to the dynamic tension of the repressed *a*-social tendencies in decent people, occasional features of their behaviour may be strange, and logically hard to reconcile with their general character and fundamental creed.

2. The writer was present at a conversation which took place in 1940 in the house where an acquaintance of his—a refugee with a lot of troubles and of not very good health—had found a home at a moderate charge a few days earlier. It was almost inevitable that the discussion turned to conditions on the Continent, and it was natural that, for my friend, at that period, there was nothing more important than the racial and political persecutions as well as economic exploitation carried out by the German State. The hosts listened for a few minutes, and then the man, a person of quite a good education, explained to their new guest: "You must realize that our people here just tolerate you, but they do not like your race." The refugee—embarrassed and with a harassed look—meekly said: "We are grateful for all you are doing for us." Then, apparently wishing to carry the conversation to a point where all might agree, he explained that there is a marked difference between the brutality of the German regime on the one hand and the dislike of some foreigners

[1] Cf. Appendix II, The Social Sense and the Libido, p. 273.

in Great Britain on the other. To this the hostess replied: "Do not think for a moment that what we are doing we would do only for you. Should those who are your present persecutors at a later time be defeated and in need of help, we are prepared to stand by them. This is how we feel." (The plural referred to a certain charitable body much opposed to the war.)

Unpleasantly though this unexpected information struck my acquaintance, he certainly benefited by it; it demonstrated to him, the gifted writer, a type of attitude he had never met with before. Moreover, it brought him back to a more realistic outlook, which is so easily dropped by people who are deprived of the feeling of security and in this situation feel impelled to make unfounded optimistic interpretations of what might only be a formal politeness on the part of their fellowmen. It is also probable that through this experience he was later able to appreciate much more the numerous instances of friendliness afforded to him by other people in a different, more personal way.

3. The writer later had the opportunity of meeting the couple quite a few times. They appeared to be really harmless people, deeply religious, and hospitable as far as their very limited means permitted. The husband was a teacher, well informed on current affairs, and very embittered about the inequities of the "capitalistic world". He professed to be "an enemy of the imperialistic British Empire" and a blind admirer of all that was Russian (1940). His wife was a kind-hearted and industrious person, and likewise a qualified teacher; in addition, she had some gift for painting to which, because of being poor and a mother of four children, she could not devote herself. To all appearances the family had to be content with a very modest standard of life. No wonder that, in spite of their honest intentions and basically sweet nature, they were not free of prejudice; they displayed more than one of these irrational sentiments. Their children followed in the wake of the parents; they entertained the visitors with discussing the "great amount of money spent by the British Government on armaments, the means of killing". (The reader might remember the greatly insufficient defences available when the war started, and the large-scale preparations made for years by contemporary Germany for conquering the world and exterminating groups and nations for the sake of economic gains.)

4. Here there was a family of six members, with a certain taste for the higher standards of life, but without the means for actually having it and with no personal gifts for attaining it through the competitive struggle required by existing circumstances. On the other hand their religious disposition, as well as their dread of the sufferings that war might bring them, made them uncompromising pacifists, whatever the real conditions of their lifetime might be. The assuming of a strict ethical ideology and attitude, beyond the average current one, implies, as suggested, for the subject an additional amount of psychoaffective repression ; this, however, cannot occur without some subconscious regret about the limitation of spontaneity as compared with that in other people. Very few, indeed, are capable of being ethical to any exceptional degree without developing some rather unpleasant reactive features of their personality. The life of the family described here consisted of mere duties and restrictions ; their means were too limited as to allow any luxury ; their membership of an organized body enforced the carrying out of certain principles to an extent beyond what their personal liking would prefer ; there was a lack of opportunity for spontaneous outlet of the psychoaffective spheres. Thus they could hardly present the picture of personalities that strikes average people as sufficiently harmonious and pleasant.

*Note.*—It is well known that average people, and also those whose moral-social behaviour is below the average, may take a passionate pleasure in discovering some weaknesses in clergymen or persons who apparently strictly adhere to religion as well as conservative ethics. No doubt, this reaction betrays, amongst other things, concealed hatred of the " good " ; perhaps also an envy of it. Certainly, the indignation expressed by this type of people is not based simply on their disapproval of the inconsistence between creed and its violation ; it is too strong, and also too peculiar on the part of some critics, to be explained so simply. It appears that people at large grudge the exceptional position of the " pious " and " ethical " they hold in the minds of many ; perhaps the critics also hate the tacit claim of these exceptional persons to be looked at with some awe. But, as suggested, the phenomenon would require a more thorough analysis for its satisfactory understanding.

The British reader may be interested to know that in certain regions of the world a similar attitude is displayed towards deficiencies of this country's policy and social system, as if Great Britain were the only country which must not fail or sin in any respect. To my mind, the reason for this type of criticism is the fact that religious-ethical principles as well as non-partisan fairness are, explicitly and implicitly, proclaimed as the foundations of public life of this country ; no doubt the people of Great Britain have manifested on many occasions in history these principles. However, all that is human is imperfect ; and those who influence the process of actualities are not always guided by pure ethics and pure logic. Moreover, it is difficult to carry out power- and economic politics, and at the same time to adhere to lofty principles. Thus, there is sufficient occasion for criticism clothed in the peculiar passion mentioned. But, undoubtedly, it is not without the risk of inviting impassioned criticism if a nation wishes to appear " moral " and assume " moral leadership " of others ; in particular, if such a nation is envied for its assets, whether material or spiritual, as for instance influence in the international world.

It is not unlikely that whole problem mooted here is explainable by the contempt cherished by most people towards weakness and limitation. Moral ideology implies

## SOCIAL PSYCHOLOGY OF UNCOMPROMISING PACIFISM

1. The writer wishes to add a few paragraphs about the psychology of intransigent pacifism. No reference will be made to the doctrine and formulated principles of this creed as set out in publications of representative bodies and individual writers. It is rather the *impression* the phenomenon makes on the uninitiated as well as a tentative interpretation of it which is the main object of this brief discussion.

Emphatic affirmation of the uniqueness and sacredness of human life appears to be the central feature of the pacifist's attitude. In his conscious motivation the life of all fellowmen—that of the dangerous enemy or criminal included—is given the emphasis. But we were uncritical by ignoring the subject's deep concern for his own life and for that of those near and dear to him.[1] No doubt there is hardly anything more human than the love of life in the healthy-minded. Firm as may be the avowed belief in the continued existence after death, the overwhelming majority of intransigent pacifists behave as if the so brief and imperfect earthly life were nevertheless of absolute, if not sole, significance. This attitude they share with masses of other people, believers and non-believers alike.

Clearly, when the concern for one's own life and the associated horror of warfare has led to the creed of uncompromising humane pacifism, the whole personality may become adjusted to this outlook, and hardly anything may overtly indicate the primary selfish motive. In this structure the attitude of " pacifism " is not different from the psychoaffective background of a large number of other ethical principles. Here, too, a distinctly subjective motive may create secondary elements of a higher ethical order, and the resulting attitude may be too complex as to permit an easy recognition of its components without psycho-analysis based on genuine free associations and the study of dreams.

2. For the non-dogmatic outsider it is difficult to forget that not all wars were aggressive ; in some, indubitably, the defence of

fetters ; those who profess it would feel uneasy without it. Thus, their activities are from the outset limited ; they cannot afford easily a practical approach to things without any regard to their own principles. This amounts, in the eyes of many, to being weak ; but weakness evokes, as it has been stated earlier in this work, some measure of contempt.

[1] Objection to military service in times of peace is a secondary sentiment associated with the horror of warfare.

human values was seriously in question. In regard to the last so terrible war now many people think that it would have been better to sacrifice a few millions, those civilians who were tortured and murdered by the past German regime and its voluntary satellites; and that through appeasing treaties it would have been possible to save the lives and comparative comfort of other millions who suffered and perished only because of the "total war".

This argument must not be brushed aside. It is *not unlikely* that such a course of events might have been feasible; that is to say, if those responsible for Government in several countries were able to think on such "revolutionary" lines, and were ready to stake so many human values and interests for which defensive wars are fought. We must not deny that wars, and even defensive wars, are frequently fought for material interests; and then it is *not* simply so that a few privileged, whose lives are comparatively safe, sacrifice for their class-interests the millions of "exploited" gullible fellow-nationals. The latter *was* indubitably the case several times in history; and frequently it was not even material interests, but hysterical concern for international political power that made national leaders enter into war. But it is equally true that enthusiastic participation of the masses in war fought for freedom, or the good of humanity, was not a rarity. The Governmental force in conscription clouds this fact; and, admittedly, most of those drafted into the army would not have volunteered for the battlefield—and left their families behind—if not for the fact of legal compulsion reinforced by the pressure of public opinion. Who dares to deny that this "public opinion" is only partly impelled by patriotism and the concern for the common good, and that it is, substantially, envy of those who do not partake of the calamity that is the lot of the others.

3. All this, however, does not solve in itself the question whether bloody wars—even though with a defensive or moral purpose—are justifiable or not; nor does it decide whether the pacifists are fundamentally "better" than their average fellowmen with a comparable standard of individual behaviour. There are many things in social life regarded as a duty or as a voluntary moral conduct that might not be upheld if not for the pressure of public opinion and explicit law. In vain would some people assert that *their* morality is firm and *their* dutifulness absolute,

being based on a deep conviction. Their and other people's sincerity is not questioned. The reader of this work knows that on whatever ground ethical principles develop, ultimately they may be genuinely liked by the subject. The problem of the firmness of individual moral conviction is, in fact, more complex than assumed by the non-psychologist. All persons who are sure of themselves have been brought up in the existing social and cultural atmosphere; hence, they cannot imagine, and believe, that their morality and humanity would not have equally developed if they had been living in full individual autonomy, entirely free from prevailing social influences. Certain peculiarities of many of them suggest that they are as little free from potential aggressiveness, envy, and narrow-minded selfishness as the vast number of average citizens who are law-abiding and humane though not so sure of their morals.

It is even very probable that the intensity of anomalous social conditions is greatly responsible for so many ideas and plans concerning the amelioration of social life. The greater the gap between actual conditions on the one hand and our ideas of a fair amount of comfort in life on the other, the stronger is the incentive to create over-optimistic social programmes. And the less conspicuous or painful the anomalies, the greater is the danger of complacency. The accumulation of historical experiences and the increasing independence of the broad masses in having, and voicing, their own opinion has given rise to the development of large-scale social and ethical programmes; but, unfortunately, it is the pressure of hardships weighing on human beings that makes people think of improvements as well as critical of the existing mode of administration. For all these reasons the social psychologist, particularly if experienced in practical psychoanalysis, is not so sure about the autogenesis and autonomy of ethics in the masses of average persons who now are admittedly beyond reproach or even exceptional in their concepts of social and Governmental morality.

4. At any rate, if war is already in progress, and millions fight and suffer, the intransigent pacifism of a small minority, exempting many of them even from non-combatant service, may seem irrational rather than logical. But this impression reflects only *one* aspect of the phenomenon. It remains nevertheless a fact that, by dint of a firmly held attitude, these people do not participate in war; that is, on the one hand they do not cause,

or contribute to, injury or death, and on the other hand the majority of them do not suffer the risks and deprivations that members of the armed forces do, being thus enabled to live normally.

Ordinary thinking revolts against privileges enjoyed by some at a time when millions are in a worse and even precarious position. We understand fully this feeling. But the decision of a Government in a well-administered country to make allowances, even amidst the grimmest war, to uncompromising pacifism is not so senseless as the mind's first reaction makes it appear. Even in a state of emergency it is necessary to have a certain fraction of the nation free from the risks of violent and premature death. For this end provision is made by exempting persons before and beyond the military age, as well as a number of people deemed important for certain occupations. Why not add to these groups another small group of people if there is some acceptable motive for their exemption. To save lives, and spare a number of decent people suffering, is also an act of humanity and civilization. Moreover, a number of conscientious objectors are otherwise helpful and useful members of the community; some of them even exceptionally valuable for relief work.

The writer is not sure that this reasoning will be appreciated by all readers. But it is nevertheless a fact that a certain proportion of the population *has* to continue its rôle in the civilian life of the nation. Therefore, we should not be very perturbed because of the privileged position of pacifists, as long as the vast majority of the nation is ready to submit to what is considered by responsible and practical men the inevitable task of the day.

5. Admittedly this whole reasoning holds only true when the group of those seeking exemption is not too large. It is also a fact that a substantial number of people become pacifists—genuine pacifists—because the law acknowledges conscientious objection to military service. That is to say, were the legal system of a country entirely opposed to such a liberal practice, and the danger to the objector's social or physical life greater than to that of the soldier, many of those who under prevailing circumstances do become conscientious objectors, would not have developed in such a direction. In this respect the general psychological rule is true that great obstacles may stifle potential inclinations, whereas the prospect of some advantage implied by an ethical attitude is apt to further its development. It is

not a chance that a large number of conspicuous " idealists " are at the same time somewhat peculiar, solitary, and unpractical. A vague realization of psychoaffective weakness in themselves makes them escape into an ideology that, apart from giving them spiritual uplift, justifies their isolating themselves from the large world of competitive fellowmen on account of deep differences in ideology.

It may seem a pity to analyse and question the purity of ethical attitudes. To this we are able to answer that whatever the deepest motives of an overt ethical attitude, its obvious values remain undoubted and untouched by any analysis. On the other hand, clear knowledge on this matter may have only beneficial results in the long run. In the wake of increasing knowledge the public's support of obviously useful ethical attitudes may increase, whereas the unpractical and apparently mentally deficient " idealist " may be deprived of his persuasive influence on credulous but normal people.

6. It may be asked whether there is any sense in this discussion, in view of the decided wish of nations not to engage in war any more ; whether it would not be wiser to write and preach uncompromisingly in favour of absolute pacifism, and to proclaim the attitude of the conscientious objector as the only humane and justifiable. This, in the opinion of the writer, might be pleasing rather than realistic, scientific, and fair.

It is a fact that in the last war millions fought, and sacrificed their comfort and life, for what was deemed—and proved to be—the good of mankind. If for no other reason, then in the retrospective analysis we must not ignore their deeds and declare their sacrifice as useless, unless it is perfectly certain that it has been useless. This we cannot state as long as we think realistically. To a substantial extent conscientious objectors and their families have enjoyed the immediate results of their fellowmen's fighting. Certainly the groups of objectors all over the world have been too small to prevent wars, aggression, and brutal intimidation. Consequently it may be said that if not for the defensive attitude of others or their manifested readiness not to avoid service, there might have been more destruction of human happiness than there actually is.

To this and similar arguments put forward in a discussion at a course of psychology, a number of objectors have answered that they rely on Heaven's help. " Whatever God pleases to do with us, we are ready to bear"—was the answer of a mother, a retired teacher, who was fortunate enough to know that her son was exempt from service on account of his pacifistic upbringing. Another small group seemed to hold the view that "to them" no aggressor would wish to do any harm.

7. Apart from this retrospective view of the problem the writer thinks that in the present pacifistic attitude there is an element that would manifest itself in other spheres if there were no question of war. It is not easy to foresee clearly the form of this future dissension; and the writer feels it is unfair to outline his own admittedly subjective prediction. This fundamental element, which is largely independent of the concrete question of wars, justifies the discussion of the social psychology of what has manifested itself in the present as uncompromising pacifism.

8. Nevertheless, it is possible to imagine a logical sequence of events in the wake of intransigent pacifism adhered to by a whole nation. Clearly, such an attitude will inevitably invite some form or degree of pressure, and even aggression, by a stronger or decidedly military power. The "enemy" might march in unopposedly, and seize control of all the wealth and administration. The masses of conscientious objectors would, for a considerable time, offer some passive resistance; but before too long the instinct of positive life would have the upper hand, and fraternization with the "conqueror" would take place. After all why should it matter very much whether our affairs are administered by our own people or by foreigners, possibly with the co-operation of our civil servants? Of course, these foreign people will, at first, send home all the materials they deem unnecessary for the elementary life of the conquered nation and desirable for their own country. But with the passage of time more or less friendship may develop between the two parties. The "enemy" may be impressed by the humane and insistent pacifistic attitude of the invaded nation, and may seek genuine union. Indeed, why not speak two languages, and think on various matters in a fashion that is a combination of the native way and that of the foreign nation. In a few decades, or perhaps only in a century, the two people may have become one . . . and what is uppermost, there has been no bloodshed, whether defensive or aggressive, and no violence apart from the

first phase of the conquest. Obviously, the life of other neighbouring nations is bound to become involved in this process of intermingling and evolution. Well, we may say, why should such a development be rejected from the outset, why such an experiment made impossible? Why should traditional nationalism and economic sovereignty be inviolable sacraments, or unalterable natural phenomena? And above all, why should blood, innocent human blood, be shed and human lives lost prematurely, and under suffering caused by planned action and provoked by irrational stubborn resistance? . . . Indeed, why should national boundaries and ideologies of narrow patriotism continue for ever to exist?

The writer finds it impossible to elaborate further this trend of thought, and leaves it to the various readers to go deeper into the matter and discover both the merits and weaknesses of the hypothetical picture presented here.

## Degree of Responsibility in the Offender

1. In Chapter III reference is made to the close relationship between inborn (organic) intellectual deficiency and the constitutional moral deficiency. There are persons who from early youth appear unable to abide by the code of approved behaviour, even though the atmosphere of their upbringing was not unsimilar to that of other people. In a number of them routine intelligence tests reveal no appreciable deficiency; in other cases the intelligence test does show that the recurrently criminal youth has a somewhat lower intelligence quotient than that which is considered normal, and here it is considered unquestionably right to correlate the two deficiencies. No essential difference results in our conception by realizing that *a*-social behaviour need not be based on intellectual deficiency in the narrower sense, but rather on disorders of impulses and emotions. No doubt should exist that certain persons are characterized by innate emotional difficulties, even though their intellect may be otherwise average or even higher. It ought to be difficult for the psychologist with a fair clinical training to avoid the conclusion that the capacity for moral conduct is in part based on an inborn factor the deficiency of which may, in some cases, render futile educational efforts. This is actually the same as with all other innate dispositions of the human individual that are developed to a full capacity only through education and

training. We know that no amount of musical tuition and practice can result in an appreciable playing technique if the subject does not possess a certain measure of musical talent. Even though one may wish to believe that regarding social morals the position is different, it is difficult to see the objective validity of such an assumption.

2. It appears that ideological bias as well as the unquestioned acceptance of legal conceptions in force, prevents a large number of psychiatrists and psychologists from seeing clearly the " organic factor " in *a*-moral behaviour. The writer feels that several members of this group merely do not dare, if one may say so, to recognize the truth which is vaguely known to them ; and this only because society in general, and the representatives of the law in particular, do not wish that the significance of the organic factor in morality should be acknowledged by official psychiatry. The average human being is too much attached to the medical profession, and the value of modern psychiatry in bringing relief to sufferers becomes increasingly recognized. Hence, a revolutionary view on this problem by serious psychiatrists may exert an influence on public opinion that could not well be disregarded.

The legal profession as well as the clergy and other ethical bodies intelligibly dislike a psychology that finds objectionable phenomena explainable and thus apparently excusable. They *have* to feel grave concern on account of the fact that so much struggle is required for the maintenance of social morality. From this angle, a public attitude that is rather severe than lenient towards crime appears expedient and even indispensable. In the ultimate result, however, a large number of offenders are judged by a legal measure that is arrived at as an outcome of ideologies rather than of a true attempt to assess rightly the psychological laws of self-control by will. Apparently, in our social system, not much can be done to spare offenders the excess of suffering imposed upon them by current sentences. No doubt the deterrent influence of the arbitrary hypothesis that assumes unconditional free will in the non-psychotic might turn the scale of decision in some persons away from offending and towards the respect for the law. Perhaps this gain derived from exaggerating volitional responsibility justifies some excessive severity in judgment meted out to offenders. On the other hand, from the angle of individual life such a mode of justice is entirely out of place. No one ought to be made to suffer more than is avoidable, since each day of life is unique and pain once suffered may be forgotten but cannot be undone. The individual may deserve to claim a more accurate assessment of his volitional power and responsibility, if retributive punishment *has* to exist for the sake of social order. Those who believe in the reformatory aspect of current punishments may retort that an excess of punitive education ought not to be taken as absolute injustice, and should be put up with because of the necessity to safeguard social peace. Yet such a philosophy is not entirely free of irony since the *reformatory* effect of punishment is on the whole hardly worthy of serious consideration.[1]

3. The recidivist, that is the offender who commits the same type of illegal act, is looked upon by public and judges alike as someone who merely *does not choose* to repent and improve, though he easily could. But in most cases—if not in all—the reason for recidivism is an accentuated constitutional moral weakness. What appears as improvement after a long term of imprisonment might be the result of ageing of the offender's brain, or a premature senescence brought about through the oppressive effect of imprisonment and all that goes with it. From the practical point of view this may be satisfactory; indeed, there is no possibility of sparing the physical and mental vitality of a person who is really dangerous to others *if* the interests of social security cannot be attained otherwise than by harming the offender. But such results do not justify the conclusion that the offender was a recidivist because before his term of imprisonment he had not chosen to become decent and law-abiding. There are a few cases of adults, and a larger number of juveniles where one has to admit that some improvement of the personality has taken place after a period of detention. But these cases do not invalidate, in the slightest, the general conception of the writer.

A stereotyped recurrence of the first offence is—except in

[1] Approximately 20 per cent of offenders sent to prison return there after the first time, in most cases before long. A large number of those who "have learnt the lesson" of punishment, would have improved at any rate, without actually serving their sentences. They have become involved in unlawful activities in an exceptional frame of their mind, and no tangible events in their external life need account for this. Another substantial proportion of imprisoned offenders become "reformed" to a sufficient extent to be careful about the letter of the law in the future. But they continue to struggle with the anti-moral factor in their psyche, and very few remain free from observable manifestations of this mental difficulty. If such an individual has reached the age of 35–40 without an open conflict with the police, he may have had the chance of altering genuinely. Such an improvement of the personality later in life is observed also in psychopaths in the narrower sense. Genuine improvement that is due to imprisonment is, in the opinion of the writer, infrequent.

the rare cases of psychoneurotic symbolic crime—a sure sign of the presence of an unfavourable constitutional factor. Logic itself must lead to this conclusion. An offender who repeatedly exposes himself to the inconveniences of being caught and sentenced cannot be a person with a fair amount of self-control or a fairly normal outlook. What he gains by his theft, fraud, or other types of offence cannot be significant enough for life if compared with the pains inflicted by punishment and the fact of being an outcast.

It has been pointed out that the habitual criminal ignores the opinion of decent society and prefers to enjoy the approval and admiration of his fellow-criminals. This is certainly not an important stimulus of his criminality, but a secondary trait of his personality. After all, the habitual offender has to come to some terms with his unfortunate inclination, since he is unable to alter it. Thus he derives pleasure from his battle against law and order, and it is only natural that he accepts, with gratitude, the approval and praise afforded to him by the group of criminal outcasts.

4. The present trend in educational psychology is to attribute a large rôle to environmental influences in moulding the youth's personality. This concept is not identical with the traditional belief in the power of personal education by adults and in free volition to act accordingly. It is increasingly recognized that it is not enough to teach a youth moral concepts and expect him to develop into a decent personality irrespective of the quality of environmental impressions. There must also be an appropriate psychic structure capable of assimilating moral principles. Success in this respect is not a matter of a conscious moral outlook and readiness to behave decently. In view of the self-restraint involved in approved conduct and the necessity to like rules and restrictions, even though they are originally a strain, psychic health in general is required for the accomplishment of this task. It is intelligible that when the personality cannot derive an adequate measure of satisfaction from its psychoaffective processes, there is no sufficient capacity for enduring the self-restraint implied by unimpeachable conduct.

Unpleasant memories referring to childhood in general and the child's relationship to adults in particular may decrease the capacity for adhering to socially approved principles. Apart from these acquired elements there is an innate factor deciding the capacity for self-restraint. Probably, if the deep psycho-affective processes in general imply too much struggle, and too little satisfaction, a weakness of volition may ensue, making difficult the task of resisting temptations. The student is referred to the discussion in Chapters XI and XII [1] regarding the more or less satisfactory quality of the intrapsychic processes as well as their interpretation on higher mental levels. There we have dealt mainly with the aspect of aggressiveness. But in fact the phenomenon discussed there has a close bearing upon the problem of moral capacity. If the deeper mental processes suggest to the subject the idea of "difficulty" and undue lack of psycho-affective harmony, then he may find the restrictive order of society an added burden beyond endurance; and this may manifest itself in a deficient moral strength.

It is true that the practical administration of society's affairs cannot yet dispense with the hypothetical belief in absolute freedom of will as far as moral conduct is concerned. But there ought to be psychiatrists who continue to search and observe without being influenced by this current and indeed indispensable hypothesis. They may ultimately succeed in directing the development towards a society that is primarily concerned with making life easier, and the temptation to offend lesser. This appears more promising than to continue trying to increase the individual's moral resistance, as well as to improve the security-service. Even though realistic knowledge will fail for the time being to bring about concrete improvements, lawyers and moralists, if they are at the same time lovers of mankind, may receive much comfort from progressing research. They may be able to abandon the distressing but popular idea that so many people are really wicked, and merely stubborn in not choosing the path of peaceable life and mutual help.

If in the condition of psychopathy there is an organic element that interferes with social conduct, then there must be in all normals an organic factor that makes the acceptable quality of conduct possible. The writer intentionally refrains from referring to the anomalous moral behaviour found in psychosis. In this condition the anomaly in conduct is largely due to a substantial loss in the sense of reality. A distorted picture about oneself and the world results in wrong actions. In psychopathy, on the other hand, the psychoaffective harmony is unsatisfactory in that it affords less intra-mental gratification than is required for average

[1] Pages 165, 187 and 190.

normality. Hence, the subject has difficulties in accepting external limitations.

5. From my experience as psychoanalyst I take a serious view of the prognosis if a young person of sufficient intelligence, and brought up in an average family environment, is repeatedly unable to resist a certain type of temptation in spite of firm and still encouraging attempts to alter him. It is true that through friendly education and psychological approach such a youth may greatly improve ; he may even give up his particular type of offence. But I have found that later in life the inevitable disappointments and hardships evoke in such a person some type of *a*-social conduct, and may even bring him into conflict with the written law. I base this discussion on the close knowledge of the lives of a number of individuals, and on the comparison of their early conduct with their adult life. It was difficult for me to avoid the conclusion advanced. It is, of course, possible to assume that another even larger group of persons, who in their youth have committed similar offences, have still managed to develop into personalities with average moral strength to such an extent that they have never been before court or in need of a psychologist. However, the number of my observations is sufficiently large, and amongst my patients there were several offenders who had decidedly a decent and appropriate upbringing. Nothing can, therefore, cloud my impression that the organic factor in moral conduct is more important than we like to admit. Even if several of these offender-patients had neurotic parents, particularly hysterical mothers, the outcome of these unspecific impressions resulting in *a*-social weakness shows clearly the presence of an organic, or let us say, unalterable factor interfering with moral conduct. It is true that the neurotic home atmosphere did not influence favourably the personality of these patients ; but it alone did not create their criminal propensities. The innate element that has appeared in the mother as hysteria, or in the father as irritability, may manifest itself in the son or daughter as a weak moral capacity.

The study of monozygotic twins likewise illustrates the innate factor in the moral difficulty. Simultaneity of criminal tendencies in such pairs is more frequent than in ordinary siblings. Cf. O. D. Maguinness, *Environment and Heredity*.

## SUMMARY

1. FRIENDLY interest in fellow-beings is a fundamental trend in the human individual. The operation of this positive attitude is, however, modified by the competitive complex with its implications. Resentment of the fellow-being, and fear of the human environment, coupled with the feeling of personal inadequacy, are the basic components of this complex. The ethical elements of the mind are, likewise, offsprings of human contact and its complexities.

2. Degeneration of the religious-ethical function of the mind is the fundamental generator of aggressive prejudice. The latter is one of the manifestations of difficulties in the deep moral process.

3. Freud's superego is partly congruent with the moral process as conceived in the present work ; but this process is a more comprehensive, and at the same time a less circumscribed, phenomenon than that which is covered by the idea of the superego. The moral process is concerned with the general capacity for self-limitation for the sake of social life, as well as the capacity for deriving genuine satisfaction from this self-limitation and social co-operation. It is not fundamentally concerned with a particular pattern of approved behaviour, nor with particular decisions in conduct ; and basically, it is not generated by the fear of environment, but rather by the elementary social interest in each other, referred to above.

4. The moral process is as deep and unconscious as are, for instance, the complex processes of assimilation both physical and psycho-affective.

5. Tolerance in the broader sense is a function associated with the moral process. It is closely linked up with self-tolerance ; but the latter function is likewise dependent on the general function of tolerance and mental assimilation. Conspicuously deficient

tolerance of fellow-men suggests difficulties in toleration of the self or its components.

6. Projection (externalization) of intramental conflicts is a propensity of the human race, based on archaic inheritance. The extent to which this mechanism is employed by the mind in the service of psychoaffective economy, is largely dependent on early education, as well as on the general social-cultural atmosphere surrounding the individual. Educational conditioning of the mind may be of the type that encourages, or of that which discourages the too ready turn of conflicts towards externalization, and thus towards aggressive prejudice. Social approval or disapproval of prejudice affects not only the conscious, logical spheres but equally strongly the deeper mental processes. Hence, the particular social atmosphere has an influence on the extent to which " irrational " psychic reactions operate in life.

It is, thus, a function of environmental forces on a large scale whether the individual's mind avails itself of the relief by projection more, or less, extensively. Accordingly, it is not so much the individual as society that is responsible for the amount of prejudice-delusions at work in human relationships. Ethnic elements acting almost imperceptibly in the formation of the social atmosphere are difficult to modify ; only international influences of a substantial impact might be capable of interfering. This, however, appears at present a rather remote possibility.

7. Aggressiveness is not merely a reactive tendency in the service of self-preservation. There is a substantial amount of elementary aggressiveness (not reactive in the ordinary sense) ; it is a correlate and product of the constant " struggle " of elements and processes in the biochemical and psychoaffective spheres. If the individual's environment suggests to him that harmony rules in society, and that each individual is significant, then the higher level of the mind interprets the afore-mentioned biological struggles merely as vitally necessary processes, serving the organism's homeostasis. Yet, in so far as the social atmosphere emphasizes the effective significance of power, exploitation, and aggression, as well as the normality of discord, the higher psychic levels interpret the deep psycho-biological processes in terms of aggressiveness ; this creates the tendency which we conceive as elementary aggressiveness. It is easy to realize that, in fact, this

aggressiveness is likewise reactive, being a secondary result of the discordant social atmosphere.

8. Direct appeal to the individual's good will, as well as the activity of various ethical societies alone, has no chance of influencing, to a substantial extent, the social atmosphere and combating its anomalous factors. People at large respect much more the organized state-power and social authority ; and only unequivocal disapproval from this side is capable of affecting the deeper automatisms of the psyche. On the other hand, any social organization that fails to cultivate, and favourably direct, people's metaphysical (anagogical) life contributes to chaos and aggressiveness.

9. The fact that dreams represent the subject's mental elements by objects, persons, and actions, suggests that the human individual is unable to conceive of himself without reference to his external environment. No doubt, dreams objectify much more frequently the disapproved and unpleasant elements of the psyche than its virtuous and peaceful aspects. This may suggest that fear of the environment is very strong.

The current conception of state—all recent brands included—is not sufficiently free of archaic, oppressive features. Further progress is necessary, and to an extent feasible, even though elements of ethnic prejudice make this task rather difficult.

10. Difficulties in the moral process constitute a fundamental factor in the genesis of psychoneuroses and characterneuroses. In the course of individual psychoanalyses, in most instances, this causal relationship does not appear clearly, because such deep processes are not capable of being recognized by the average person, and thus they are not directly expressed in free associations and dreams.

It is, perhaps, a great mistake that current psychopathological theories ignore the primary etiological significance of factors that are not " thinkable " in the ordinary sense, or do not appear in dreams and free associations. The writer thinks that what is considered, frequently, the " primary etiological agent " may be a secondary element, potent enough to dominate the scene for the observer's eye, but nevertheless not be the primary factor. There may be a few, or even numerous cases, where it would be better to devote some thought to the " intangible ", or less concretely conceivable factors in the genesis of psychic disturbances. The writer has in mind no metaphysical mysteries, nor such vague notions as psychoneurotic constitution.

11. Symbolic perception by the psyche of impressions seems to be an intrinsic propensity of the human being, as if a means of enriching the mental function through imparting several meanings to any single impression. In general, psychologists have taken notice of this phenomenon only in so far as pathological phenomena result. Should society ever be able to purge the " imperceptible environmental atmosphere " of most of its archaic and aggressive elements, the symbolic perception of concrete impressions would very likely occur on more agreeable lines, and result indeed in more mental satisfaction and less psychoneurotic stimulation.

# INDEX

For Product Safety Concerns and Information please contact our EU
representative GPSR@taylorandfrancis.com
Taylor & Francis Verlag GmbH, Kaufingerstraße 24, 80331 München, Germany

www.ingramcontent.com/pod-product-compliance
Ingram Content Group UK Ltd.
Pitfield, Milton Keynes, MK11 3LW, UK
UKHW021501240926
475702UK00035B/36
*9780415211208*